GENERAL
HOSPITAL PSYCHIATRY

GENERAL HOSPITAL PSYCHIATRY

Michael Alan Taylor, M.D.
Professor and Chairman

Frederick S. Sierles, M.D.
Associate Professor and Director of Undergraduate Medical Education

Richard Abrams, M.D.
Professor and Vice-Chairman

Department of Psychiatry and Behavioral Sciences
University of Health Sciences/The Chicago Medical School

THE FREE PRESS
A Division of Macmillan, Inc.
NEW YORK

Collier Macmillan Publishers
LONDON

FOREWORD

This is an unusual and important book. With clarity and detail it guides the reader through the diagnosis and treatment of the severely mentally ill. Its organization and illustrative case examples make it an essential textbook for medical students, residents, and others in psychiatric training programs. It will also be of significant practical value to neurologists, other physicians who consult regarding psychiatric inpatients, psychologists, social workers, nurses, hospital administrators, and anyone who deals with the inpatient care of the mentally ill.

This unique contribution to psychiatry derives much of its strength from the authors' long-standing research program. Since 1971, Drs. Taylor and Abrams have collected data on a sample of inpatients. Drawing on this rich data and on their examination of other diagnostic criteria, such as psychological testing, EEG, and neurologic examination, they have defined and explored the borders between schizophrenia and manic depressive illness.

Following an original approach, Taylor, Sierles, and Abrams cross the borders between psychiatry and neurology and treat psychiatric patients as sufferers of specific brain disorders. They are neuropsychiatrists in the oldest and best tradition. Thus, they highlight the value of neuropsychological and behavioral neurologic examination, and in descriptions of patients they include a section on behavioral neurologic diseases: epilepsy, delirium, dementia, and headaches, among others.

Part I, entitled Patient Evaluation, discusses the importance of making the correct diagnosis and demonstrates how to confirm the diagnosis by appropriate mental status and neurologic examination. While emphasizing history taking as "gathering data," the authors also delineate an approach to patient care when information is incomplete. The reader is immediately engaged by the case histories used to illustrate specific points.

Part II deals with Patient Management. Not only does it cover the usual principles of treatment with drugs, and the use of specific drugs for specific diagnoses, but, in addition, this section includes a long discussion on the use of ECT, an area in which the authors have done significant research. Here, they review the efficacy of the treatment and provide instructions on how to do it, including pre-ECT tests and orders, equipment, and post-ECT advice. The authors also cover verbal intervention and behavioral techniques.

The final three chapters of this section (psychiatric emergencies, the inpatient unit, and consultation/liaison psychiatry) are especially noteworthy. The inpatient chapter must be read. It is a guide for all psychiatry departments trying to develop short-stay inpatient psychiatric units consistent with the knowledge and advancement of therapies today. The acute inpatient unit, with its emphasis on diagnosis, specific and timely interventions, and short-term stay, becoming *the* model of general hospital patient care, is very different from the standard long-term inpatient facility. When the new short-stay unit is developed, the orientation of the entire staff must be redirected so that the physician/psychiatrist, the psychologist, and social worker, nurses, and activity therapists take on new roles and responsibilities. To aid all concerned in making this transition, the authors describe in detail an inpatient unit and outline the roles and responsibilities of each of the mental health professionals working there.

In part III the authors explain how to treat specific diagnostic disorders such as affective disorder, schizophrenia, delusional disorder, behavioral neurologic disease, substance abuse, anorexia nervosa, anxiety disorder, somatization disorder, conversion disorder, and sociopathy; and specific patient problems such as malingering, suicidal or violent tendencies, catatonia, postpartum disorders, and symptoms associated with old age. This section, which does not always follow *DSM-III*, is, like the others, a joy to read. Throughout, the authors reemphasize a modern, straightforward approach to psychiatric patients, stressing the need for sensitivity, awareness, and practicality in handling both the patient and his or her family and friends. This commonsense, direct approach to the staff's dealing with patients has been all too rare in psychiatric textbooks.

General Hospital Psychiatry is a guide for psychiatric inpatient care, full of general and specific information. The advice is priceless. With unmatched thoroughness and clarity, all the essential elements for providing this care are reviewed. This volume sets a new standard by which all similar texts must be judged.

Dr. Paula Clayton
Professor and Head
Department of Psychiatry
University of Minnesota

PREFACE

In the present renaissance of biological psychiatry, increasing numbers of psychiatrists are practicing in general hospitals and treating an increasingly diverse patient population with a variety of pharmacologic agents. In concert with this developing general hospital practice style, the stereotype of the psychiatric inpatient has metamorphosed from the permanently impaired, edentulous, baggy-clothed, dyskinetic state hospital schizophrenic into a pleasant-looking but depressed individual spending a few weeks in the living room atmosphere of a general hospital psychiatric unit while receiving the latest miracle from an elaborate pharmacopoeia. In fact, neither stereotype reflects the reality of modern hospital psychiatry, in which today's psychiatrist, like his colleagues in internal medicine and surgery, faces complex clinical problems requiring expertise about behavior, neuroscience, pharmacology and laboratory assessment and a better than passing knowledge of general medicine. The stethoscope and reflex hammer are, once again, tools of his trade, and electrophysiologic monitoring, computerized brain tomography and cognitive testing are his standard diagnostic tools. Today's hospital-based psychiatrist is called upon to treat deliria, dementias and psychomotor states as well as psychoses, anxiety disorders and dysthymias of traditional practice. Anticonvulsants, monoamine oxidase inhibitors, B-adrenergic and calcium channel blockers are his to use

along with neuroleptics and cyclic antidepressants, and his day-to-day activities are much like those of a busy internist.

Most psychiatrists approach this modern practice armed solely with a
brief experience based primarily on the role modeling gained during residency training. Although there are books galore on psychopharmacology
and the various psychiatric syndromes and a few texts dealing with the
treatments of hospitalized psychiatric patients, there is little practical help
for the psychiatrist in the form of a book that presents the principles and
strategies of hospital psychiatry.

As practitioners and teachers of biologic psychiatry and researchers of
the more severe mental disorders often requiring hospitalization, we have
been fascinated and frustrated by the vicissitudes of hospital psychiatric
practice and have long felt a practical guide to the diagnosis and treatment of
psychiatric patients within a general hospital to be sorely needed. We believe
this book, in part, fills that need for the practitioner, for the psychiatrist-in-
training, and for all physicians and students concerned with the modern
treatment of the patient with serious mental illness.

GENERAL
HOSPITAL PSYCHIATRY

PART I

PATIENT
EVALUATION

CHAPTER 1

Principles of Diagnosis

Introduction

Prior to the 1970s reliable psychiatric diagnosis was often a hit-or-miss affair leading to the standard joke, particularly in the United States, that where there were three psychiatrists, there would be four different diagnoses. Studies correlating changes in patterns of diagnoses with the availability of novel treatments (1,2), cross-national studies comparing diagnosis in Europe and the United States (3–5), and investigations of the diagnostic decision-making process provided overwhelming evidence of the capricious and unreliable nature of how individuals with mental illness were classified (6–8).

The 1970s witnessed a recrudescence of research and clinical interest in psychiatric diagnosis, and from that interest developed several sets of reliable research criteria for psychiatric disorders. *DSM-III*, the first official diagnostic system in the United States with known reliability and operationally defined criteria (9), is the clinical counterpart of that process.

No matter how carefully diagnostic criteria are defined, however, they are useless unless properly implemented. Experience and skill are required to use the criteria and to relate dry definitions to flesh-and-blood patients. The clinician also must have a command of the relevant data base and a clear understanding of the clinical principles of diagnosis.

The Diagnostic Process

Until reliable, specific, sensitive diagnostic laboratory tests for psychiatric illness are developed, diagnosis will remain a probabilistic process of exclusion and inclusion. Each diagnosis derives from many possibilities. Initially all diagnoses are equally probable. As the clinician collects data, the probability of any one diagnosis changes. For example, patient A is referred for evaluation. Without the additional information of age, sex, and chief complaint every diagnosis is equally probable. As the clinician collects more information, however, the probability that patient A is suffering from some disorders diminishes, eventually reaching zero, while the probability favoring other diagnoses increases. This continuing process of exclusion and inclusion eventually leaves the clinician with the most likely diagnosis. Using this model again, patient A is referred for evaluation. If patient A is male, the possibility of obstetrical/gynecological conditions is zero. If patient A is a male who has trouble walking, slurs his speech, and smells of alcohol, the probability of an acute intoxication increases and the probability of other conditions decreases. More information of the right sort is essential for furthering the process of exclusion/inclusion by probability, until the most likely diagnosis is reached. This is as true for the psychiatrist as for any other clinician.

Diagnostic success derives from the clinician's ability to collect accurate information and to relate this information to specific disorders. In the example of patient A, the diagnosis would have been wrong if the clinician failed to detect slurred speech or the smell of alcohol or if he did not know that these signs correlated with an acute alcoholic state.

The integration of accurate data with the process of exclusion/inclusion by probability is a powerful diagnostic tool. One of the earliest clinical axioms taught in medical school is that a woman of childbearing age who has missed two consecutive menstrual periods is considered pregnant until proved otherwise. Virtually every physician will diagnose "possible pregnancy" based solely upon the information: female, age twenty-five, two missed menstrual periods. Psychiatric phenomena can be equally suggestive. For example, a forty-three-year-old woman, who has never been ill before and whose physical examination and laboratory tests are normal, states that for the past three months she has felt "anxious, mildly irritable, and out of sorts." Her age, sex, general good health, and late onset episode of dysphoria strongly suggest depression. Should one hundred such patients all be diagnosed "depressed" solely upon the above information, diagnostic validity would exceed 90 percent (10). Other diagnostically powerful data patterns are displayed in Table 1–1.

TABLE 1-1   Some Examples of Diagnostic Patterns

SYMPTOM PATTERN	MOST LIKELY DIAGNOSIS(ES)
1. Typical depressive features (insomnia, anorexia, psychomotor retardation), but without the profound unremitting sadness of depression	a. Coarse brain disease b. Systemic illness c. Bipolar patient switching from depression to mania or euthymia
2. Typical and constant anxiety features (anxious mood, air hunger, tachycardia) beginning after age thirty-five in a male patient	Systemic illness (e.g. endocrinopathy, hypertension)
3. Irritability, broad affect, rapid/pressured speech, no coarse brain disease	Mania
4. Transient and episodic visual hallucinations and first-rank symptoms, but no thought disorder or affective blunting	Seizure disorder
5. Diffuse cognitive impairment, ataxia, urinary incontinence	Normal pressure hydrocephaly

Principles of Clinical Diagnosis

The proper collection of data and the bits of information that most influence diagnostic probabilities are discussed in detail elsewhere in the text. However, to diagnose the patient's illness correctly so that definitive treatment can be administered requires the clinician to adhere to the principles of clinical diagnosis. The simplicity of these "rules of thumb" belies the extraordinary difficulty most clinicians have in adhering to them in actual practice.

The fundamental principle of clinical diagnosis is to observe the patient prior to instituting treatment. Observing behavior and obtaining laboratory results uncontaminated by psychotropic medication is critical for valid diagnosis. Except for certain emergency situations or a patient who is well known to the clinician, this rule should never be violated. Unfortunately, it almost always is—in the irrational rush to treatment so much a part of our culture. This need not be the case despite our indoctrination to the immediate purchase of remedies for each new ache or discomfort (e.g. "Headache? Take aspirin. Nervous? Take Compoz"). Most patients are reassured by a clinician who conducts a careful, thorough examination and diagnostic evaluation, explains the rationale for each procedure to be administered, empathizes with the patient and his family, and educates them about the patient's illness. The few days taken to evaluate the patient properly may prevent years of suffering and minimize the risk of iatrogenic disorder, such as tardive dyskinesia often induced by needless or prolonged neuroleptic administration. The following vignette illustrates the point:

A thirty-year-old-man, without prior psychiatric history, suddenly became violent at home, destroying several pieces of furniture. One month later he again became violent and destroyed more furniture. He was hospitalized and, although calm, was immediately given chlorpromazine 400 mg. daily. During the next seventy-two hours he became increasingly agitated and irritable and often spoke in a loud and stilted manner as if he were "an angry robot." His frightening behavior resulted in his transfer to a locked unit, where chlorpromazine was discontinued and sodium amobarbital ordered if he became agitated or destructive. His frightening behavior quickly resolved, and he was subsequently observed to have transient episodes of automatic behavior, forced speech, and right-sided hypertonicity during a period of altered consciousness, for which he was amnesic. An EEG confirmed a seizure disorder. Anticonvulsant medication was administered, and he remained well for the next two years.

The initial failure to observe the patient before definitive treatment was administered could have had tragic consequences. The hasty administration of chlorpromazine lowered the patient's seizure threshold resulting in paradoxically increased pathological behaviors, which could have resulted in serious injury to the patient and staff. The chlorpromazine also masked his transient seizure phenomena, particularly the hypertonicity (which could have been misinterpreted as an extrapyramidal drug side effect), preventing an accurate diagnosis. Ultimately he might have been labeled "psychotic" and treated with high and prolonged doses of neuroleptics, with minimal therapeutic effects, prolonging hospitalization and increasing his risk for tardive dyskinesia. On the other hand, the neuroleptic-free observation period permitted adequate observation, accurate diagnosis, and specific, effective treatment.

The appropriate delay in starting definitive treatment optimizes the evaluation process. The phenomenological clinical method (11,12) is best utilized during this observation period. It incorporates the basic diagnostic principles of *objective observation* without interpretation; description using *precise terminology* and consideration of the *form* of behavior separately from its *content*. This approach forms the basis of modern research criteria and *DSM-III*.

Objective observation without interpretation is essential to the diagnostic process. Clinicians too frequently make interpretations rather than observations and undermine the reliability and validity of their diagnoses. For example:

A forty-six-year-old man sits on the floor of a hospital day room. He masturbates publicly and repeatedly places nonedible objects in his mouth. He is said to "chew on everything," swallowing foreign objects which require surgical removal. Despite constant turmoil in the dayroom, he remains placid and unconcerned. This patient's behavior could easily be summarized by the term "regressed," but this would prematurely terminate the diagnostic process. "Regression" implies a theoretical notion of return to a less mature level of psychosexual development or acting more childlike, and has no power to discriminate groups of seriously ill psychiatric patients. The term is not observational and lacks demonstrated reliability and validity. The proper phenomenologic observation of this patient would be: He is placid and calm amidst turmoil. His sexual behavior, public masturbation, deviates from the norm. He has repetitive, oral behaviors: putting nonedible objects in his mouth, and chewing and swallowing them.

To a diagnostician aware of the specific diagnostic correlates of various disorders, the interpretation "regression" is not helpful. In contrast, the observations "placidity . . . deviant sexual behavior . . . and increased oral behavior" suggest the Kluver-Bucy syndrome, a manifestation of bilateral temporal lobe dysfunction (13). Indeed, the patient also exhibited visual agnosia (visual nonrecognition of objects that can be properly identified tactilely), which completes the syndrome. Objective observation enabled the clinician not only to make a diagnosis but also to localize anatomically the involved brain regions.

Precision of language has been stressed by all phenomenologists. Often clinicians disagree about the meaning or usage of common psychiatric terms. Some use the term "paranoid" to mean delusional, others to mean suspicious or having referential ideas or delusions with persecutory content. Some clinicians use "paranoid" as a synonym for schizophrenia. A term with so many meanings is unreliable for diagnosing psychopathology. It is preferable to characterize a suspicious person as "suspicious" and a delusional person as "delusional" rather than use the global term "paranoid."

Table 1–2 displays some commonly used descriptive terms without precise definition or with too many meanings. They should be avoided, as they are unhelpful in discriminating homogeneous patient groups.

Theoretical terms such as narcissism, introjection, ego-boundary, transference, libidinal fixation, reaction-formation, and superego, have meaning only within a psychoanalytic framework, have no demonstrated reliability, often substitute for objective observation, and should not be used in clinical diagnosis.

The separation of the *form* of psychopathology from its *content* is the final general principle of diagnosis. The subject matter a patient is discussing, the words spoken by a hallucinated voice, and the specific delusional idea are all content. The way a person uses language; the clarity and duration of a perception without a stimulus (hallucination); whether the delusional idea develops fully formed or is secondary to other psychopath-

TABLE 1-2   Imprecise Descriptive Terms and Suggested Alternatives

IMPRECISE TERM	PREFERRED TERM OR DESCRIPTION DEPENDENT UPON PATIENT'S BEHAVIOR
Confusion	Disoriented, perplexed, in an altered state of consciousness
Ambivalence	The ambitendency of catatonics, opposite feelings toward the same object
Irrational	Illogical, exhibiting hallucinations and/or delusions, exhibiting thought disorder, acting strangely
Paranoid	Suspicious, delusional, having persecutory delusional ideas
Nervous	Anxious (the lay terms "upset," and "having symptoms of mental illness" should not be used by professionals)
Unintelligible, incoherent or irrelevant speech/ looseness of associations	Flight of ideas, driveling speech, tangentiality, rambling speech, paraphasias and neologisms

ology—all these constitute form. Generally the form of psychopathology has more diagnostic power than its content. The fact that a person is perceiving without external stimulation alters the probabilities of diagnosis more than the content of that false perception. The content of psychopathology reflects the individual patient's past experience, cultural and socioethnic background, whereas the form of psychopathology reflects the illness itself. Cross-cultural studies (14–16) have demonstrated that although the content of psychopathology varies dramatically across cultures, the form of major psychiatric disorder is strikingly similar from one culture to another. Thus, the depressive in India may have guilty ruminations about past transgressions of caste injunctions and dietary laws, whereas the depressive in the United States may have guilty ruminations about childhood masturbation and petty cheating on paying income tax. However, both individuals will exhibit the typical form of major depression with its characteristic profound sadness, insomnia, anorexia, psychomotor retardation, and feelings of guilt.

Although often elaborate, the content of delusional phenomena is also of minimal diagnostic importance. For example, a patient states, "The FBI is after me." If the clinician is to determine whether this is a true or false belief, he must determine its form (he already knows its content) by asking questions designed to elicit the source of knowledge, e.g. "How do you know?" The patient may then respond with verifiable statements that reflect reality or with statements having a psychopathological form. A pervasive feeling that "something is wrong," that people and events are not what they seem, of being observed, or of being followed all constitute a *delusional mood*, which may occur in individuals who are extremely anxious and shy, or who have dissociative states, drug-induced psychosis, epilepsy, endogenous depression, or schizophrenia (12). The conclusion that things are "not right," that there is a plot afoot, and that "the FBI is after me," if based on observing the milkman coming late, a light being left on in the apartment, and furniture seemingly out of place is termed a *delusional idea* and indicates major psychiatric disorder (12). However, the conclusion that a fork placed on the wrong side of a dinner plate means "the FBI is after me" is so arbitrary and personalized that there is no meaningful connection between the event and the conclusion. Such an experience is termed a *delusional perception* and, although not pathognomonic, is most commonly observed in schizophrenia (17–20). The terms delusional mood, delusional idea, and delusional perception each denote a specifically different form of psychopathology, despite, in the above example, their identical content.

Decision-making and the Concept of Illness

The diagnostic process that progresses from all illness possibilities to the single most probable illness proceeds by a series of decisions, each of which increases the likelihood of the final diagnosis. *DSM-III* presents a series of "decision trees" illustrating this process.

The most important decision undoubtedly is the first, in which the clinician decides if the patient is ill. Despite the multitude of diagnostic criteria in *DSM-III* and in all other major classification systems, none has an agreed-upon definition of illness. This lack of definition results in part from the overwhelming concern of clinicians with practical day-to-day patient care, including many problems not defined as "illnesses" (e.g. pregnancy, childbirth; monitoring normal childhood development, preventive weight and diet control). The definition of mental disorder is further confounded by social forces which have led to the inclusion or exclusion of conditions from our nosology based upon political rather than scientific considerations. A striking example of this was *DSM-III*'s redefinition of homosexuality as a sexual orientation preference rather than a disease. For all its advantages over its predecessors, *DSM-III* is replete with listings of "mental disorders," which are unconfirmed by empirical data (e.g. tobacco and caffeine dependence, academic and occupational problems, noncompliance with medical treatment).

Definitions of mental illness also reflect the biases and theoretical models of their proponents (21). Some behaviorists, for example (e.g. Skinnerians) conclude that disturbed behaviors are learned "bad habits," which bring the patient into conflict with himself or society. The learned inappropriate behavior is the illness, while the brain is presumed to be functioning normally. In this paradigm the obvious treatment is nonreinforcement of the bad behavior and reinforcement of good habits. Although useful in the study of and as the primary treatment of some behavioral disorders (e.g. simple phobias) and in the shaping of some social behavior of seriously ill psychiatric patients, the behaviorist approach (with its assumption of normal brain functions) is not applicable to the understanding and primary treatment of the severely mentally ill who have demonstrable brain dysfunction (e.g. EEG and CT scan abnormalities) and significant genetic liability for their disorder (23).

Other theorists, such as Thomas Szasz (24), have concluded that mental illness is the label attached to a deviant member of society in order to justify isolating and ignoring him. The label is the illness and the brain is again considered to be functioning normally. The obvious "treatment" in this paradigm is not to label patients but to deal with their deviations as individual differences rather than conditions requiring medical treatment.

In the psychoanalytic model deviant behavior is considered merely symptomatic, symbolizing an intrapsychic conflict. This disturbance is the illness. Although some analysts, including Freud, suggest that a biological (i.e., brain dysfunction) basis may accompany the emotional disturbance, they conclude that appropriate treatment must focus upon the intrapsychic conflict rather than on the behavioral or biological dysfunction, both of which are expected to return to normal with resolution of the intrapsychic emotional disturbance (21).

The medical model is the theoretical framework of this book. It posits that the brain is the organ of behavior and that mental disorders are diseases or syndromes reflecting brain dysfunction. In this paradigm the primary treatment modality is biological.

Thus, the initial clinical question—Does the patient have an illness? —will be answered by a definition of illness based upon a theoretical model of mental disorder. Adherents of the medical model traditionally diagnose a patient as ill if his condition is associated with high risk for death or disability or if he complains of pain, discomfort, or loss of function. Organ pathology is either identified or implied. Among mental disorders, the involved end organ is always the brain.

The vast literature delineating structural (25–27), electrophysiological (28–30), and biochemical abnormalities (31) in psychiatric patients clearly suggests that conditions such as schizophrenia, delusional disorders, and affective disorders are expressions of brain dysfunction. Although more subtle in pathophysiology, they nevertheless should be conceptually grouped with mental syndromes (e.g. dementias) that result from coarse brain dysfunction. Although the data are less compelling (32,33), some anxiety disorders (e.g. neurasthenia, phobic-anxiety-depersonalization syndrome), also appear to reflect brain dysfunction.

The nature of other mental syndromes, such as somatoform, psychosexual, and dissociative states and personality disorders, is not clear. Future research may well demonstrate that some of these conditions are also expressions of brain dysfunction, whereas others may reflect individual variations, which, although statistically deviant (abnormal), do not result from functional or structural brain pathology. This concept is illustrated by the distribution of height in the general population. The majority of individuals fall within an arbitrarily defined height range and are considered "normal." Those individuals who are outside this range are statistically deviant or "abnormal." Although their variation in height does not result from any illness process, most basketball players are abnormally tall in that they differ significantly in height from the majority of the population. On the other hand, some individuals are abnormally tall because of pituitary dysfunction. These individuals are more than statistically deviant because their abnormality reflects organ pathology. Mental syndromes also may be considered statistical deviations from the norm, reflecting either simple individual variations or organ (brain) pathology. Schizophrenics and individuals with affective disorders, delusional states, and some anxiety disorders are analogous to people whose abnormal height results from organ pathology. Individuals with somatiform, psychosexual, dissociative, and personality disorders may be analogous to the person whose abnormal height is simply an individual variation.

This concept of disease and deviation is theoretically and practically important. Theoretically it implies that behavioral deviance might result from both environmental and biological factors, just as height is determined by multiple factors, including individual variation and organ pathology. It is of practical importance because individuals with presumed organ pathology as well as individuals whose behavior is at variance with the norm are behaviorally abnormal, but only those with organ pathology are likely to respond to biological treatment. It is not surprising that somatic treatments have demonstrable efficacy for the major psychoses and for some anxiety disorders, whereas individuals with personality disorder and related conditions respond to no treatment, physical or psychological. To expect such individuals to alter their personalities dramatically would be as realistic as expecting some tall people to shrink to normal height.

This does not mean that people with deviant behavior do not suffer or require professional help. Many do, as society demands normal behavior. Individuals with deviant behavior are often unhappy with their deviance, or society is unhappy with them. What this concept of illness suggests is that behavioral deviance should not be treated any differently from "physical" deviance. Those with organ pathology require somatic treatments, in addition to social and psychological support, whereas those without pathology rarely benefit from biological treatment yet require guidance for the problems of living arising from their deviant behaviors.

References

1. Baldessarini, R. Frequency of diagnosis of schizophrenia versus affective disorders from 1944 to 1968. *Am. J. Psychiat. 127:* 759–63, 1970.

2. Kurionsky, J. B.; Gurland, B. J.; Spitzer, R. L.; *et al.* Trends in the frequency of schizophrenia by different diagnostic criteria. *Am. J. Psychiat. 134:* 631–36, 1977.

3. Kramer, M. Cross-national study of diagnosis of the mental disorders: Origin of the problem. *Am. J. Psychiat. (Suppl.) 125:* 1–11, 1969.

4. Sandifer, M. G.; Hordern, A.; Timburg, G. C.; *et al.* Similarities and differences in patient evaluation by U.S. and U.K. psychiatrists. *Am. J. Psychiat. 126:* 206–12, 1969.

5. Leff, J. International variations in the diagnosis of psychiatric illness. *Br. J. Psychiat. 131:* 329–38, 1977.

6. Spitzer, R. L.; Fleiss, J. L. A re-analysis of the reliability of psychiatric diagnosis. *Br. J. Psychiat. 125:* 341–47, 1974.

7. Beck, A. T. Reliability of psychiatric diagnosis 1. A critique of systematic studies. *Am. J. Psychiat. 119:* 210–16, 1962.

8. Kreitman, N. The reliability of psychiatric diagnosis. *J. Ment. Sci. 107:* 876–86, 1961.

9. APA Committee on Nomenclature and Statistics. *Diagnostic and Statistical Manual of Mental Disorders. 3d ed. (DSM-III).* Washington, D.C.: American Psychiatric Association, 1980.

10. Usdin, G. (ed.). *Depression: Clinical, Biological, and Psychological Perspectives.* New York: Brunner/Mazel Publishers, 1977.

11. Taylor, M. A.; Heiser, J. P. Phenomenology: An alternative approach to diagnosis of mental illness. *Comp. Psychiat. 12:* 480–86, 1971.

12. Taylor, M. A. *The Neuropsychiatric Mental Status Examination.* New York: SP Medical and Scientific Books, 1981.

13. Pilleri, G. The Kluver-Bucy syndrome in man. *Psychiat. Neurol. 152:* 65–103, 1966.

14. Fava, G. A.; Kellner, R.; Munari, F.; *et al.* The Hamilton Depression Rating Scale in normals and depressives: A cross-cultural validation. *Acta Psychiat. Scand. 66:* 26–32, 1982.

15. Jablensky, A.; Sartorius, N.; Gulbinat, W.; *et al.* Characteristics of depressive patients contacting psychiatric services in four cultures: A report from the WHO collaborative study on the assessment of depressive disorders. *Acta Psychiat. Scand. 63:* 367–83, 1981.

16. Orley, J.; Wing, J. K. Psychiatric disorders in two African villages. *Arch. Gen. Psychiat. 36:* 513–20, 1979.

17. Mellor, C. S. First-rank symptoms of schizophrenia: 1. The frequency in schizophrenics on admission to hospital. 2. Differences between individual first-rank symptoms. *Br. J. Psychiat. 117:* 15–23, 1970.

18. Carpenter, W. T., Jr.; Strauss, J. S.; Muleh, S. Are there pathognomic symptoms in schizophrenia? *Arch. Gen. Psychiat. 28:* 847–52, 1973.

19. Taylor, M. A.; Abrams, R. The phenomenology of mania: A new look at some old patients. *Arch. Gen. Psychiat. 29:* 520–22, 1973.

20. Abrams, R.; Taylor, M. A. The importance of schizophrenic symptoms in the diagnosis of mania. *Am. J. Psychiat. 138:* 658–61, 1981.

21. Eysenck, H. J. Classification and the Problem of Diagnosis. In Eysenck, H. J. (ed.), *Handbook of Abnormal Psychology.* London: Pitman Medical, 1960, pp. 1–31.

22. Flor-Henry, P.; Gruzelier, J. (eds.). *Laterality and Psychopathology.* Amsterdam: Elsevier Science Publishers, 1983.

23. Taylor, M. A. The Genetics of Behavior. In Sierles, F. (ed.), *Clinical Behavioral Science.* New York: SP Medical and Scientific Books, 1982, pp. 3–10.

24. Szasz, T. S. *Law, Liberty and Psychiatry.* New York: Macmillan, 1963.

25. Weinberger, D. R.; DeLisi, L. E.; Perman, G. P.; *et al.* Computed tomography in schizophreniform disorder and other acute psychiatric disorders. *Arch. Gen. Psychiat. 39:* 778–83, 1982.

26. Tanaka, Y.; Hazama, H.; Kawahara, R.; *et al.* Computerized tomography of the brain in schizophrenic patients: A controlled study. *Acta Psychiat. Scand. 63:* 191–97, 1981.

27. Nasarallah, H. A.; McCalley–Whitters, M.; Jacoby, C. G. Cerebral ventricular enlargement in young manic males: A controlled CT study. *J. Aff. Dis. 4:* 15–19, 1982.

28. Abrams, R.; Taylor, M. A. Differential EEG patterns in affective disorder and schizophrenia. *Arch. Gen. Psychiat. 36:* 1355–58, 1979.

29. Vianna, V. The electroencephalogram in schizophrenia. In Lader, M. H. (ed.), *Studies of Schizophrenia. Br. J. Psychiat.* Special pub. ser. no. 10. Kent, England: Headley Bros. 1975, pp. 54–58.

30. Rockstroh, B.; Elbert, T.; Berbaumer, N.; *et al. Slow Brain Potentials and Behavior.* Baltimore: Urban & Schwarzenber, 1982, pp. 199–210.

31. Van Praag, H. M.; Lader, M. H.; Rafaelson, O. J.; *et al. Handbook of Biological Psychiatry,* pt. 4, *Brain Mechanisms and Abnormal Behavior Chemistry.* New York: Marcel Dekker, 1981.

32. Goodwin, D. W.; Guze, S. B. *Psychiatric Diagnosis.* 2d ed. New York: Oxford University Press, 1979, pp. 51–69.

33. Lader, M.; Marks, I. *Clinical Anxiety.* New York: Grune & Stratton, 1971, pp. 124–44.

CHAPTER 2

The Neuropsychiatric Examination

The neuropsychiatric examination is part of every complete physical examination of every patient seen by a physician. No physician would think his examination complete unless he listened to the patient's heart or recorded vital signs. The brain as a body organ deserves no less attention. Each patient, whether suffering from cardiovascular disease, or liver disease, or simply requesting a routine annual "physical," exhibits behavior. Many have deviant behaviors, some reflecting brain dysfunction. Each patient's behavior, normal or abnormal, must be noted and recorded systematically. Studies indicate that 10 to 15 percent of hospitalized acute medical or surgical patients are suffering from deliria of varying severities (1–3), that 50 to 80 percent of patients seeing general practitioners do so for signs and symptoms of anxiety (4), and that 15 to 20 percent of the general population is at risk for major psychiatric disorder (5,6). The odds are great that a significant proportion, if not the majority, of patients seen by the average clinician will exhibit some form of psychopathology.

The neuropsychiatric or mental status examination conducted by a psychiatrist is analogous to a cardiologist's examination of the heart. It is presumably more elaborate and skilled than that of the average clinician, but it is only a part of the complete physical examination, without which it has limited meaning. A physical examination without a mental status evaluation is also incomplete.

The goals of the neuropsychiatric examination are (1) to establish a reasonable doctor–patient relationship and (2) to make a thorough evaluation of the patient's present behavior so that a probable (working) diagnosis can be made and a treatment plan developed, executed, and monitored. Historical information, an integral part of the global evaluation of the patient, does not belong in the mental status examination, which deals only with the "here and now." This separation of past from present behaviors can be critical when dealing with a patient whose condition fluctuates. A patient may not have been suicidal or confused yesterday, but today—now—he could be both. Some patients, particularly those with affective disorder, can shift rapidly from stupor to excitement to depression within hours. Moods can shift within minutes. Multiple daily mental status examinations may be necessary to document such changes, and confusion will result unless each evaluation is clearly limited to the patient's behavior during that particular examination.

It is also important to understand what the neuropsychiatric examination does not do. Most lay people and many students and novice psychiatrists conceptualize all interactions with psychiatrists as the stereotype of an implacable, stone-faced, Viennese-accented psychoanalyst making interpretations of the putative symbolism in the comments and behaviors of neurotic patients. In fact, such psychoanalytic sessions are uncommon nowadays, with most psychiatrists practicing psychological intervention in a more animated, face-to-face, interactive manner. Still, this more prevalent interactive psychotherapeutic approach is not a neuropsychiatric mental status examination. The goals of a psychotherapy session are treatment-oriented, whereas the goals of the mental status evaluation are diagnostic. This does not mean that the mental status examination cannot be "therapeutic"; patients are often comforted by an examiner who does his job well and is knowledgeable about the patient's condition. What it does mean is that the goals of the examination require a specific clinical approach and specialized techniques that facilitate the establishment of the doctor–patient relationship, the acquisition of information, and the elicitation of behaviors necessary to make an accurate diagnosis.

Novice clinicians often have the misconception that they must remain impersonal with patients. The "Freudian blank screen" approach to interviewing was rarely used by Freud, let alone by modern psychoanalysts, and is not appropriate to the mental status examination. A warm, supporting, yet firm manner, creating a positive doctor–patient relationship, is the most fruitful approach.

It is often helpful to explain to the patient the reasons for the interview and what he can expect during the examination. Patients have a right to know about their condition and treatments, and about their physician's opinions concerning their illness. Within the limits of good judgment this right should be upheld. Often the best approach for obtaining the information needed in a mental status examination is to engage the patient in a pseudo-conversation. No matter how structured an interview, the maintenance of the conversational approach will increase the chances of acquiring sufficient and reliable information to make the high probability (working) diagnosis. In our society normal conversation between strangers or acquaintances has certain rules. The inexperienced examiner often suspends these rules during a mental status examination. He omits an initial "Hello, I'm Dr. So-and-so" in favor of a more clinical but less effective opening, such as "What's today's date?" Questions that are socially inappropriate, non-sequitive, or jarring will increase the patient's anxiety and often decrease his cooperativeness.

The examiner's comments and questions must relate to the patient's behavior. "Hello, I'm Dr. So-and-so" is an appropriate opening for the patient seated calmly in the waiting area. It is not appropriate for the agitated patient who is standing in the hall beating his face with his hands. A firm "Stop that. Sit down. I want to talk with you," followed by an introduction, is more to the point.

Patients with psychiatric illness often ask direct and personal questions. Although responses to personal questions must be limited, and patients should not be allowed to control the interview, patients do have the right to know something about the person examining them. Truthful responses to questions about education, experience, or professional role (e.g. student, resident, practitioner) or other reasonable questions are often helpful in maintaining a good relationship. In addition to their direct questioning of the examiner, patients often say or do things that are quite humorous. The examiner should not be afraid to laugh. If humor and responses to questions help achieve the goals of the examination, they are appropriate.

A good mental status examination should not be haphazard. Some structuring is important, and questions and testing procedures should proceed in a logical pattern while remaining responsive to the specific needs and behaviors of the patient. The examiner should be prepared to cover every area of the examination and develop a standardized manner of eliciting each form of psychopathology. Open-ended questioning during which the examiner is passive and nondirective, permitting the patient to control the topics of the interview, is rarely a useful mental status examination strategy. Sequences of questions can vary, and "lead-ins" to questions must be individualized, but a basic sequence of topics and a tactical approach for each symptom area should exist throughout the examination. Specific tactics for eliciting psychopathology will be discussed in succeeding sections.

Behavioral Sections of the Neuropsychiatric Examination

The mental status examination can be divided into *eight* broad symptom areas (Table 2-1).

GENERAL APPEARANCE AND MOTOR BEHAVIOR

Acquiring information that correlates with specific diagnoses is essential to the mental status examination. All too frequently, obvious patient behaviors and/or characteristics of general appearance helpful in diagnosis (e.g. sex, age) are overlooked by the examiner. The fact that women have greater risks than men for affective disorder, anxiety states, and Briquet's syndrome and that neuroses rarely develop for the first time after age thirty-five or sociopathy after age fifteen may be critical in determining the most probable diagnosis (6, 7).

The patient's *general appearance* is the first area to be evaluated. This evaluation requires no speech, no manipulation, no testing—just objective observation. Whenever possible, the examiner should greet the patient outside the examining room and walk with him to the area chosen for the interview. This initial outwardly informal introductory period permits the examiner to observe the patient's general motor coordination, gait, and manner. Observations of the patient's behavior on the ward are also extremely helpful. The examiner should deliberately review the patient's apparent age, sex, race/ethnic background, body type, nutrition, personal hygiene, and state of consciousness. No detail should be overlooked: A short, stocky, hirsute, "depressed" woman might have adrenal hyperplasia; an unkempt,

TABLE 2-1   The Neuropsychiatric Mental Status

SYMPTOM AREAS	EXAMPLES
1. General appearance	Race, apparent age, sex, hygiene, body type, level of consciousness
2. Motor behavior	Gait, motor overflow, frequency of movements, catatonic features
3. Affect	Range, intensity, quality of mood, lability, relatedness
4. Speech and language	Rate, rhythm, pressure, language (thought processes), thought content (suicidal thoughts)
5. Delusions	Delusional mood, delusional ideas
6. Perceptual function	Hallucinations, illusions
7. First-rank symptoms	Thought broadcasting, complete auditory hallucinations
8. Cognition	Practic/gnostic/mnestic functions

dazed, ataxic man with urine-stained pants might have normal pressure hydrocephalus. Physical constitution should also be noted. Large-framed, heavy people with a high fat/muscle ratio (endomorphs) are over-represented among individuals with affective disorder. Small-framed linear people with low fat and muscle mass (ectomorphs) are overrepresented among individuals with schizophrenia. Although by no means absolute, the presence of one of these body types alters the clinical probabilities and is thus helpful in the diagnostic process (8). Table 2–2 further illustrates some correlations between major psychiatric conditions and observations of general appearance.

Motor behavior, like general appearance, is observed upon meeting the patient. Observations of motor behavior should include a description of gait, abnormal movements, frequency of movement, rhythm, coordination, and speed. Walking with the patient to the examining room is an excellent opportunity to begin observing these behaviors. The wide-based or ataxic gait of the alcoholic, the hesitant gait of the Huntington's chorea patient, the stooped shuffle of the patient with frontal lobe disease, and the manneristic hopping and tiptoe gaits of the catatonic are but a few of the unusual motor behaviors that can be observed while walking to the office.

One of the more common motor disturbances seen in seriously ill patients is *agitation*. Agitation, or an increase in the frequency of non-goal-

TABLE 2–2 Some General Appearance Diagnostic Correlations for Major Psychiatric Illness

ITEM	EXAMPLE OBSERVATION	CONDITIONS AT RISK
1. Age and sex	male under 20	Character and behavior disorder; drug-related conditions
	female over 40	Unipolar affective disorder
	female	Affective disease; neuroses; Briquet's syndrome
	male	Sociopathy; schizophrenia
2. Body type	endomorph	Affective disorder
	ectomorph	Schizophrenia
3. Nutrition	recent weight loss, chronic malnutrition	Depression, dementia
4. Personal hygiene	unkempt/dirty	Coarse brain syndrome (acute or chronic); schizophrenia
5. State of consciousness	clouded	Acute coarse brain syndrome (delirium)
6. Manner	hostile and suspicious	Delusional psychosis; coarse brain disease
7. Dress	head decorations, bright colors, scant clothing	Mania

directed motor behavior, is the expression of an intense mood and can reflect anxiety, sadness, anger, or euphoria. Pacing, hand-wringing, head-rubbing, constant shifting of body position, playing with one's fingers, and picking at bed sheets are all examples of agitation.

Because of chronic ingestion of neuroleptics, many psychiatric patients will exhibit constant jerky finger movements, foot-tapping, pelvic thrusts, and/or repetitive oral movements such as lip smacking or moving the torgue in and out of the mouth. These movements are manifestations of a coarse brain disorder and have been given the global term *tardive dyskinesia* (9, 10). Although tardive dyskinesia typically exacerbates with stress, it is also frequently observed in patients who are calm. It should not be confused with agitation.

Adventitious motor overflow—small, uncontrollable, and jerky hand, head, and shoulder movements (e.g. chorea)—must also be distinguished from agitation. Motor overflow can be observed as the patient walks toward the examining room. Patients with chorea often exhibit sudden involuntary hand movements, which they try to "cover up" by transforming the movement into a socially accepted action (e.g. smoothing hair, fixing a tie). Adventitious motor overflow can be tested by asking the patient to hold both arms straight out in front of him for twenty seconds, during which choreiform jerks may appear. Adventitious motor overflow, unlike agitation, is not an expression of an intense mood and can be observed in perfectly calm individuals (11–13).

Global, usually goal-oriented activities of psychiatric patients are often altered. The extremes of these activity changes are termed *hyperactivity* and *hypoactivity*. A patient who is engaged in too many things at the same time, talks to several people one after the other, and goes from one place to another in quick succession is said to be hyperactive. The patient who does nothing, who sits for long periods in a chair, rarely moving or responding to surrounding events, is said to be hypoactive. In its extreme form, hyperactivity appears as frantic, constant, impulsive, and incomplete multiple activities, which may appear non-goal-directed. It is invariably associated with an intense *excitement* state in which the patient is constantly talking and often shouting. Extreme importunate and intrusive behavior and intense irritability and/or euphoria are usually present (7). Prior to the availability of electroconvulsive treatment, patients experiencing extreme excitement were reported occasionally to suffer cardiovascular collapse and even death (14). Extreme hyperactivity or excitement is most frequently observed in individuals who satisfy modern diagnostic criteria for mania (15, 16).

Extreme hypoactivity is termed *stupor*. A stuporous patient may stay motionless for hours, staring fixedly or following the examiner about the room with his eyes, yet mute and unresponsive to spoken comments and even to painful stimuli (general analgesia) (17). When associated with coarse disease, particularly of the brainstem, the syndrome is termed *akinetic mutism* (18). When coarse disease cannot be demonstrated, such stuporous patients most frequently satisfy diagnostic criteria for affective disorder (19–21). Stupor is also a feature of the catatonic syndrome (see Chapter 14).

AFFECT

Affect is the emotional tone underlying all behaviors. Affect can be understood quantitatively as having a range, intensity, and stability and qualitatively as having appropriateness of mood, quality of mood, and relatedness. Mood is the content of affect. They are not synonymous terms.

Mood refers to expressions of sadness, happiness, anger, and anxiety. Patients will often spontaneously relate the quality of their mood (e.g. "I am anxious"). Their appearance and manner will also reflect their mood and provide reliable information for assessing its quality. Facial expression is particularly useful in this regard. Two outstanding facial characteristics of depression, for example, are the *omega sign* and *Veraguth's folds*, both shown in Figure 2–1. The omega sign is the furrowing between the eyebrows that resembles the Greek letter *omega*. Veraguth described eyelid folds in depressives that formed an upward angle at the inner canthus of the eye. Both the omega sign and Veraguth's folds have been used to predict a good response to electroconvulsive treatment (22, 23).

In mental illness the quality of mood may become constant despite changes in the patient's immediate surroundings (7). Patients with affective disorder express a constant mood of sadness, elation, or irritability. Patients with anxiety states may be in a constant state of panic, and patients with schizophrenia may have no expression of mood and appear *emotionally blunted* and apathetic. Variability of emotional expression over time is the *range of affect* and can be compared to the variations and modulation in music. In each of the above examples of constant mood, the range of affect is *constricted*. A person with a constricted affect essentially expresses only one mood over a period of time regardless of surrounding events. Thus, a depressed patient who expresses only sadness and a manic patient who expresses only euphoria both have a constricted affect.

In contrast, some patients have rapid shifts in their mood (7), moving quickly from tearfulness to laughter, and then to angry outbursts. Often these outbursts occur with minimal or no provoking stimuli. This instability of emotional expression is termed *lability of affect*. Constricted affect and lability of affect are opposite extremes in the variability of emotional expression. Regardless of the underlying pathophysiology, most mentally ill individuals have some disturbance in their affective variability.

Moods can vary in *intensity* as well as quality (7). Intensity of mood

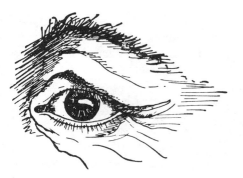 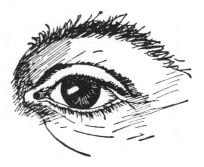

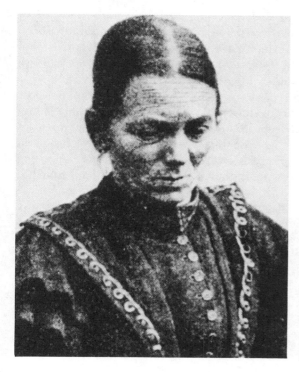

Figure 2-1 *Above left:* An eye exhibiting Veraguth's folds. *Above right:* An eye with normal folds. (Both are left eyes.) *Bottom left:* A woman whose face shows the omega sign. Reproduced from Eugen Bleuler's *Textbook of Psychiatry* (1924) with thanks to Edmund R. Brill.

refers to the degree or amplitude of emotional expression. Thus anger is more intense than irritability and euphoria more intense than happiness. In many patients affectivity can be constricted in range (restricted to a single quality of mood) but with great intensity. The psychomotor epileptic, for example, can shout and rage with great force, never varying his mood until overcome by exhaustion. His range of affect is severely constricted, but the amplitude of his affect is great.

Mood appropriateness has been given great diagnostic weight in past official nosologies. Its definition and meaning have been generally misconstrued. Mood appropriateness refers *only* to the patient's moods expressed during the mental status examination and is determined, in part, by the examiner's own mental state and empathic understanding of the patient's behavior ("What's appropriate for me is appropriate for the patient"). Inappropriateness of mood (laughing in a sad situation) is not a pathognomonic sign and may reflect normal anxiety (e.g. gallows humor), as well as serious illness. For example, a patient who is angry at being hospitalized against his will has an appropriate mood by the standard of our "empathic understanding." We would be angry too in the same situation. A patient who shows no sadness in stating that a parent died ten years ago has an appropriate lack of mood, because normally intense grief does not last that long. A patient who laughs uproariously when exhibiting a significant injury has an inappropriate mood, since by the standard of "empathic understanding" we would not think such a situation humorous.

Using this scheme, it becomes possible to categorize patients' emotional behavior precisely. A manic who emits prolonged bellylaughs at only mildly humorous situations has an appropriate mood but an inappropriately increased amplitude of mood and probably constriction of affect (decreased range). A schizophrenic who is apathetic and shows no emotion when seeing his parents for the first time in months has an inappropriate mood, constriction of affect, and decreased mood intensity. The pattern of emotional behaviors (Table 2–3) has diagnostic correlation and must be carefully observed and recorded. These patterns will be discussed in more detail in the chapters dealing with the major psychiatric syndromes.

The most difficult facet of affect to evaluate is *relatedness*, or the ability of an individual to express warmth, to interact emotionally, and to establish rapport. Schizophrenics are notoriously unable to respond in this manner

TABLE 2–3   Patterns of Affect Responses

RANGE	INTENSITY OF MOOD	MOOD APPROPRIATENESS	RELATEDNESS	QUALITY OF MOOD
1. Increased (labile)	1. Increased	1. Appropriate	1. Related	1. Euthymia
2. Normal	2. Normal	2. Inappropriate	2. Unrelated	2. Happiness
3. Decreased (constricted)	3. Decreased			3. Sadness
				4. Anxiety (dysphoria)
				5. Anger
				6. Apathy

and often appear cold and unfeeling. They are said to have *emotional blunting*.

Emotional blunting has been considered a core sign of schizophrenia since the earliest descriptions of the syndrome (24, 25). More recently a reliable measure (Table 2-4) for determining the presence of emotional blunting has been reported (26) and confirmed (27). High scores (above 20) on this rating scale are consistent with significant coarse brain disease (dementia) and schizophrenia.

Patients with *emotional blunting* have a paucity of emotional response. Thus their characteristic pattern of affective response is a constricted affect,

TABLE 2-4   Rating Scale for Emotional Blunting

ITEM	RATING[a]		
Affect			
1. Absent, shallow, incongruous mood	0	1	2
2. Constricted affect (narrow range)	0	1	2
3. Unvarying affect (lacks modulation)	0	1	2
4. Unrelated affect (lacks warmth, empathy)	0	1	2
Behavior			
5. Expressionless face	0	1	2
6. Unvarying, monotonous voice	0	1	2
7. Seclusive/withdrawn, avoids social contact	0	1	2
8. Lacks social graces (negligent dress, ill-mannered, unbathed)	0	1	2
9. Difficult to excite emotions/unresponsive	0	1	2
10. Lacks spontaneity	0	1	2
11. Causeless, silly laughter/silly disposition	0	1	2
12. Indifferent to surroundings (staff and visitors, patients, physical environs)	0	1	2
Thought Content			
13. Indifference/lack of affection for family, friends	0	1	2
14. Indifference/unconcern for own present situation	0	1	2
15. Indifference/unconcern for own future (lacks plans, ambition, desires, drive)	0	1	2
16. Paucity of thought (unable to elaborate on answers	0	1	2
☐ Total score			

[a]0 = absent; 1 = slight or doubtful; 2 = clearly present
Relationship to Psychiatric Disorder

Score	Illness
0–5	No illness
6–10	Personality disorder, neuroses, depression
10–15	Affective disorder, acute coarse brain disease
20	Schizophrenia, chronic coarse brain disease

SOURCE: "A Rating Scale for Emotional Blunting," by R. Abrams and M. A. Taylor, in *The American Journal of Psychiatry* 135:2 (1978), Table 1, p. 227. Copyright © 1978 by the American Psychiatric Association. Reprinted by permission.

a decreased intensity of mood, apathy, inappropriateness of mood, and unrelatedness. They are expressionless in facial movements, tone of voice, and social behaviors. They are seclusive, avoiding social contact, and are indifferent to hospital staff, visitors, relatives, and their physical environs. They express little affection for their families and friends and are unconcerned about their present situation. They are without plans or desires for the future. When asked how they feel about being in the hospital or how they would feel if they had to remain hospitalized for many months, emotionally blunted patients respond:

"Well, I guess I'll have to."
"Its okay being here."
"Well, I don't like to, but what can I do?"

When asked if they miss their family, they respond:

"They're okay. They can take care of themselves."
"They have their own lives to lead."

The following exchange took place between one of us and a patient whose facial expression remained blank and whose voice remained monotoned and stilted throughout the examination:

E: Do you miss your wife?
P: (Pause) Yes.
E: What do you miss about her?
P: (Pause) Meals.

Occasionally patients with emotional blunting will make silly jokes and will express a fatuous but shallow mood, incongruous to the situation. This is termed *Witzelsucht* and will be discussed in the chapters on coarse brain disease.

Speech and Language

The organization of language and language disorder, although recognized as essential aspects of normal and pathological human behavior, have received insufficient attention in most discussions of the mental status examination. Indeed, one set of modern research criteria for schizophrenia (28) simply uses the phrase "verbal production that makes communication difficult because of a lack of logical or understandable organization" as an all-encompassing thought (language) disorder, thus ignoring the different processes of language function. In contrast, the neuropsychiatrist and the aphasiologist should consider the form of language (e.g. thought processes) fundamental to the examination, as different forms of language disorder are associated with different diagnostic conditions and dysfunction in different brain regions.

Thought processes are inferred from a person's speech and use of language. The form of speech and language differs from thought content. The form of speech is characterized by its rate, pressure, rhythm, idiosyncrasy of word usage, grammar, syntax, and associational linkage. The way a patient speaks is *process;* what he is talking about is *content* and primarily reflects cultural and personal life experience rather than the disease process in question. Thought content is rarely of diagnostic importance. Possible exceptions to this rule are the thoughts of suicide, guilt, and hopelessness often expressed by depressed patients, or the grandiose ideas of great wealth, power, or high birth expressed by manics. These too, however, can be conceptualized as the content of a profound unremitting sadness and dysphoria, which is the essential psychopathological form of major depressive illness or the content of an intense euphoric mood, a cardinal feature of mania. Strange or "bizarre" ideas are never diagnostic and can occur in many conditions (7, 16, 29, 30).

The evaluation of speech and language is the most difficult aspect of the neuropsychiatric examination to master. It demands considerable concentration and practice. The speech of psychiatric patients is often filled with unusual and fascinating content upon which unwary clinicians can focus to the exclusion of form recognition. Skill in determining speech and language dysfunction can be developed only by consciously asking oneself questions about how the patient is using language. For example:

"What is the rate and rhythm of this patient's speech?"
"Is his speech fluent or halting and dysarthric?"
"Is he using precise words?"
"Does his speech make sense and, if not, how precisely are his associations linked?"

It is also helpful to allow the patient to talk for a bit while the examiner listens, not to the content, but to the patient's use of language.

Although the rate of speech can reflect cultural patterns, severe deviations are commonly observed in mentally ill patients. Slow and/or hesitant speech is characteristic of depression, altered states of consciousness, and several coarse brain disorders (19, pp. 77–80; 23, 31–33). Rapid, pressured speech is characteristic of anxiety and mania (19, 24, 31–33). The rhythm or cadence of speech can also be disturbed in the mentally ill patient. Hesitant speech is often heard in patients with Huntington's chorea (34); scanning speech (where word sounds are stretched, producing a slow, sliding cadence) is characteristic of multiple sclerosis (33); and staccato (abrupt and clipped) speech is often a sign of psychomotor epilepsy (30).

During the past century and a half psychiatrists have been concerned with the precise definition of the differing patterns of the spoken language of the mentally ill. A definitive classification of these phenomena does not exist, but many of the traditional definitions have moderate reliability (35) and are valid to the extent that they tend to discriminate patient groups (36), predict outcome, and relate to differences on electrophysiological measures (37). All abnormal patterns of the spoken language of the mentally ill, traditionally, are termed thought disorder. Those patterns which classically have been related to schizophrenia and are reminiscent of aphasic speech are specifically termed formal thought disorder.

The presence of certain thought disorders suggests particular syndromes (7). For example, rambling speech is characteristic of acute coarse brain disorders (e.g. intoxications); driveling speech, perseveration, non sequiturs, derailment, paraphasias, and tangential speech are more often associated with chronic coarse brain disorders (e.g. dementia) and schizophrenia; and flight-of-ideas is the classical speech pattern in mania. Table 2–5 displays the various types of thought disorder, their definition and associated conditions. Each will be presented in greater detail in discussions of specific syndromes. The specific evaluation of language function will be discussed in Chapter 3, "The Behavioral Neurologic Examination."

Delusional Phenomena

Delusional phenomena are characterized by false or arbitrary ideas developed without adequate proof. These phenomena, each of distinct psychopathological form, include delusional mood, delusional ideas (primary and secondary), autochthonous delusional ideas, and delusional perceptions (7). Delusional phenomena are frequently observed in severely ill psychiatric patients. They are not pathognomonic of schizophrenia, however, and are frequently found in patients with affective disorder and coarse brain disease (7, 15, 16; 19, pp. 18–22, pp. 84–85; 22, 38).

When delusional ideas are accepted as real by patients, they may readily reveal these ideas, because they feel them to be obvious to everyone. Some patients, aware that other people might think them crazy, will be reluctant to reveal strange but—to them—true ideas. When they do, however, describe plots against their lives, special relationships with God, or national and international intrigues, the examiner must express an immediate interest in "these happenings," acquire more specific information about the situation as any concerned person about a friend's problems, and ultimately determine the form of the delusion by asking the patient for proof, i.e., "How do you know?"

TABLE 2-5 Thought Disorders

DISORDER	ASSOCIATED ILLNESS	DEFINITION
Rambling	Acute coarse brain disease	Non-goal-directed speech in which meaningful connections between phrases or sentences are lost
Flight-of-ideas	Mania	Jumping from topic to topic, often in response to external stimuli. Multiple lines of thought can occur. Line of thought often fails to reach goal
Clang associations	Mania	Associations by the sound rather than the meaning of words
Circumstantial speech	Mania; inter-ictal temporal lobe epilepsy; alcoholism	Tightly linked associations but with extra, nonessential associations interspersed. The speech takes a circuitous route before reaching the goal
Formal disorders	Schizophrenia, chronic coarse brain disease	
Driveling		Associations are tightly linked and syntax appears preserved but the meaning (content) of speech is lost. Similar to double talk. Word salad is its most severe form
Perseveration		The repetition of stock words and phrases automatically placed into the flow of speech
Nonsequiturs		There is no evidence of flight-of-ideas and the patient's responses are totally unrelated to the examiner's questions.
Paraphasia		The use of words or phrases without precise meaning (word approximations), new words often formed by the improper use of the sound of words (neologisms)
Derailment		The sudden switch from one line of thought to a new parallel line of thought
Tangential speech		Tightly linked associations that bypass the goal. Responses are vague, allusive, and beside the point
Verbigeration		A verbal stereotype in which the patient repeats associations, particularly at the end of a thought, in an automatic manner

The simplest delusional experience is termed a *delusional mood*. This phenomenon is characterized by the intense and persistent "feeling" that "something is wrong," that "things are not right" and are perhaps sinister. It is akin to, but more severe than, the feeling of being watched or the common experience of self-consciousness felt by sensitive people entering a noisy room full of people who, for the moment, become quiet to observe the newcomer. When the patient describes his belief that something "bad" is taking place that will adversely effect him and the examiner asks "How do you know?" the patient suffering from a delusional mood will respond, "Well, I don't know, I'm not sure. I just feel it." Delusional moods can be observed in almost any serious psychiatric condition, following serious viral illnesses, and in association with coarse brain disorders. It does not have diagnostic specificity (7).

Delusional ideas have been defined as (1) "fixed false beliefs not in keeping with one's own cultural environment" (39), and (2) "the making of a relationship without adequate proof" (40). When the delusional idea develops from other psychopathology (e.g. an altered mood, a hallucination), it is derivative in sequence of occurrence and is termed a *secondary delusional idea*. These phenomena are particularly common in patients with affective disorders and certain psychomotor states. When the delusional idea forms without obvious development from previous psychopathology, it is termed a *primary delusional idea*. An *autochthonous delusional idea* is a particular type of primary delusional idea that develops suddenly and fully formed (rather than insidiously). Except for the fact that an autochthonous delusional conclusion is fixed and arbitrary, it is similar to the "eureka" phenomenon (7).

Although primary and secondary delusional ideas are conclusions reached arbitrarily and without adequate proof, the patient can often identify "evidence" to support his notion. For example, a patient who repeatedly received recruitment material from the Army concluded that there was a dangerous government reorganization and a plot was "afoot" to "silence" him. He cited real problems with electrical blackouts in his neighborhood as confirmatory evidence of the plot. This patient's sequence of thought from recruitment material and electrical blackouts to a plot, although arbitrary, has an understandable connection—i.e., it is delusional, but most observers can follow how he reached his conclusion. *Delusional perceptions* on the other hand, are ideas for which no meaningful connection can be found between the "evidence" and the conclusion. Delusional perceptions are based upon real perceptions that are then given great significance and personalized by the patient. For example, a patient concluded a neighbor was going to kill him because a yellow cab drove down the street. Delusional perceptions are primary, because they do not develop from any other obvious psychopathology.

PERCEPTION

Perceptual disturbances are very common among psychiatric patients. Perceptions without external stimuli (hallucinations) and misperceptions of real external stimuli (illusions) are most frequently observed (7).

Hallucinations can occur in all sensory modalities—visual, auditory, olfactory, gustatory, tactile, and visceral—and can occur in a variety of nonpathological conditions, such as fatigue, distractability, and falling asleep and awakening. Nearly 50 percent of people without any mental disorder have hallucinated at some time in their lives (41). Anyone who has heard his name paged when no sound came from the loudspeakers has hallucinated. Table 2-6 displays the different forms of perceptual disturbances, their definition, and the disorders to which they best correlate. None is pathognomonic.

When examining a patient for delusional phenomena, we ask him about "trouble with neighbors, co-workers, or relatives" that might reveal his delusional ideas. Hallucinatory experiences can be elicited in a similar manner with such questions as: "Have people been bothering you or trying to harm you in anyway? Have you seen them following you or plotting against you? Do you overhear their conversations about you? Do they say things to you through electronic devices, such as the TV or radio? Can they touch you even when they are not in the room? Can you feel them? Do they do anything to your food? Do they try to harm you with gas that smells bad?"

The development of good rapport with the patient is vital if adequate information is to be obtained about delusional and perceptual phenomena. Patients will converse more readily if they feel the examiner is concerned, interested, and knowledgeable about such phenomena. Frequently a statement such as the following is helpful: "I have spoken with other people with similar experiences [feelings, situations] to yours and they also experienced . . ." Examples of delusions and hallucinations can then be given, and many patients will respond with "yes, I've had that happen to me too." Details usually follow. On rare occasions a fruitful question might be, "Have you recently had any frightening experiences or experiences you couldn't explain?" Examples of "voices and visions" can then be given. Some chronic patients will respond to the direct: "Do you hallucinate? Do you hear voices?"

Occasionally, during a discussion of his delusional ideas, a patient will ask, "Do you think I'm right?" The best response is, "I understand what you're saying and I know you feel these experiences are true, but I wonder if there isn't another explanation." If the patient says, "No, there isn't," go on to the next logical topic. If the patient insists on an opinion, the examiner should offer the explanation that the experiences are signs and symptoms of an illness. After going "on the record" the examiner should not argue. Many

TABLE 2-6 Perceptual Disturbances

DISTURBANCE	MOST COMMON ASSOCIATION	DEFINITION
Pseudo-hallucination	Can occur in the non-ill	Any vague, poorly formed hallucination
Hypnagogic/ hyponopompic hallucination	Can occur in the non-ill	Pseudo-hallucinations occurring respectively upon falling alseep and awakening
Incomplete auditory hallucination	Nonspecific	Most common perceptual disturbance. A muffled or whispered voice limited to a few words
Complete auditory hallucination	Schizophrenia	Most common first-rank symptom. A clear, sustained voice perceived as originating from outside the patient's subjective inner space
Elementary hallucination	Toxic and epileptic states	Unformed hallucinations such as flashes of light unidentified voices, smells and taste
Functional hallucination	Toxic and epileptic states	A hallucination that occurs only immediately after ordinary stimulation in that particular sensory modality (e.g. hearing voices only when the water faucet is turned on)
Extracampine hallucination	Toxic, epileptic states and schizophrenia	A hallucination outside the normal sensory field (e.g. seeing people behind you)
Dysmegalopsia	Epileptic states	Perceiving objects as becoming larger (macropsia) or smaller (micropsia)

patients will trust a truthful examiner far more than one who appeases them, treats them as if they were crazy, or disregards their feelings and debates the validity of their experiences.

First-Rank Symptoms of Schneider

The late Kurt Schneider, a German psychiatrist, who was the first to describe systematically clinical phenomena he termed first-rank symptoms (42), wrote that "when any of these modes of experiences is undeniably present, and no basic somatic illness can be found, we may make the decisive clinical diagnosis of schizophrenia." Schneider regarded these symptoms as "first-rank" only in the diagnostic sense. They were correlative assumptions formed purely from clinical experience and were without relationship to any theoretical concept. Even though his descriptions and definitions have generated great interest in the phenomenologic study of schizophrenia, investigations have demonstrated that, although first-rank symptoms occur in 60 to 75 percent of rigorously defined schizophrenics, they are also experienced by individuals with affective disease, particularly during manic episodes (15, 16, 19, 39, 43).

Schneider listed eleven first-rank symptoms, which can be conveniently categorized under five headings: (1) thought broadcasting, (2) experiences of influence, (3) experiences of alienation, (4) complete auditory hallucinations, and (5) delusional perceptions (described above under "Delusional Phenomena").

Thought broadcasting refers to the relatively uncommon phenomenon of a patient's literally experiencing his thoughts escaping from his head. The patient "feels" his thoughts diffusing out of him and then hears them in the external world. Patients will often have secondary delusional ideas involving telepathy, electronic surveillance, or metaphysical intervention to explain the phenomenon. The examination for thought broadcasting often begins with questions focusing on the associated secondary delusional ideas. Once the form of these ideas has been established, the examiner can proceed to such questions as: "Do you feel people know what you're thinking?" "Can others really hear your thoughts?" "You mean, if I were standing next to you, I could hear your thoughts coming out of your head, as loud as my voice?" "Come on, you mean to say it's as if your head were a radio and everyone here can hear what you're thinking?" When a patient expresses the feeling that others can read his mind or says he believes people know what he's thinking by the expression on their faces, he most probably has delusional ideas. Only affirmative responses to the above questions satisfies the definition of thought broadcasting.

Some patients describe the experience that their body sensations, feelings, impulses, thoughts, and actions are controlled and manipulated by some external agency and that they must passively submit to the experience, which is literally felt on or within their bodies. Schneider termed this phenomenon *experience of influence*. Patients often develop secondary delusional ideas as explanations of the nature of these experiences.

In contrast, *experiences of alienation* are the subjective disowning of one's feelings, thoughts, or movements. The patient experiences (feels) his mental activity or actions literally to belong to someone else. Some patients with large parietal lobe lesions will also deny any relationship to certain of their body parts (usually those contralateral to the lesion). Although this phenomenon is similar to the Schneiderian experience of alienation, cerebral localization has never been demonstrated for any first-rank symptom.

Schneider also described hallucinated voices that occur in clear consciousness, are clearly audible, are experienced as coming from outside the patient's subjective space, and are sustained in duration. He termed these voices *complete auditory hallucinations*, including in this category prolonged voices continually commenting upon the patient's actions, multiple voices discussing the patient among themselves, or a voice repeating the patient's thoughts (thought echo). Complete auditory hallucination is the most common first-rank symptom (7).

A complete neuropsychiatric evaluation includes a thorough evaluation of cognitive function. Numerous investigators have demonstrated significant cognitive impairment in as many as 60 percent of severely ill psychiatric patients. This part of the mental status examination will be covered in Chapter 3, "The Behavioral Neurologic Examination."

References

1. Morse, R. M.; Litin, E. M. Post-operative delirium: A study of etiologic factors. *Am. J. Psychiat. 126:* 388–95, 1969.
2. Wells, C. Chronic brain disease: An overview. *Am. J. Psychiat. 135:* 1–12, 1970.
3. Wells, C. Delirium and Dementia. In Abram, H. (ed.), *Basic Psychiatry for the Primary Care Physician.* Boston: Little, Brown, 1976.
4. Sierles, F. Behavioral Medicine. In Sierles, F. (ed.), *Clinical Behavioral Science.* New York: SP Medical and Scientific Books, 1982, pp. 159–77.
5. Weissman, M.; Meyers, J.; Harding, P. Psychiatric disorders in a US urban community 1975–1976. *Am. J. Psychiat. 135:* 459–67, 1978.
6. Goodwin, D.; Guze, S. *Psychiatric Diagnosis.* 2d ed. New York: Oxford University Press, 1979.
7. Taylor, M. A. *The Neuropsychiatric Mental Status Examination.* New York: SP Medical and Scientific Books, 1981.
8. Parnell, R. W. *Behavior and Physique: An Introduction to Practical and Applied Somatometry.* London: Edward Arnold, 1958.
9. Asnis, G. M.; Leopold, M. A.; Duvoisin, R. D.; *et al.* A survey of tardive dyskinesia in psychiatric outpatients. *Am. J. Psychiat. 134:* 1367–70, 1977.
10. Crane, G. E. Persistent dyskinesia. *Br. J. Psychiat. 122:* 395–405, 1973.
11. Quitkin, F.; Rifkin, A.; Klein, D. F. Neurologic soft signs in schizophrenia and character disorders. *Arch. Gen. Psychiat. 33:* 845–53, 1979.
12. Cox, S. M.; Ludwig, A. M. Neurologic soft signs and psychopathology: 1. Findings in schizophrenia. *J. Nerv. Ment. Dis. 167:* 161–65, 1979.

13. Hertzig, M.; Birch, H. Neurologic organization in psychiatrically disturbed adolescents: A comparative consideration of sex differences. *Arch. Gen. Psychiat. 19:* 528–37, 1968.

14. Derby, I. M. Manic–depressive "exhaustion" deaths. *Psychiat. Quart. 7:* 436–49, 1933.

15. Taylor, M. A.; Abrams, R. The phenomenology of mania: A new look at some old patients. *Arch. Gen. Psychiat. 29:* 520–22, 1973.

16. Carlson, G. A.; Goodwin, F. K. The stages of mania. *Arch. Gen. Psychiat. 28:* 221–28, 1973.

17. Kahlbaum, K. L. *Catatonia.* Baltimore: Johns Hopkins University Press, 1973.

18. McCusker, E. A.; Rudick, R. A.; Honch, G. W.; *et al.* Recovery from the 'locked-in' syndrome. *Arch. Neurol. 39:* 145–47, 1982.

19. Kraepelin, E. *Manic–Depressive Insanity and Paranoia.* New York: Arno Press, 1976.

20. Abrams, R.; Taylor, M. A. Catatonia: A prospective clinical study. *Arch. Gen. Psychiat. 33:* 579–81, 1976.

21. Taylor, M. A.; Abrams, R. The prevalence and importance of catatonia in the manic phase of manic–depressive illness. *Arch. Gen. Psychiat. 34:* 1223–25, 1977.

22. Hamilton, M.; White, J. M. Factors related to the outcome of depression treated with ECT. *J. Ment. Sci. 106:* 1031–41, 1960.

23. Roth, M. The phenomenology of depressive states. *Can. Psychiat. J. 4:* 532–53, 1959.

24. Kraepelin, E. *Lectures on Clinical Psychiatry.* Johnstone, J. (trans.). London: Bailliere, Tindull & Cox, 1904.

25. Bleuler, E. *Dementia Praecox or the Group of Schizophrenias.* Zinkin, J. (Trans.). New York: International Universities Press, 1950.

26. Abrams, R.; Taylor, M. A. A rating scale for emotional blunting. *Am. J. Psychiat. 135:* 225–29, 1978.

27. Andreasen, N. C. Affective flattening and the criteria for schizophrenia. *Am. J. Psychiat. 136:* 944–47, 1979.

28. Feighner, J. P.; Robins, E.; Guze, S. B.; *et al.* Diagnostic criteria for use in psychiatric research. *Arch. Gen. Psychiat. 26:* 57–63, 1972.

29. Bleuler, M. Acute Mental Concomitants of Physical Diseases. In Benson, D. F.; Blumer, D. (eds.), *Psychiatric Aspects of Neurologic Disease,* vol. 1. New York: Grune & Stratton, 1975, pp. 37–61.

30. Blumer, D. Temporal Lobe Epilepsy. In Benson, D. F.; Blumer, D. (eds.), *Psychiatric Aspects of Neurologic Disease,* vol. 1. New York: Grune & Stratton, 1975, pp. 171–98.

31. Benson, D. F. Disorders of Verbal Expression. In Benson, D. F.; Blumer, D. (eds.), *Psychiatric Aspects of Neurologic Disease,* vol. 1. New York: Grune & Stratton, 1975, pp. 121–36.

32. Brown, J. W. *Aphasia, Apraxia and Agnosia: Clinical and Theoretical Aspects.* Springfield, Ill.: C. C. Thomas, 1972.

33. Levin, N.; Switzer, M. *Voice and Speech Disorders: Medical Aspects.* Springfield, Ill.: C. C. Thomas, 1962.

34. McHugh, P. R.; Folstein, M. F. Psychiatric Syndromes of Huntington's Chorea: A Clinical and Phenomenological Study. In Benson, D. F.; Blumer, D. (eds.), *Psychiatric Aspects of Neurologic Disease,* vol. 1. New York: Grune & Stratton, 1975, pp. 267–86.

35. Andreasen, N. C. Thought, language and communication disorders: 1. Clinical assessment, definition of terms and evaluation of their reliability. *Arch. Gen. Psychiat. 36:* 1315–21, 1979.

36. Andreasen, N. C. Thought, language and communication disorders: 2. Diagnostic significance. *Arch. Gen. Psychiat. 36:* 1325–30, 1979.

37. Abrams, R.; Taylor, M. A. Psychopathology and the electroencephalogram. *Biol. Psychiat. 15:* 871–78, 1980.

38. Abrams, R.; Taylor, M. A. The importance of schizophrenic symptoms in the diagnosis of mania. *Am. J. Psychiat. 138:* 658–61, 1983.

39. Hamilton, M. (ed.). *Fish's Outline of Psychiatry.* 3d ed. Bristol: John Wright & Sons, Ltd., 1978.

40. Hinsie, L. E.; Campbell, R. J. *Psychiatric Dictionary.* 3d ed. New York: Oxford University Press, 1960.

41. Hamilton, M. (ed.). *Fish's Clinical Psychopathology: Signs and Symptoms in Psychiatry.* Rev. repr. Bristol: John Wright & Sons, Ltd., 1974, pp. 18–22.

42. Schneider, K. *Clinical Psychopathology.* Hamilton, M. W. (trans.). New York: Grune & Stratton, 1959.

43. Carpenter, W. T., Jr.; Strauss, J. S.; Muleh, S. Are there pathognomonic symptoms in schizophrenia? *Arch. Gen. Psychiat. 28:* 847–52, 1973.

CHAPTER 3

The Behavioral Neurologic Examination

Significance

Behavioral neurology is the clinical discipline in which normal and abnormal behaviors are linked to functioning of specific areas or regional systems of the brain (1). For example, the ability to perform skilled fine motor tasks (e.g. typing) is associated with the frontal lobe of the dominant hemisphere, and the loss of such abilities is usually the product of dominant frontal lobe dysfunction.

In the traditional, "routine" evaluations of neurologic function, examiners focus almost exclusively upon brain areas such as the brainstem, cerebellum, basal ganglia, motor and sensory strips, and the "long tracts." In contrast, the associational areas of the cortex and their related subcortical structures (areas primarily associated with behavior) are often overlooked. This attitude is in part due to past unreliability of clinical testing procedures and the consequent difficulty in localizing lesions that result in defects of higher cortical functions.

In fact, testing of these higher cortical functions can be reliable, valid, and sensitive (2–12). On occasion, a behavioral neurologic examination can identify a lesion before it is noted on CT scan or electroencephalogram, as in the following example:

A fifty-five-year-old man was admitted to a medical service because of disorientation, impaired memory, and irritability. A psychiatric consultation was requested. The psychiatrist identified prominent functional deficits in all cortical regions. A CT scan identified a solitary brain mass thought to be a tumor. The patient underwent a craniotomy with removal of the tumor. The patient died several days postoperatively and, as predicted by clinical examination, metastatic nodules were found on postmortem examination in every lobe of his brain.

The significance of behavioral neurology extends beyond the identification and localization of coarse brain disease. There is a high frequency of signs of cortical dysfunction in several of the major psychiatric syndromes (10, 13–21). For example, two-thirds of patients with schizophrenia (as against 20 percent of normals) and half of patients with major affective disorders have at least one abnormality on a standard aphasia screening test (20). Some syndromes traditionally associated with psychiatric illness can sometimes be localized to particular portions of the brain. For example, the syndrome of catatonia may result from frontal lobe dysfunction (22), and Capgras' syndrome is often associated with nondominant parietal dysfunction (23–25).

Historical Development

Neuropsychology, the basic science of behavioral neurology, is concerned with understanding the relationships among cognitive functions, behavior, and brain structure (26, 27). Until the middle of the nineteenth century, it was thought that cognitive—specifically, higher cortical—functions could not be localized to regions of the brain, each of which was viewed as functionally equipotential (28, 29). In 1861 Broca reported on a series of patients who had slow, labored, dysarthric, telegraphic speech. These patients had disease in what is now called "Broca's area" in the frontal cortex. In 1874 Wernicke described a group of patients with fluent but jargon-filled, often incomprehensible speech. These patients had pathology in the posterior portion of the superior temporal gyrus (Wernicke's area). These observations began an "era of localization," in which behaviors were overassociated with locations in the brain. Modern researchers and clinicians view the brain as anatomically and functionally regionalized but think more in terms of "systems" extending beyond limited sections of specific lobes (26, 27). Also within the past decade the importance of the connections (e.g. the corpus callosum) between hemispheres has been elucidated by researchers such as Roger Sperry.

Currently a number of reliable and valid neurophysiological tests may be employed in identifying and localizing brain malfunction (2–12). These include extensive instruments such as the Luria battery (3, 26, 30), the

Halstead–Reitan battery (6, 8, 31–33), and the Wechsler Intelligence Scales (34–37), and screening tests such as the Aphasia Screening Test (12) and the "Minimental State" examination (10, 38). The discussion that follows is based upon data obtained from such tests as these, as well as from clinical neuroradiology and neurosurgery (4, 10, 34, 35).

Central Concepts

PRIMARY, SECONDARY, AND TERTIARY CORTEX

According to Luria (26), the cerebral cortex can be divided into primary, secondary, and tertiary areas. Primary cortex, such as the transverse auditory gyrus of Heschl or the visual cortex in Brodmann's area 17, is organized to receive uninterpreted stimuli such as light or sound. Secondary cortex, occupying such areas as Brodmann's areas 18 or 19, organizes incoming sensations into recognizable patterns. For example, the light comprising the image of a flower is organized by secondary visual cortex into a pattern that a preverbal child would find familiar. In tertiary cortex, which comprises such areas as the angular gyrus, the speech areas of the cortex, or much of the frontal lobe, sensory patterns are interpreted, linked to other cortical regions, and acted upon. For example, the statement "What a sweet-smelling daisy" reflects the linkage of olfactory and visual sensations, the identification and explanation of what is perceived, and the communication of the idea to another person.

DOMINANT AND NONDOMINANT HEMISPHERES

By definition the term "dominant hemisphere" refers to the cerebral hemisphere that is organized functionally to express language. For 97 percent of people the dominant hemisphere is the left. For 3 percent the dominant hemisphere is the right, or dominance is mixed. Hemispheric dominance is not synonymous with hand preference, although there is a relationship. Ninety percent of people are right-handed (dextral), and in 99 percent of right-handers, the left hemisphere is dominant for language. Ten percent of people are left-handed (sinistral). Among left-handers, 60 percent have language organized in their left hemisphere (it is "dominant") and 40 percent have mixed dominance for language or language organized in their right hemisphere. Thus the clinician should be more alert to the possibility of mixed or right hemispheric dominance for language in sinistrals (39–43).

There is a considerable body of evidence that the two hemispheres process information differently and have different functional specializations.

The dominant hemisphere, usually the left, appears to process information in a sequential, analytic, linear fashion and is particularly efficient at processing language and other symbolic information. The "nondominant" hemisphere, the right, appears to process information in a gestaltic, holistic, parallel fashion and is particularly efficient at processing visual spatial information (26, 40–43).

The determination of a patient's preferred hand for writing is a crude but clinically useful strategy for determining which of his hemispheres is organized for language, i.e., is dominant (44). To confirm that the patient's hand preference for writing is a natural tendency and not the product of having been required as a child to write with the nonpreferred hand, the patient should be asked to state his hand preference and then demonstrate with which hand he pours liquids, holds his knife to cut food, holds scissors, throws a ball, and holds a thread when threading a needle.

Most individuals who write with their right hand will use their right hand for these purposes. Left-handers often give a mixed response.

INTERHEMISPHERIC CONNECTIONS

The corpus callosum and other deep cortical structures are responsible for communicating and integrating information between the two hemispheres. Although sensory and motor long tracts do not pass through the interhemispheric structures, messages from one secondary or tertiary cortical region to another secondary or tertiary region in the opposite hemisphere do pass through these structures. For example, in a left-brain-dominant patient, the instruction, "With your left hand, show me how you would hit a nail with a hammer" is processed by the tertiary cortex for speech in the left hemisphere and by the tertiary cortices of the left parietal and frontal lobes, and a "message" is then transmitted to the right hemisphere to initiate the motor response in the left hand. The pathway from right frontal lobe motor areas to the spinal cord and left upper extremities does not pass through the corpus callosum (45). (See Figure 3–1.)

Techniques for Testing of Cognitive Functions

ORGANIZATION

A behavioral neurologic examination, which is an extension of the mental status examination, should be performed on every patient. As in any portion of physical diagnosis, it should be done thoroughly and systematically. One

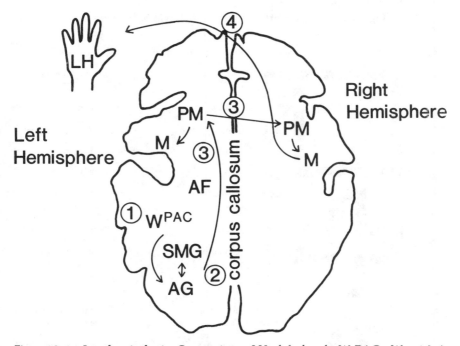

Figure 3-1 Interhemispheric Connections. LH, left hand; W-PAC, Wernicke's area—primary auditory cortex; SMG, supramarginal gyrus; AG, angular gyrus; AF, arcuate fasiculus; PM, premotor area; M, motor area; 1—patient decodes information "With your left hand, show me how you would use a hammer"; 2—control of ideokinetic praxis; 3—transmission of ideokinetic information from dominant parietal area to dominant frontal area and then across corpus callosum to nondominant frontal area; 4—transmission of motor sequencing (i.e., hammering) along pyramidal tract to spinal cord and then to left upper extremity.

strategy is to employ screening tests such as the Aphasia Screening Test (Figure 3–2) and the "Minimental State" Exam (Table 3–1). Another tactic is to proceed regionally (e.g. frontal, dominant temporoparietal, nondominant temporoparietal, occipital). We prefer this examination sequence:

1. Motor behavior
2. Language
3. Frontal lobe
4. Memory
5. Soft neurologic signs
6. Dominant parietal lobe
7. Nondominant parietal lobe
8. Nondominant temporal lobe
9. Occipital lobe

Figure 3-2   The Reitan-Indiana Aphasia Screening Test

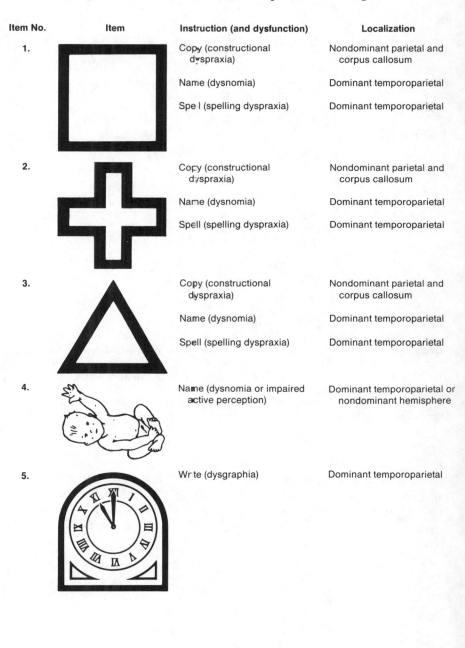

Item No.	Item	Instruction (and dysfunction)	Localization
1.		Copy (constructional dyspraxia)	Nondominant parietal and corpus callosum
		Name (dysnomia)	Dominant temporoparietal
		Spel l (spelling dyspraxia)	Dominant temporoparietal
2.		Copy (constructional dyspraxia)	Nondominant parietal and corpus callosum
		Name (dysnomia)	Dominant temporoparietal
		Spell (spelling dyspraxia)	Dominant temporoparietal
3.		Copy (constructional dyspraxia)	Nondominant parietal and corpus callosum
		Name (dysnomia)	Dominant temporoparietal
		Spell (spelling dyspraxia)	Dominant temporoparietal
4.		Name (dysnomia or impaired active perception)	Dominant temporoparietal or nondominant hemisphere
5.		Write (dysgraphia)	Dominant temporoparietal

Item No.	Item	Instruction (and dysfunction)	Localization
6.		Name (dysnomia)	Dominant temporoparietal
7.	7 SIX 2	Read (number agnosia, dyslexia)	Dominant temporoparietal
8.	M G W	Read (letter agnosia)	Dominant temporoparietal
9.	SEE THE BLACK DOG.	Read (dyslexia)	Dominant temporoparietal
10.	HE IS A FRIENDLY ANIMAL, A FAMOUS WINNER OF DOG SHOWS.	Read (dyslexia)	Dominant temporoparietal
11.	SQUARE	Write (dysgraphia)	Dominant temporoparietal
12.	SEVEN	Read (dyslexia)	Dominant temporoparietal
13.	85 – 27 =	Compute (dyscalculia)	Dominant parietal
14.		Name (dysnomia)	Dominant temporoparietal
		Demonstrate use (ideokinetic dyspraxia)	Dominant parietal, corpus callosum
		Draw (constructional dyspraxia)	Nondominant parietal, corpus callosum
15.	PLACE LEFT HAND TO RIGHT EAR.	Read (dyslexia)	Dominant temporoparietal
		Place (left-right disorientation)	Dominant parietal

Modified by permission from R.F. Heimburger and R.M. Reitan, "Easily Administered Written Test for Lateralizing Brain Lesions," in *Journal of Neurosurgery* 18:301–312 (1961). The test booklet may be purchased from Ralph M. Reitan, Ph.D., Department of Psychiatry, University of Arizona-Tucson 85721.

TABLE 3–1   The Minimental State Examination of Folstein, Folstein, and McHugh

SPECIFIC TEST	FUNCTION AND AREA TESTED[a]	POINTS SCORE
1. What is the year/season/day/date/month?	Orientation (frontal)	5
2. What is the state/county/town/hospital/floor?	Orientation (frontal)	5
3. Repeat three items.	Registration (frontal)	3
4. Serial subtraction of sevens *or* spell "world" backwards.	Concentration (frontal)	5
5. Name wristwatch and pen.	Naming (dominant temporoparietal)	2
6. Say "No ifs, ands, or buts."	Expressive speech (dominant frontal)	1
7. Take this paper in your right hand, fold it in half, and put it on the table.	Three-stage command (frontal)	3
8. Read "close your eyes" and do it.	Reading (dominant temporoparietal)	1
9. Remember the three items from part 3.	Short-term memory (dominant hippocampal)	3
10. Write a sentence.	Writing (dominant temporoparietal)	1
11. Copy intersecting pentagons.	"Construction" (nondominant parietal)	1

[a]Suggested cortical localization only. Score < 24 suggests coarse brain disease.
SOURCE: Modified from "Minimental State: A Practical Method of Grading the Cognitive State of Patients for the Clinician," by M. F. Folstein, S. W. Folstein, and P. R. McHugh, in *The Journal of Psychiatric Research* 12 (1975), pp. 189–98. Reprinted by permission of the copyright holder.

The various examination strategies can be cross-checked with each other by using Tables 3–2 and 3–3. For example, if motor testing reveals echopraxia and language testing shows expressive aphasia, both abnormalities can be seen as manifestations of frontal lobe dysfunction (see Table 3–3).

THE MEANING OF CORRECT RESPONSES AND ERRORS

Most tests in the behavioral neurologic examination are designed to "zero in" on specific higher cortical functions and secondary and tertiary cortical regions and systems. Nevertheless, intactness of multiple primary, secondary, and tertiary cortical regions is required for the correct performance of a given test.

For example, in the usual manner for testing for constructional ability (which is a tertiary cortical function often affected by lesions of the nondom-

TABLE 3-2 Cortical Mapping of Normal Function

	FRONTAL	DOMINANT TEMPOROPARIETAL	DOMINANT PARIETAL	NONDOMINANT PARIETAL	NONDOMINANT TEMPOROPARIETAL	OCCIPITAL	CORPUS CALLOSUM
Motor behavior	Motor persistence Initiation and stopping Rapid sequential movement Resistance to stimulus binding Learned complex motor behavior	Writing	Ideokinetic (ideomotor) praxis Kinesthetic praxis	Constructional praxis Dressing praxis Kinesthetic praxis			Tying shoelace with eyes closed Ideokinetic praxis in hand ipsilateral to dominant hemisphere
Language	Verbal fluency Spontaneous prosody and gesturing[a] Ability to repeat with prosodic affective variation[a]	Comprehension of spoken language Reading Relevance and word usage Naming Writing Letter gnosis Number gnosis	Symbolic categorization		Auditory comprehension of affective components of prosody Visual comprehension of affective components of prosody		Writing Reading

(Continued)

43

TABLE 3-2 (*Continued*)

	FRONTAL	DOMINANT TEMPOROPARIETAL	DOMINANT PARIETAL	NONDOMINANT PARIETAL	NONDOMINANT TEMPOROPARIETAL	OCCIPITAL	CORPUS CALLOSUM
Memory	Short-term memory store	Rehearsed consolidated memory (30 sec. –30 min.)			Musical memory	Visual memory	
Other	Concentration Global orientation Judgment Problem-solving Abstracting ability Right spatial recognition		Finger gnosis Calculation Right–left orientation Stereoagnosis Graphesthesia	Stereognosis Graphesthesia Recognition of familiar faces and other things East–west orientation		Visual pattern recognition (visual gnosis)	Stereognosis Graphesthesia

[a] Nondominant frontal lobe.

TABLE 3-3 Cortical Mapping for Brain Dysfunctions

	FRONTAL	DOMINANT TEMPOROPARIETAL	DOMINANT PARIETAL	NONDOMINANT PARIETAL	NONDOMINANT TEMPOROPARIETAL	OCCIPITAL	CORPUS CALLOSUM
Motor abnormalities	Motor impersistence Inertia Impaired rapid sequential movements Stimulus-bound behavior (e.g. echopraxia, gegenhalten)	Dysgraphia	Ideokinetic (ideomotor) dyspraxia Kinesthetic dyspraxia	Constructional dyspraxia Dressing dyspraxia Kinesthetic dyspraxia			Inability to tie shoes with eyes closed Ideokinetic dyspraxia in hand ipsilateral to dominant hemisphere Constructional dyspraxia in hand contralateral to dominant hemisphere
Language abnormalities	Broca's aphasia Transcortical aphasia Motor aprosodia[a] Verbigeration	Wernicke's aphasia Pure word deafness Driveling, word approximations, neologisms, stock phrases, phonemic paraphrasias, private use of words		Sensory aprosodia			Alexia without agraphia

(*Continued*)

TABLE 3-3 (*Continued*)

	FRONTAL	DOMINANT TEMPOROPARIETAL	DOMINANT PARIETAL	NONDOMINANT PARIETAL	NONDOMINANT TEMPOROPARIETAL	OCCIPITAL	CORPUS CALLOSUM
		Dysgraphia Dyslexia Dysnomia Letter agnosia Number agnosia					
Memory abnormalities	Impaired short-term memory store	Impairment of rehearsed consolidated memory			Impaired musical memory	Impaired visual memory	
Other abnormalities	Impaired concentration Global disorientation Impaired judgment Impaired problem-solving Impaired abstraction Right spatial neglect		Finger agnosia Dyscallulea Right–left disorientation Astereognosis Graphanesthesia Impaired symbolic categorization	Astereognosis Graphanesthesia Anosognosia Prosopagnosia Paragnosia Reduplicative paramnesia Left spatial neglect East–west disorientation			Astereognosis of hand ipsilateral to dominant hemisphere Graphanesthesia of hand ipsilateral to dominant hemisphere

[a]Nondominant frontal lobe.

46

inant parietal lobe), whereby the patient is asked to copy the outline of a simple geometric shape with his preferred hand, the following must be intact: (1) hearing—primary auditory cortex, (2) comprehension of speech—secondary and tertiary cortex of the dominant hemisphere, (3) vision—primary visual cortex, (4) visual gnosis/pattern recognition—secondary occipital cortex, (5) attention and concentration—frontal lobes, (6) visual-motor coordination—nondominant parietal lobe, (7) interhemispheric connection—corpus callosum and other deep cortical structures, (8) motor regulation—frontal lobe, and (9) motor strength of upper extremities—frontal motor strip, pyramidal tracts, spinal cord, and peripheral nerves.

When a patient makes an error, then, the examiner must put the error in the context of what is already known about the patient from the testing already completed and may need to perform other tests to localize the dysfunction (6, 8, 12, 27, 46). For example:

A patient is unable to copy the outline of a simple geometric shape with his right hand. His hearing, vision, visual gnosis, comprehension of speech, attention, concentration, motor regulation, and muscle strength are already known to be intact. The examiner then asks the patient to copy the outline of the shape with his left hand. The patient cannot copy the outline of the shape with his left hand either, suggesting that the dysfunction is in the nondominant parietal lobe, not the corpus callosum or left hemisphere structures. Had the patient been able to copy the outline with his left hand but not his right hand, a presumption might be made of abnormal functioning of corpus callosal or dominant hemisphere structures regulating the right hand. To verify the latter possibility, the patient could be asked to tie his shoelaces with his eyes closed, a task requiring grossly intact corpus callosal function.

If a patient gives an incorrect or unduly slow response, he will usually be asked to repeat the response. This helps the examiner to determine whether the patient understands the question and to assess further the severity of the dysfunction. If the instructions were not clear or if the patient is foreign-born or insufficiently fluent in the examiner's language, the test may not be valid. In the latter case the patient should be questioned in his native language. For example, a Puerto Rican patient could not name a Greek cross "a cross," but readily called the cross "cruz."

A final source of error may be a product of the patient's being uncooperative or poorly motivated. A notation should be made of the patient's level of motivation and cooperation.

General Strategies

The examining room should be well lighted and quiet, and the patient should be in a reasonably comfortable position for writing. A hard surface (e.g.

desk, dining cart) should be used for testing of writing and drawing. Instructions should be given with the utmost clarity.

Findings should be reported objectively; any error should be recorded as such. An examiner's statement, "Well, he got that wrong only because he was tired, so I won't report it" is an interpretation, not an observation. The examiner must be prepared to "judge" the normal speed and correctness of the patient's responses against a normal standard, usually his own performance. For example, when the doctor instructs the patient, "Touch your *left* hand to your *right* ear," the patient should be able to do so immediately.

The patient may require supportive comments from the examiner, e.g. "Try your best; there's no penalty if you make an error." The examiner must be patient with individuals whose brain dysfunction makes them slow to reply.

Observation and Testing of Specific Functions

MOTOR FUNCTIONS

In the mental status examination (Chapter 2), motor behavior plays a prominent part, with the examiner expected to note the general level of motor activity, the gait, the presence of tremors, choreo-athetoid movements, intrusiveness, agitation, and inertia. The behavioral neurologic examination requires further testing of motor functions, to include the following:

Motor Persistence

The examiner should note whether the patient is able to sustain a motor action. He should ask the patient to perform each of four tasks and note whether the patient is able to continue at the task for at least twenty seconds:

1. "Hold out your arms."
2. "Make a fist with both of your hands."
3. "Stick out your tongue."
4. "Raise your legs off the ground" (or "Close your eyes tightly").

Inability to persist with both extremities with eyes open may be due to the frontal lobe dysfunction called motor impersistence or to motor weakness of one or both upper extremities (46–48). To distinguish between the two, motor strength is tested as in the general neurologic examination.

Patients with normal motor persistence and strength should then be asked to close their eyes and again hold out their arms for twenty seconds. If one or both arms drift downward before twenty seconds, the parietal lobe contralateral to the drifting hand may be affected (46, 49).

Termination of Motor Actions

The frontal lobe is associated with the decision to start and stop motor actions and the ability to begin and stop once the decision is made (26). One abnormality of this function is called *perseveration,* which is the unnecessary repetition or maintenance of action. It can present itself or be elicited in a number of ways:

1. The patient can be asked to copy or spontaneously draw a design or shape that "lends itself" to unnecessary repetition (Figure 3–3).
2. The patient can be asked to perform a three-stage command such as, "Take this piece of paper in your right hand, fold it in half, and return it to me." A common perseverated response is for the patient to fold the paper in fourths or eighths.
3. The patient is asked to perform a task such as, "Place your left hand to your right ear," and despite precise instructions to lower his hand once the task is completed, he maintains the posture.
4. Occasionally a patient is asked to perform a sequence of tasks. If, following a request to do a new task, he continues to perform an action that had been requested earlier in the examination, he has perseverated (50–52).

Because of dysfunctions such as perseveration, frontal lobe abnormalities often produce false positive findings on testing of functions of other regions of the brain. For example, a patient is asked to draw the outline of a Greek cross (constructional praxis, a nondominant parietal function) after having been asked to draw a square. He again draws a square, which to the untrained examiner could be mistaken for a severely dyspraxic response (46, 50). In such a case the patient is asked to do a number of drawings. Sometimes the ability to copy the outline of a geometric or other shape will then become manifest. A behavior related to motor perseveration is diffi-

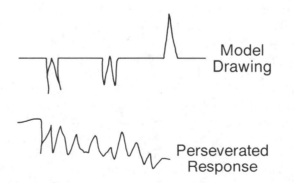

Model Drawing

Perseverated Response

Figure 3–3　A Drawing Which Lends Itself to Perseveration

culty in initiating motor tasks. Some patients will be virtually immobile, moving extremely slowly and hesitantly. The combination of difficulty initiating motor tasks and difficulty stopping the task once started (perseveration) is termed motor inertia (26).

Stimulus-Resistant Motor Behavior

The ability willfully to control one's motor actions based on thinking or reasoning, despite the presence of visual, tactile, or other stimuli that might lead a person with brain dysfunction to lose control over those actions, is called stimulus-resistant motor behavior. It is principally a frontal lobe function (26, 46). Abnormalities of stimulus-bound motor regulation include echopraxia and Gegenhalten (22).

1. *Echopraxia:* This occurs when the patient copies an action of the examiner, even after receiving specific instructions not to do so. In its severest form, which is rare, the patient will mimic an action of the examiner without any effort by the examiner to elicit this. Echopraxia usually must be elicited, in any or all of the following ways: At any point in the interview, the examiner may elevate his hands above his head and maintain this position for several seconds while he has the patient's attention. If the patient elevates his hands, he has manifested echopraxia, unless this has followed testing in which the patient has been asked to mimic the doctor's action. At this point the doctor should say, "You don't have to do that; you don't have to raise your arms." If the patient keeps his arms elevated, or if the patient again elevates his arms when the examiner next raises his, the echopraxia is severe.

The examiner may also instruct the patient, "When I touch my nose, you touch your chin." The doctor then touches his nose. If the patient then touches his own *nose*, he has manifested echopraxia. Several trials may be needed to assess (1) whether the patient understood the request and (2) how severe the echopraxia is.

The examiner might also ask the patient to extend his upper extremities in an anterior direction and then state, "I'd like you to do with your right hand what I do with my right hand." Once he thinks that the patient has shown he understands the question, he then places the fingers and palm of his right hand in various positions. If the patient copies these hand positions with his *left* hand (regardless of what he does with his right hand), he has echopraxia. To *verify* that this latter error is the product of echopraxia, and not left–right disorientation (a dominant parietal dysfunction) (49), the patient should then be tested for right–left orientation (see page 65).

2. *Gegenhalten:* The examiner instructs the patient to relax his arms and then attempts to flex and extend the patient's hand, forearm, or arm. If the patient's muscles give equal and opposite resistance to the examiner's maneuvers, the patient has manifested gegenhalten. Gegenhalten can occur

with the patient offering equal and opposite resistance to gentle pressure exerted against *any* part of his body. Although Gegenhalten often localizes to the frontal lobe, it is also considered a neurologic "soft sign" (53) (see pages 63–64).

3. *Catatonia:* In the syndrome of catatonia (see Chapter 14) the patient may show echopraxia or Gegenhalten or any of the following signs of motor dysregulation: (1) stupor with mutism, (2) automatic obedience, (3) catalepsy, (4) mannerisms, (5) stereotypy, (6) Mitgehen, and (7) posturing. Catatonic behaviors are often seen in patients with frontal lobe dysfunction (see Chapter 14) (22, 26, 46).

Another example of stimulus-bound motor dysregulation due to frontal lobe dysfunction is the following: Tell the patient "Don't shake my hand." When the examiner is convinced that the patient understands the question, he then extends his hand in a handshaking position. If the patient then shakes the doctor's hand, he has manifested stimulus-bound behavior.

Rapid Sequential Finger Movements

The examiner asks the patient to mimic his hand movements. He then proceeds to wiggle each finger, one at a time (little finger, ring finger, middle finger, forefinger, thumb), rapidly and in sequence. The patient should be able to mimic these rapid sequential finger movements; if not, he has probably revealed contralateral frontal lobe dysfunction (22, 26, 46).

If, as the examiner tests one hand for sequential finger movements (or for the ability to tap his fingers repeatedly against his knee or on a table), the fingers of the other hand start to wiggle or tap, the patient has manifested *adventitious motor overflow* (choreiform movements is another example). Although this sign sometimes localizes to the frontal lobe, it is considered a neurologic "soft sign."

Ideokinetic (Ideomotor) Praxis (26, 27, 30, 49, 52, 54)

Ideokinetic praxis is the ability to perform an action from memory upon request without props or cues. Primary motor and sensory function must be intact. To rule out the effect of interhemispheric dysconnection, the nonpreferred hand is tested first, and then the preferred hand is tested. For the same reason, the patient should not be allowed to cue himself by restating the instruction. The patient is asked to "Make believe you have a key in your left [nonpreferred] hand, and show me how you would use it." Other tests of ideokinetic praxis include: "Make believe you had a comb in your left hand, and show me how you would use it"; "Imagine you had a coin in your left hand, and show me how you would flip it"; and "Make believe you had a hammer in your left hand, and show me how you would use it." The patient should be able to mime these actions well. Common errors include awkward performance of these actions, miming only with proximal movements while distal movements (hand and wrist) are stiff or absent, use of the hand *as* the object itself (e.g. combing the hair by running the hand into the hair, hitting the imaginary nail with the fist itself) instead of as the bearer of the object, or the inability to perform the task without verbalizing the action (verbal overflow) (1, 26, 27, 30, 49, 52, 54).

In patients with interhemispheric dysconnection, ideokinetic praxis will be normal in the hand (usually the right) contralateral to the dominant (usually the left) hemisphere, and abnormal in the other hand. In patients with dominant parietal lobe dysfunction, ideokinetic dyspraxia will be manifest with both hands (49, 54).

Kinesthetic Praxis

Kinesthetic praxis is the ability to duplicate hand, finger, and other limb positions presented to the patient by the examiner (26, 43, 45). The examiner says to the patient, "What I do with my right hand, you do with your right hand, and what I do with my left hand, you do with your left hand." He then presents a variety of hand positions to the patient and asks the patient to mimic these. If the patient cannot reproduce these hand positions, he is manifesting kinesthetic dyspraxia, reflecting malfunction in the parietal lobe contralateral to the hand being tested (22, 30, 46, 49, 54).

Constructional Praxis

Constructional ability is generally tested by asking the patient to copy the outline of a shape (e.g. a square, a triangle, a Greek cross, a key) (1, 26, 30, 46, 49, 52, 54). To eliminate facilitating (e.g. straight lines) or distracting (e.g. other drawings) cues, each drawing should be done on a separate blank 8-by-11-inch sheet of unlined paper. The examiner should present the shape to be copied to the patient with the instructions, "I'd like you to copy the *outline* of this shape, without taking your pen (or pencil) off the paper. Your drawing should be the same size as the shape I am presenting to you, and should be in the center of the page." The shape to be copied should remain in full view of the patient. If the patient lifts the pen during the task, he must repeat the drawing. If the drawing is inaccurate, the dysfunction is called constructional dyspraxia. If the patient cannot complete the drawing unless he lifts his pen in mid-task, this may mean that he has dyspraxia. If he draws incorrectly with his preferred hand, he should repeat the drawing with the other hand. If the preferred-hand drawing is incorrect and the drawing with his nonpreferred hand is accurate, the dysfunction is likely the product of interhemispheric dysconnection (55). If both drawings are inaccurate, the dysfunction is most likely in the nondominant parietal region (1, 26, 30, 46, 49, 52, 54).

The reason the patient is asked to copy only the outline of the drawing is that accurate copying of the small details within the object's boundaries may require verbal reasoning (dominant hemisphere) as well as nondominant parietal lobe functioning.

Dressing Praxis

Dressing praxis is the ability of the patient to dress and undress himself efficiently. When patients make errors such as putting on clothes inside out or putting their feet in their shirtsleeves, they probably have nondominant parietal dysfunction (49, 54, 56).

LANGUAGE FUNCTIONS

Language is the use of symbols, usually in the form of spoken or written words, to convey meaning. Assessment of language is an extension of the "thought processes and content" section of the mental status examination. Language functions include spontaneous speech, naming, reading, and writing. Language functions are by definition primarily served by the dominant hemisphere, but the "affective components" of speech (called prosody) are served by the nondominant hemisphere (57–61).

Speech

The function of speech localizes primarily to the parasylvian areas of the frontal, temporal, and parietal lobes of the dominant (for words and word usage) and nondominant (for the "affectivity" of speech) hemispheres. In the dominant hemisphere this includes Broca's area, the frontal cortex deep to Broca's area, the supplementary motor cortex, the arcuate fasciculus connecting Broca's to Wernicke's area, Wernicke's area and adjacent temporal lobe structures, and the supramarginal gyrus of the parietal lobe (1, 46, 62, 63).

1. *Speech fluency.* Fluency of speech is a function of Broca's area, the frontal cortex deep to it, and the supplementary motor cortex. Speech fluency can be grossly estimated by simply listening to the extent, continuity, and fluidity of the patient's utterances. A standardized, sensitive test of general verbal fluency should also be administered by asking the patient to name as many animals as he can (or words beginning with a specific letter) as fast as he can. If expressive language function is normal, the patient can

name twenty to thirty animals (or "alliterated" words) in sixty seconds. Abnormalities of speech fluency include Broca's aphasia and transcortical motor aphasia (1, 46, 62, 63).

BROCA'S APHASIA

Broca's aphasia results from damage to the posterior inferior region of the left frontal lobe area. Patients with Broca's aphasia often understand spoken language reasonably well but are unable to express themselves fluently and are occasionally totally mute. Most can speak, but struggle to "get the words out." Even when they are able to verbalize, their sentences are often missing words, most commonly small words such as "the," "to," or "a." Speech without these small words resembles the language of telegrams (e.g. "Don't write, send money.") and is hence called "telegraphic." Broca's aphasia patients are often dysarthric, with labored words or mispronounced syllables (e.g. "Messodist Epistopal" for "Methodist Episcopal").

Sometimes a mild Broca's aphasia is not immediately recognized by the examiner, who should routinely test for it in all patients by having the patient repeat sentences or phrases containing small words (e.g. "The Polish Pope now lives in the Vatican" or "No ifs, ands, or buts") or phrases difficult to pronounce (e.g. "Methodist Episcopal," "Massachusetts Avenue") (27, 52, 54). Repetitive language also involves decoding and phonemic expression, so dysfunction in posterior language areas must be ruled out if a patient has difficulty repeating sentences. Sometimes the facility of expression of individual words can be increased by prompting the patient with the first sound of a word that the examiner thinks the patient wishes to speak. For example, if the examiner knows the patient wishes to say "daughter," and the patient is struggling, the examiner may say "duh." Improvement of speech with prompting may occur with angular gyrus lesions as well as Broca's area lesions.

Because of the extent of brain tissue damage associated with most diseases producing Broca's aphasia, problems not directly related to spoken language often accompany it (46, 62, 63). These abnormalities include (1) ideokinetic dyspraxia (discussed on pages 51–52) of the ipsilateral hand, (2) buccolingual dyspraxia (the patient may have trouble puffing out his cheeks, whistling, or blowing out a match), (3) weakness or paralysis of the contralateral extremities, and (4) dysgraphia (see pages 57–58) of the ipsilateral (and sometimes the contralateral) hand. In general, many patients with aphasia of any type cannot compensate for the aphasia by writing.

TRANSCORTICAL MOTOR APHASIA

Transcortical motor aphasia results from damage to the frontal lobe deep to Broca's area. In this type of aphasia, the patient manifests a paucity of speech. Speech is labored, as with Broca's aphasia; however, it is not telegraphic.

2. *Comprehension of speech—linkage of words to visual images.* These highly complex functions of the dominant hemisphere are associated with (1) the posterior two-thirds of the superior temporal gyrus, encompassing the transverse auditory gyrus of Heschl (the medial third of the superior temporal gyrus) and Wernicke's area (the posterior third), and (2) the angular gyrus. Dysfunctions in these regions, or in tracts such as the arcuate fasciculus connecting Wernicke's area to Broca's area, can produce Wernicke's aphasia, impaired auditory comprehension, dysnomia, and conduction aphasia.

WERNICKE'S APHASIA

Wernicke's aphasia is the product of a lesion in or around Wernicke's area, which is the posterior third of the superior temporal gyrus. This language disorder is characterized by fluent jargon-filled speech and impaired comprehension of the speech of others (27, 30, 54). As is the case in Broca's aphasia, writing is usually aphasic. A synonym for jargon speech is driveling. In driveling speech, the rhythm, volume, modulation, and syntax are normal, but the content is meaningless. The following is an example of driveling: "You can't give them away, but if they plot for too many of them, usually handling it."

The individual language abnormalities that constitute jargon speech can also appear independently in patients with dominant temporoparietal dysfunction (27, 30, 54). These abnormalities include the following:

Word approximations: The patient uses one or several words whose meaning is similar to that of the correct word. For example, instead of saying "pen" a patient says "a writer" or "an ink pencil."

Circumlocutions: Instead of using a correct word, the patient employs a phrase or sentence that either defines or comes close to identifying the desired word. For example, instead of saying "The pen is on the table," the patient may say, "The pen is on that wood thing with drawers that people write on."

Neologisms are new words that are not part of the language. For example, a patient used the following "words" during an interview: ventrontal, diangle, repture, kintle, nertrontral, cassey, and diatral.

Phonemic (literal) paraphasias are neologisms which sound similar to a correctly used word. For example, instead of saying "There's a chimney," a patient said, "There's a chimley." This abnormality can usually be distinguished from the labored, dysarthric productions of a Broca's aphasic patient (e.g. "Messodist Epistopal").

Private use of words: The patient uses real words or phrases in an idiosyncratic way. For example, a patient stated, "I was able to *industrialize* him and then I understood what was happening."

Stock words or phrases can be observed with frontal lobe dysfunction as well as with Wernicke's area dysfunction. They are words or phrases which are repeatedly inserted in conversations out of context. For example, a patient said, "I'll tell you why I was admitted here. *Don't take the cake.* They thought I was having a nervous breakdown. And I think I was. *Don't take the cake.*"

The poor comprehension of speech of a Wernicke's aphasia patient may be immediately apparent in his not responding appropriately to simple requests (e.g. "Would you sit down, please?"), or it may have to be elicited. Aphasiologists present requests of gradually increasing complexity. Sometimes a patient who can respond properly to a simple request ("Show me the picture of the baby") will be unable to respond to a more complex one ("Show me all the pictures that contain white or black or red").

On occasion a lesion of the middle third of the superior temporal gyrus will produce a solitary *defect of auditory comprehension.* Here the patient's speech is fluent, clear, and understandable, but the patient has grossly impaired comprehension of the speech of others.

3. *Other abnormalities of speech.* In addition to those abnormalities of speech seen in Broca's transcortical, and Wernicke's aphasias, other abnormalities of speech also exist.

DYSNOMIA (OR ANOMIA)

The patient with dysnomia has difficulty naming objects. The examiner asks the patient to name a series of objects, a list of which commonly includes a square, a cross, a triangle, a clock, a baby, a pen, and a wristwatch, and may include any other item in the room. The choice of items used in testing should be commensurate with the patient's level of education. For example, following a stroke a physician had little problem naming mundane objects; however, he was unable to name medical instruments whose function he could still describe. Dysnomia can be the product of a dominant temporal or dominant parietal lesion (54). Some neuropsychologists believe that if the patient's naming ability improves when he is prompted with the first syllable of the word to be named, it is more likely that the dysfunction is in the angular gyrus of the parietal lobe (54).

VERBIGERATION

The patient who verbigerates, automatically repeats words or small phrases. For example, the statement, "My brother gave me the pen, pen, the pen, and then he took it away" contains verbigeration. Verbigeration is most often seen with frontal lobe dysfunction, but it can probably be seen with dysfunction elsewhere in the dominant hemisphere. It is different from stuttering in that stutterers usually struggle and usually repeat only syllables, and usually at the beginning of sentences. Stutterers are also less likely to have serious brain dysfunction, and they do not evidence localized dysfunction.

ECHOLALIA

In echolalia the patient, without being told to do so, repeats the examiner's words, phrases, or sentences. It is commonly seen in catatonic patients.

Other Language Functions of the Dominant Hemisphere

In addition to speech, there are a number of other language functions, all associated with the dominant temporoparietal region (27, 30, 46, 54, 56, 62, 63).

1. *Pointing to named objects.* The examiner asks the patient to point to various items that the examiner names (e.g. "Point to your belt," "Show me a button"), or to nod yes or no to whether the patient is wearing a certain item (e.g. "Do you have a collar?" "Do you have a button?").

2. *Letter gnosis.* The patient is asked to identify several letters (e.g. MGW), which are shown to him. Although this is usually associated with the dominant temporoparietal region, there are several case reports linking letter agnosia to frontal lobe dysfunction.

3. *Number gnosis.* The patient is asked to identify numbers (e.g. 7, 2) that are shown to him.

4. *Reading.* The patient is asked to read several words (e.g. SEVEN) and sentences (e.g. SEE THE BLACK DOG. HE IS A FRIENDLY ANIMAL, A FAMOUS WINNER OF DOG SHOWS). He should also be asked to demonstrate reading comprehension. For example, he can be instructed, "Read this sentence and then do what it says to do," then shown the sentence, TOUCH YOUR LEFT HAND TO YOUR RIGHT EAR (also a test of right–left orientation) or CLOSE YOUR EYES. Impaired reading ability is called dyslexia; when the disability is profound, it is called alexia.

5. *Writing.* The patient is asked to write one or several words (e.g. square, cross, triangle, clock) from memory, to write a word (e.g. SQUARE) that is presented to him, and to "Write a sentence, it can be about anything you want." The doctor asks the patient to use cursive writing ("Write in script. Use your handwriting") rather than printing, as this may permit detection of a subtle dysgraphia that would not be noticed if the patient

printed. If the patient cannot write in script, which itself would represent dysgraphia or agraphia, he may print. The examiner evaluates what is written for letter construction, syntax and word usage.

Prosody and Emotional Gesturing: Language-Related Functions of the Nondominant Hemisphere (57–61)

Recent studies of regional blood flow during spontaneous speech have revealed changes in the parasylvian regions of the nondominant hemisphere. During speech, activity in these regions "mirrors" changes in homologous regions of the dominant hemisphere, serving the functions of prosody and emotional gesturing (the "affective components" of language). Patients with normal dominant hemispheric functioning and lesions in the nondominant hemisphere manifest normal spontaneity, clarity, and comprehension of speech. But they have impairments of range, modulation, and melody of voice, of gesturing with speech, or of comprehension of the emotional tone of the speech of others. These abnormalities are analogous to aphasic disturbances due to dominant hemisphere dysfunction. For example, in an anterior (frontal) prosodic disturbance, there is impaired spontaneous emotionality and gesturing with speech; in posterior (temporal) prosodic disturbance, there is impaired comprehension of the prosody and gesturing of others. The following observations should be made on all patients:

1. *Spontaneous prosody and gesturing.* As he speaks spontaneously, does the patient manifest normal range, modulation, and melody of voice? Is the tone of voice appropriate to what he is saying? Does the patient gesture sufficiently to convey the feeling associated with what he is saying? The examiner must look and listen especially hard when affectively important subjects are being discussed. This is akin to the evaluation of spontaneity and fluency of speech.

2. *Prosodic-affective repetition* is akin to presenting the patient with a sentence to repeat (e.g. "The Polish Pope lives in the Vatican"). Here the patient is asked to repeat a sentence with the same *affective* quality as the examiner. Then the examiner presents statements using a happy, sad, tearful, disinterested, angry, or surprised voice, and expects the patient to repeat these statements the same way.

3. *Prosodic-affective comprehension.* While standing behind the patient, the examiner presents the patient with sentences devoid of emotion-laden words, with varying affective tones. The patient is then asked to state whether the sentence was spoken with an "angry, sad, happy, indifferent, surprised, or tearful tone." This is analogous to the assessment of the comprehension of speech.

4. *Comprehension of emotional gesturing.* Here the examiner faces the patient and mimes a facial expression to convey one of the above-mentioned

moods. The patient is then asked to describe the mood portrayed. If he is unable to do this, he is given the possible choices and asked to choose which one is correct.

Sometimes dysprosodia can be distinguished from emotional blunting by the patient's stating that he experiences moods normally but is unable to convey them, and is troubled by this problem. Also, emotional blunting is, by definition, associated with other affective incompetence, whereas dysprosodia can be, and often is, a solitary affective dysfunction.

FRONTAL LOBE FUNCTIONS (1, 5, 22, 26–30, 32, 45, 46, 50, 52)

Following the testing of motor and language functions, the examiner tests frontal lobe functioning. The assessment of the following frontal functions has already been described:

Motor Behavior
>Motor persistence
>Initiation and termination of movement
>Rapid sequential movements
>Resistance to stimulus binding

Language
>Expressive language and verbal fluency
>Spontaneous prosody and gesturing
>Ability to repeat with prosodic-affective variation

There are, however, additional important frontal lobe functions. Among the most important is the frontal lobe's *executive* function, that is, decision-making, problem-solving, and planning occur in the frontal lobe. These are observed by (1) listening to how the patient describes his handling of his own life situations (his *judgment*) and (2) presenting him with hypothetical problems to solve.

Judgment

The following is an example of impaired judgment:

A twenty-three-year-old unemployed man tells his doctor that after he is discharged from the hospital he is going to become a major league baseball player. The doctor then asks him the following questions: "Are you a good baseball player?" "Were you ever on a baseball team?" "Are you a good athlete?" The patient responds "no' to each. Then the doctor says, "Then what makes you think you can make the major leagues?" The patient says, "Well, I just will."

Judgment should *not* be tested by presenting the patient with hypothetical situations: "What would you do if you found a stamped, sealed, addressed envelope lying on the street?" "How would you find your way out of a forest?" This is because the typical answers are very stereotyped ("I'd mail the letter") and not usually the product of problem-solving and reflection.

Solving of Complex Problems

If the examiner were to ask, "How much is six times three?" he would primarily be testing memory and secondarily be testing calculating ability. However, if he presents the same numbers in the context of a more complex "algebraic" problem, he is testing frontal functioning: "If you had eighteen books and had to put them on two shelves so that one shelf had twice as many books as the other, how many books would you put on each shelf?" Another such test would be, "If I had three apples and you had four more than I, how many apples would you have?"

Verbal Thinking

Reasoning and thinking abilities should also be assessed as part of the evaluation of frontal lobe functioning. Proverb interpretation is the most widely used mental status strategy for assessing thinking. Unfortunately, responses to proverbs do not correlate well with deficits in abstract thinking (64–66), and fewer than 22 percent of non–brain-damaged adults fully understand them (36). As thinking is also not a monolithic function, no single test spans the various cognitive processes subsumed under that rubric. A clinical assessment of "thinking," however, can be obtained by specifically assessing a patient's *comprehension, concept formation,* and *reasoning.* The extent of this assessment will be determined by the individual clinical situation.

Some of the nonproverb items from the comprehension subtest of the WAIS (5, 36), such as "Why do we wash clothes?" "Why does a train have an engine?" and "Why does land in the city cost more than land in the country?" can be used to assess clinically a patient's *comprehension.*

Verbal concept formation can be tested by asking the patient to state how two items are similar or dissimilar. For example, "In what way are an airplane or a bicycle similar?" "In what way are paint and concrete the same?" Although there are many possible "abstract" responses to such questions, correct answers are those which reveal the most important, usually functional, characteristics of the items. For example, the answer, "The plane and the bicycle are both means of transportation" is better than "Both have wheels."

Verbal reasoning can be tested by asking the patient to listen to a statement and then tell the examiner what is "foolish" about the statement (5, 36). Such statements include:

1. A man had flu twice. The first time it killed him, but the second time he got well quickly.
2. In the year 1980 many more women than men got married in the United States.

Concentration

The patient is asked to subtract sevens serially from one hundred (16) thus: "I'd like you to subtract seven from one hundred, and then keep subtracting seven from what you have left." If he has trouble understanding the question, the examiner can give an example by subtracting another number, such as five, serially from one hundred. While this is also a test of calculating ability (a dominant parietal function), it is principally a test of concentration, a frontal function (30, 67). If the patient cannot perform "serial sevens," he should be given other tests of concentration and of calculation. Another useful test of concentration is to have the patient spell a five-letter word (earth, world, money). This tests spelling ability, a dominant temporoparietal function. If he does this correctly with one of these (or any other) five-letter words, he should be asked to spell that word backward, a test of concentration, a frontal lobe function.

Global Orientation

Global orientation is orientation to time, place, and person. It is a frontal function (2, 30, 67). Other types of orientation (left–right orientation, east–west orientation, and spatial orientation) are not frontal functions.

Occasionally a patient will be so patently disoriented that global orientation need not be formally tested (e.g. an elderly woman in an intensive care room walked frantically into adjacent rooms "to find my sister who lives next door to me" and could not find her way back to her room). Usually orientation needs to be formally tested. Leading questions ("What *hospital* are we in?") are unacceptable. Questions such as "What *place* are we in?" "What *kind* of work do I do?" or "What time of day is this?" are usually preferable.

Very specific questions, such as "What day of the week is this?" "What is the exact date?" or "What floor are we on?" are primarily tests of memory, not orientation.

Active Perception

Active perception is the ability "mentally" to rotate an item in one's visual field without using one's hands or tilting one's head. It is tested by asking the patient to identify a drawing of an item (e.g. a baby, a hat) presented in a sideways or upside-down position. If the patient is unable to identify the rotated object, the object is then placed in the position in which it is most readily recognized. If the patient then identifies it correctly, the abnormality is called impaired active perception, a function of the nondominant frontal lobe as well as other portions of the nondominant hemisphere. If the patient is still unable to name the object once it has been presented in its readily recognizable position, the abnormality is most likely anomia, a dysfunction of the dominant temporoparietal region.

Right Spatial Recognition

The left frontal lobe functions in the recognition of the right side of space or the right side of the patient's body. If the patient reads only the left side of printed material (e.g. he reads "MGW" as "MG"), if he doesn't shave the right side of his face, or if he bumps into objects only to his right, he manifests right spatial neglect (68).

MEMORY

Memory can be divided into five phases. (1) Sensations immediately received (without any attention needing to be paid by the person) by the primary sensory cortex are initially stored in the *sensory memory store* (sensory register, ultra-short-term store, echoic/iconic memory, precategorical store). If not attended to within one or two seconds, these sensations are not remembered. (2) When these sensations are immediately organized into patterns by the secondary sensory cortex and *attention* is paid by virtue of frontal lobe activation, the second stage has occurred. Stages (1) and (2) are not formally testable. (3) In the third stage, seven to eight items can be "held" or "retained" if the patient concentrates or makes an effort. This information, said to be in the *short-term-store* (active verbal memory, primary memory, rehearsal buffer system, working memory) is lost within twenty seconds if not processed further. This stage is tested by slowly presenting the patient with a series of five to seven digits and asking him to repeat this *digit span* immediately afterward. Another test of the short-term-store is to ask the patient to repeat three unrelated items ("book, house, yellow"; "chair, swim, glove") immediately after presentation by the examiner (1, 52, 67). While it is known that good frontal lobe functioning is required for these tests, the short-term-store has not been localized to a specific brain structure. (4) What is being remembered then becomes *consolidated* in the *transfer system* if some effort is made at rehearsal (by way of repetition or use of other mnemonic devices). This function takes place within thirty seconds to thirty minutes and requires intact function of at least one hippocampus (1, 27, 30, 46, 54, 69). It is tested by having the patient repeat, after five to fifteen minutes, the three items ("chair, swim, glove") used originally in testing the short-term-store (1, 27, 30, 46, 54, 69). When these three items were presented in testing the short-term-store, the patient should have been instructed to remember them because he would then be asked to repeat them five to fifteen minutes later. (5) In the *long-term-store* (secondary memory), information is remembered beyond thirty minutes, and sometimes (depending on many factors) for years or a lifetime. This information is probably "laid down" in secondary and tertiary cortical areas throughout the brain. While it is readily testable, it has no localizing value.

NEUROLOGIC "SOFT SIGNS" (1, 15, 50, 51, 53, 70)

Signs that indicate brain dysfunction but cannot routinely be localized within the brain, despite their association by some neurologists with frontal lobe dysfunction, are called neurologic soft signs. When present these signs are well correlated with psychiatric illnesses and other behavior disorders. The soft signs are as follows.

The Palmar–Mental Reflex

The examiner repeatedly scratches the base of the patient's thumb. If the patient's lower lip and jaw move slightly downward, and if this response does not extinguish (50 percent of the general population will exhibit this feature but will quickly extinguish it with repeated stimulation), the patient has manifested a palmar–mental reflex.

The Grasp Reflex

The examiner presses his fingers into the palm of one or both of the patient's hands. If the patient's hand grasps the examiner's fingers, the examination has revealed a grasp reflex.

The Snout (Rooting) Reflex

The examiner strokes the corner of the subject's mouth. If the patient's lips purse and the lips or head move toward the stroking, the patient has a snout reflex.

Adventitious Motor Overflow

The patient is asked to tap rapidly and repetitively with one hand on his knee or on a table. If he also begins to tap or move the other hand, he has shown adventitious motor overflow. Each hand should be tested separately.

Impaired Double Simultaneous Discrimination

With the patient's eyes closed, the examiner simultaneously brushes one of his fingers against one of the patient's cheeks and another finger against one of the patient's hands. He asks the patient where he feels the touch. When a patient has impaired double simultaneous discrimination, the touch on the hands is usually not perceived. Occasionally only stimuli on one side of body are extinguished, which suggests contralateral dysfunction. Some patients with large parietal lobe lesions (usually the right) locate the stimuli outside their body parts.

The phenomena of *motor impersistence* and *Gegenhalten* are also thought by some to be soft neurologic signs.

THE DOMINANT PARIETAL LOBE

The next group of tests is associated with functioning of the dominant parietal lobe. Two dominant parietal functions, kinesthetic praxis and ideokinetic (ideomotor) praxis, have already been discussed in the section on testing of motor functions.

Finger Gnosis (49, 54, 71–73)

The examiner points (without touching) to each of the patient's fingers and then asks him to name them. Patients fluent in English should be able to identify their thumb, index finger (forefinger), middle finger, ring finger, and pinky (little finger). Inability to do this suggests finger agnosia (a dominant parietal dysfunction) or dysnomia (49). If the patient makes significant errors, he should be asked to name other items to test his naming ability in general. Then an additional maneuver is in order: The examiner should assign a number to all ten fingers. When the patient has learned the numbering system, he should be instructed to interlock his fingers (as if in prayer) and then to rotate his wrists so that the interlocking fingers face the patient (49). If the patient is then able to identify his fingers by number, finger gnosis is intact.

Calculation (1, 49, 67)

The patient is asked to perform, on paper, several calculations in which he is asked to "carry" one or two digits. Examples: "How many nickels in $1.35?" "How much is 85 − 27?" "How much is 25 − 7?" The way the patient writes the problem on paper may reveal dysfunctions other than dominant parietal dysfunction.

For example, if the patient writes:

$$\frac{\overline{85}}{-27}\!\!\!\diagdown_{68}$$

he is perseverating, revealing frontal lobe dysfunction.

If he writes:

$$\frac{85}{-85}$$
$$\overline{85}$$

he is making an error of visual–motor coordination, revealing nondominant parietal dysfunction. Single-digit computations (e.g. 4 + 4, 5 × 3) should not be used, as they probably have become memorized, overlearned rote responses.

Right–Left Orientation (49, 72, 74, 75)

The patient should be asked to perform several tasks, each of which requires that he tell left from right *twice*. For example, he is told, "Touch your left hand to your right ear," "Touch your right hand to your left elbow," "Touch your right hand to your right knee." Commands such as "Show me your right hand" have a fifty–fifty chance of being answered correctly, so multiple trials would then have to be given.

Symbolic Categorization (26)

Another dominant parietal lobe function is symbolic categorization, which can be tested by asking the patient to identify consanguineous (blood) relationships between members of a family. For example, the patient can be asked: "What would be the relationship to you of your brother's father (or father's brother, or son's daughter)?" If the patient has trouble answering the question, he can be given an example thus: "Your father's father is your grandfather. Who would be your father's brother?" Symbolic categorization requires that the patient make a "mental diagram" in order to answer the question correctly.

Graphesthesia and Stereognosis (4, 46, 49)

Just as in the assessment of kinesthetic praxis, the evaluation of graphesthesia and stereognosis tests both (1) the parietal lobe contralateral to the hand being tested and (2) the connections between the two hemispheres.

1. *Graphesthesia.* The examiner tells the patient that he is going to print some letters, one at a time, on the palms of the patient's hands, using an implement (e.g. the cap of a ballpoint pen) that leaves no ink or graphite on the patient's hand. He then asks the patient to supinate his hands and close his eyes. Then he prints, one at a time, several letters on the palm (usually the left) ipsilateral to the side of his dominant (usually the left) hemisphere. After each letter the examiner asks the patient to name it. If the patient experiences difficulty, the examiner should then test for letter gnosis by drawing the letters on the patient's palm with the patient's eyes open or by using the test for letter gnosis mentioned previously. If letter gnosis is intact, the error is called graphanesthesia and could be due to dysfunction of the contralateral parietal lobe or of the interhemispheric connections such as the corpus callosum. Following the test of graphesthesia on the hand ipsilateral to the patient's dominant hemisphere, graphesthesia should be tested on the other hand. If the patient manifests graphanesthesia on the latter hand, the abnormality is probably in the contralateral parietal lobe.

2. *Stereognosis.* The examiner tells the patient that he is going to place several objects, one at a time, in the palms of the patient's hands. He does not specify which objects. He then asks the patient to supinate his hands and close his eyes, then places, one at a time, several items (e.g. a key, several coins of different sizes, the cap of a ballpoint pen—all items that make no noise when palpated) on the palm (usually the left) ipsilateral to the side of his dominant (usually the left) hemisphere. After each placement the patient is asked to "feel it with your fingers and then name it." If the patient experiences difficulty, and if his naming ability as previously tested was intact, the patient is manifesting astereognosis, which could be due to dysfunction of the contralateral parietal lobe or of the interhemispheric connections such as the corpus callosum. Following the test of stereognosis on the hand ipsilateral to the patient's dominant hemisphere, stereognosis should be tested on the other hand. If the patient manifests astereognosis on the latter hand, the abnormality is probably in the contralateral parietal lobe.

THE NONDOMINANT PARIETAL LOBE (1, 26, 30, 23–25, 46, 49, 76–79)

Previously discussed functions of the nondominant parietal lobe included constructional praxis, dressing praxis, kinesthetic praxis (of the contralateral hand), graphesthesia (of the contralateral hand), and stereognosis (of the contralateral hand). Additional functions can be characterized as the abilities "to recognize," "to be familiar with," or "to be aware of" people and things. Abnormalities include nonrecognition of (1) serious medical disability (anosognosia), (2) the left side of one's body or objects in the left visual field (left spatial nonrecognition), and (3) familiar people and faces (prosopagnosia).

These abnormalities, when present, are often so obvious that the examiner's questions are usually required only to reaffirm and elaborate upon his impression of the existence of such a disability. The abnormalities are as follows.

Anosognosia

Anosognosia is nonrecognition of a serious medical disability (69). For example, in *Babinski's agnosia* a patient with hemiparalysis will attempt to get out of bed and walk (and is very prone to an accident) despite evidence of paralysis from repeated failures to walk, and despite instructions not to walk from staff and visitors. In *Anton's syndrome* a blind patient believes he is able to see. It is also possible that other phenomena routinely described as "denial" are actually the product of nondominant hemisphere (usually parietal) dysfunction, and that some conversion disorders (see Chapter 24) also are the product of nondominant parietal dysfunction.

Prosopagnosia

Nonrecognition of faces that should be familiar to the patient is called prosopagnosia (77, 78). It is sometimes diagnosed when the patient accuses one or more people of being impostors. The delusion that a family member or other familiar person is an impostor is called *Capgras' syndrome*, and many people with Capgras' syndrome have nondominant parietal lobe dysfunction (23–25, 79). Some recent evidence suggests prosopagnosia extends to the nonrecognition of other nonfacial visual phenomena and that lesions are often bilateral.

A related phenomenon is called the *Fregoli syndrome* (80). Here the patient, observing another person not well known to the patient, mistakenly thinks the other person is someone very familiar (e.g. a friend, a relative, or a famous person) despite the fact that there is no resemblance. For example a patient in a psychiatric ward was convinced that Charlton Heston and Marilyn Monroe had been admitted to his ward.

Reduplicative Paramnesia (Doppelganger Phenomenon) (26, 49, 77, 80)

Another related phenomenon is reduplicative paramnesia, in which a patient with nondominant parietal dysfunction manifests a delusion that a duplicate of a person or place exists elsewhere. For example, a white woman on a psychiatric service had the delusion that she had a twin sister, and that this twin sister was a black woman. This patient also manifested Capgras' syndrome, thinking her husband was an impostor sent to spy on her.

Left Spatial Nonrecognition (26, 46, 49, 76)

Some patients with intact left–right orientation pay no attention to the left side of their body or to objects in their left visual field. This left spatial nonrecognition (a product of nondominant parietal lobe dysfunction) may reveal itself in a number of ways, including not shaving the left side of one's face, bumping into objects on the left, or reading only the right side of printed materials. For example, a man (who didn't shave the left side of his face) read "7 SIX 2" as "SIX 2", and read "SEE THE BLACK DOG" as "BLACK DOG." The patient may also ignore the left visual field when visual field confrontation testing is done. As mentioned earlier in this chapter, *right* spatial nonrecognition is a product of left frontal lobe dysfunction.

East–West Disorientation (26, 46, 49)

The examiner draws two crossed arrows to represent the directions on an imaginary map. He then asks the patient to identify which portions of the map would be north, south, east, and west.

Paragnosia (26, 49)

Occasionally patients with normal global orientation, who will select the correct answer when given a series of choices about their location, are unable to state spontaneously where they are. When asked to do so they will make a series of wild guesses (43). For example, a patient on a psychiatric ward is unable to answer correctly the question, "Where are we now?" Instead he answers in rapid succession, "At the McDonalds. At the railway station. In a high-rise building." This wild guessing is called paragnosia and is often associated with lesions in the nondominant parietal lobe.

THE NONDOMINANT TEMPORAL LOBE (26, 30, 46): MUSICAL MEMORY

In a routine behavioral neurologic examination, other than testing for comprehension of prosody, only one nondominant temporal lobe function, musical memory, can be tested. The examiner asks the patient to sing a familiar song such as "Happy Birthday" or "Jingle Bells." If the patient is hesitant to try, the examiner begins singing the song, encouraging the patient to complete the song. The examiner observes whether the words and the melody are correct.

THE OCCIPITAL LOBE (26, 30, 46)

Other than in the testing of primary occipital cortical functions such as visual fields or color vision, it is difficult to test separately for right and left hemispheric occipital lobe functioning. Thus errors on tests for secondary and tertiary occipital cortical functioning cannot readily be lateralized. These tests are (1) camouflaged objects and (2) memory for a point on a line, both of which require competent visual pattern recognition.

Camouflaged Objects

To determine whether a patient can identify a visual pattern in the presence of a distracting background, the patient is shown a drawing such as the one presented in Figure 3-4 and asked to name it. If he cannot do so, and his capacity to name objects is intact, he has manifested visual agnosia (26, 45).

Memory for a Point on a Line

The doctor draws a 3-to-4-inch line on a blank sheet of paper, places a dot on the line, and tells the patient to remember the location of the point on the line. Then he removes the first paper, replaces it with a second blank piece of paper, draws another line for the patient, and asks the patient to place a dot at the same location as the dot in the original. If the patient places the dot farther than 2 centimeters away from the site of the original dot, he may have a visual memory problem.

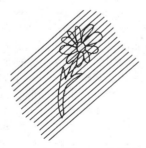

Figure 3-4   Obscured Object

The Neurologic History (81, 82) and Laboratory Examinations

The *neurologic history* and *examination* (of the spinal cord, peripheral nerves, and primary cortex) is part of a complete neuropsychiatric evaluation. Although presented toward the end of this chapter, in practice the neurologic history generally precedes the cognitive and behavioral examinations. A careful review of systems, of the patient's nutritional status, exposure to toxins and substances of abuse, history of surgical procedures, trauma, hospitalizations, seizures, and antenatal and perinatal difficulties may each provide the necessary clue to the etiology of the patient's present symptoms.

Some common symptoms of nervous system dysfunction include headache; spinal pain; pain in the extremities; disorders of memory and thinking; loss of interest, drive, and energy; clumsiness or weakness of the extremities; tremors and involuntary movements; change in speech and difficulty in swallowing; loss of balance and vertigo; loss of hearing or tinnitus; blurring or dimness of vision; diplopia; sensory distortions (paraesthesias); sensory loss; difficulty urinating; and signs and symptoms of convulsive disorder.

Despite the association of the above symptoms with neurologic disease, in the past two decades a large body of data has accumulated that makes discrimination of "neurologic" from "psychiatric" disorder difficult, if the traditional neurologic versus nonneurologic variables are used without qualification. For example, automatically to label a patient neurologically ill rather than schizophrenic on the basis of that patient's having an abnormal EEG would be to ignore the literature that demonstrates that 40 percent or more of schizophrenics have abnormal EEG findings (83–85).

IMPORTANT HISTORICAL ANTECEDENTS OF COARSE BRAIN (NEUROLOGIC) DISEASE

Although virtually any neurologic disease that affects brain functioning can lead to behavioral changes, head trauma is the most common historical antecedent of brain syndromes. To be of sufficient magnitude to result in subsequent behavioral changes, a closed head injury will probably be associated with a skull fracture, unconsciousness of thirty minutes or longer, anterograde amnesia of several hours or longer, focal neurologic signs (even if transient), or blood in the spinal fluid. "Bumps on the head," even when suturing is required, do not correlate highly with most brain syndromes (86, pp. 335–68; 87–92). Mild to moderate trauma is, however, a typical antecedent of the postconcussion syndrome (93–95).

A documented history of epilepsy is also commonly associated with behavioral syndromes (1, 98–101), as is a history of major systemic disease. Of these, those most frequently associated with behavioral change include endocrinopathies, lupus erythematosis, diabetes, extensive cardiovascular disease (particularly arrhythmias, heart failure, myocardial infarction, endocarditis, and vasculitis), cancer, nutritional deficiencies, metabolic acidosis, chronic infection, and blood dyscrasias. Exposure to toxic substances (organic solvents, carbon monoxide, heavy metals) and chronic substance abuse may also result in a brain syndrome (96, 97).

PHYSICAL SIGNS OF COARSE BRAIN DISEASE

Physical examination findings consistent with coarse neurologic disease (and relatively inconsistent with syndromes such as bipolar disorder and melancholia) include focal neurologic signs (e.g. abnormal cranial nerve signs, pathological reflexes, paralysis) and sufficient signs of a systemic illness known to produce behavioral change (86, pp. 335–68; 96, 97, 102, 103). Soft neurologic signs have been reported in 40 to 70 percent of "functional" psychotics and are not useful in discriminating neurologic from psychiatric conditions (1, 15, 51, 52, 70, 104).

LABORATORY STUDIES

The use of laboratory studies to distinguish neurologic from psychiatric disorder has been complicated by recent work that demonstrates that schizophrenics and patients with affective disorder have abnormalities on a variety of laboratory measures. Nevertheless, there are specific differences in the laboratory findings of psychiatric patients and patients with coarse brain disease, which can be diagnostically useful.

Numerous computer-enhanced tomographic studies (105–110) have found that compared to normal controls, schizophrenics have enlarged lateral ventricles, reduced cortical thickness, decreased gray matter density, greater or reversed cerebral asymmetry, and reduced cerebellar mass. Several investigators have reported similar findings in patients with affective disorder (111, 112) and psychiatrically ill children (113), while others have failed to confirm differences between patients and controls (114–117).

Although theoretically interesting, these findings are primarily based on group mean comparisons, and few individual subjects have CT scan images that would be clinically reported as abnormal. An individual scan characterized as clinically abnormal (e.g. circumscribed lesion, significant cortical atrophy) is consistent with diagnosis of neurologic coarse brain disease (86, pp. 335–68; 91, 102, 103).

Similarly, numerous studies have reported that from 40 to 50 percent of schizophrenics have clinically abnormal resting EEG findings, usually nonspecific slowing (83, 84). None of these studies, however, has been able to demonstrate a characteristic schizophrenic EEG pattern. Although less numerous, EEG studies in affective disorder (83, 118) and other psychiatric conditions (119) have also failed to identify specific abnormalities. A resting EEG with a specific clinical abnormality (e.g. spike and slow wave complexes, paroxysmal bursts of slow waves, circumscribed abnormalities) is inconsistent with a "functional" psychiatric diagnosis and indicates the patient may have coarse brain disease. Power/spectral (120–122) and evoked response studies (123), each suggesting differences between psychotic patients and normal controls, have not yet proved useful diagnostically. Evoked response studies, however, can be helpful in determining the presence of demyelinating disease (124, 125).

Neuropsychological testing of affective disorder patients and schizophrenics has captured the imagination of many investigators. Despite a common notion that schizophrenics exhibit dominant hemisphere dysfunction, while affectives exhibit nondominant hemisphere dysfunction, the data overwhelmingly show most schizophrenics to have bilateral and diffuse cognitive impairment (perhaps more profound in the anterior dominant regions), and a smaller proportion of affectives to have evidence of bilateral anterior impairment and general nondominant hemisphere dysfunction (126–128). A circumscribed neuropsychological deficit is inconsistent with the major functional psychoses and suggests the patient has coarse brain disease (27, 30, 46). There are only a few neuropsychological studies of other functional disorders (e.g. Briquet's syndrome, psychopathy, obsessive–compulsive disorder), and clear-cut patterns of dysfunction have not been reported. None of these disorders, however, appear to be associated with severe or focal cognitive impairment (128).

Any cerebrospinal fluid abnormality, any abnormal blood finding associated with causes of dementia (e.g. low serum B_{12}, low serum T_3), or other laboratory finding consistent with a systemic illness known to produce behavioral change (e.g. x-ray evidence of pneumonia, EKG evidence of a recent myocardial infarction) should strongly influence the clinician toward a diagnosis of coarse brain disease, as these abnormalities are rarely reported in the primary "functional" states (86, pp. 335–68; 91, 102, 103). In some samples of psychotic patients (96, pp. 3–9), nearly 40 percent had systemic illness, which appeared to be the most likely cause of the behavioral syndrome. Such investigative techniques as brain electrical area mapping (BEAM) (129) and cerebral blood flow studies (130–132) show promise as discriminating measures of different behavioral syndromes. Many more patients, however, will have to be studied by these techniques before consistent and clear-cut differences emerge.

References

1. Pincus, J. H.; Tucker, G. J. *Behavioral Neurology.* 2d ed. New York: Oxford University Press, 1978.

2. Golden, C. J. Validity of the Halstead–Reitan neuropsychological battery in a mixed psychiatric and brain injured population. *J. Consult. Clin. Psychol.* 43: 1043–51, 1977.

3. Golden, C. J.; Hammake, T. A.; Purisch, A. D. Diagnostic validity of a standardized neuropsychological battery derived from Luria's neuropsychological tests. *J. Consult. Clin. Psychol.* 46: 1258–65, 1978.

4. Heimburger, R. F.; Reitan, R. M. Easily administered written test for lateralizing brain lesions. *J. Neurosurg.* 18: 301–2, 1961.

5. Lezak, M. *Neuropsychological Assessment.* 3d ed. New York: Oxford University Press, 1983.

6. Matarazzo, J. D.; Matarazzo, R. G.; Wiens, A. M.; *et al.* Retest reliability of the Halstead Impairment Index in a normal, schizophrenic, and two samples of organic patients. *J. Clin. Psychol.* 32: 338–349, 1976.

7. Reitan, R. M. The comparative effects of brain damage on the Halstead Impairment Index and the Wechsler–Bellevue Scale. *J. Clin. Psychol.* 15: 281–85, 1959.

8. Reitan, R. M. An investigation of the validity of Halstead's measures of biological intelligence. *Arch. Neurol. Psychiat.* 73: 28–35, 1955.

9. Reitan, R. M. Psychological deficits resulting from cerebral lesions in man. In *The Frontal Granular Cortex and Behavior.* Albert, K., Warren, J.; (eds.), New York: McGraw-Hill, 1964, pp. 295–312.

10. Tsai, L.; Tsuang, M. T. The "Minimental State" and computerized tomography. *Am. J. Psychiat.* 136: 436–39, 1979.

11. Vega, A. J.; Parsons, O. A. Cross validation of the Halstead–Reitan tests for brain damage. *J. Consult. Clin. Psychol.* 31: 619–25, 1967.

12. Wheeler, L.; Reitan, R. M. Presence and laterality of brain damage predicted from responses to a short aphasia screening test. *Percept. Mot. Skills* 15: 783–99, 1962.

13. Donnelly, E. F.; Dent, J. K; Murphy, D. L. Comparison of temporal lobe epileptics and affective disorders on the Halstead–Reitan Test Battery. *J. Clin. Psychol.* 28: 61–62, 1972.

14. Klonoff, H.; Fibiger, C. H.; Hutton, G. H. Neuropsychological patterns in chronic schizophrenia. *J. Nerv. Ment. Dis.* 150: 291–300, 1970.

15. Rockford, J.; Detre, T.; Tucker, G. J.; *et al.* Neuropsychological impairments in functional psychiatric diseases. *Arch. Gen. Psychiat.* 22: 114–19, 1970.

16. Spear, F. G.; Green, R. Inability to concentrate. *Br. J. Psychiat.* 112: 913–15, 1966.

17. Spitzer, R.; Fleiss, J. L.; Burdock, E. I.; *et al.* The mental status schedule: Rationale, reliability and validity. *Comp. Psychiat.* 5: 384–95, 1964.

18. Spitzer, R. L.; Forman, J. B. W.; Nee, J. *DSM III* field trials: I. Initial interrater diagnostic reliability. *Am. J. Psychiat.* 136: 815–17, 1979.

19. Taylor, M. A.; Abrams, R.; Gaztanaga, P. Manic-depressive illness and schizophrenia: A partial validation of research diagnostic criteria using neuropsychological testing. *Comp. Psychiat. 136:* 1031–34, 1979.

20. Taylor, M. A.; Greenspan, B.; Abrams, R. Lateralized neuropsychological dysfunction in affective disorder and schizophrenia. *Am. J. Psychiat. 136:* 1031–34, 1979.

21. Tucker, G. J.; Campiar, E. D.; Silberfarb, P. M. Sensorimotor functions and cognitive disturbance in psychiatric patients. *Am. J. Psychiat. 132:* 17–21, 1975.

22. Abrams, R.; Taylor, M. A.; Stolrow, K. A. C. Catatonia and mania: Patterns of cerebral dysfunction. *Biol. Psychiat. 14:* 111–17, 1979.

23. Hayman, M.; Abrams, R. Capgras' syndrome and cerebral dysfunction. *Br. J. Psychiat. 130:* 68–71, 1977.

24. Abrams, R. Capgras' syndrome. *Br. J. Psychiat. 131:* 550–51, 1977.

25. Alexander, M. P.; Stuss, D. T.; Benson, D. F. Capgras' syndrome: A reduplicative phenomenon. *Neurology 29:* 334–39, 1979.

26. Luria, A. R. *The Working Brain: An Introduction to Neuropsychology.* Hough, B. (trans.). New York: Basic Books, 1973.

27. Golden, C. J. *Diagnosis and Rehabilitation in Clinical Neuropsychology.* Springfield, Ill.: C. C. Thomas, 1978.

28. Krech, D. Cortical localization of function. In L. L. Postman, (ed.), *Psychology in the Making.* New York: Knopf, 1962.

29. Lashley, K. S. *Brain Mechanisms and Intelligence.* Chicago: University of Chicago Press, 1929.

30. Christensen, A. L. *Luria's Neuropsychological Investigations Text.* New York: Basic Books, 1973.

31. Klove, H. Validation Studies in Adult Clinical Neuropsychology. In Reitan, R.; Davison, L. (eds.), *Clinical Neuropsychology: Current Status and Applications.* Washington, D.C.: Winston, 1974, pp. 211–35.

32. Halstead, W. *Brain and Intelligence: A Quantitative Study of the Frontal Lobes.* Chicago: University of Chicago Press, 1947.

33. Wheeler, L.; Burke, C.; Reitan, R. An application of discriminant functions to the problem of predicting brain damage using behavioral variables. *Percept. Mot. Skills 16:* 417–40, 1963.

34. Anastasi, A. *Psychological Testing.* New York: Macmillan, 1976.

35. Wechsler, D. *The Measurement of Adult Intelligence.* Baltimore: Williams & Wilkins, 1944.

36. Matarazzo, J. *Wechsler's Measurement and Appraisal of Adult Intelligence.* New York: Oxford University Press, 1972.

37. Honzik, M.; MacFarlan, J.; Allen, L. The stability of mental test performance between two and eighteen years. *J. Exp. Ed. 17:* 309–24, 1948.

38. Folstein, M. F.; Folstein, S. W.; McHugh, P. R. "Minimental State": A practical method of grading the cognitive state of patients for the clinician. *J. Psychiat. Res. 12:* 189–98, 1975.

39. Geschwind, N. The Anatomical Basis of Hemisphere Differentiation. In Diamond, S.; Beaumont, J. (eds.), *Hemisphere Function in the Human Brain*. New York: Halstead Press, 1977, pp. 7–24.

40. Levy, J. The Origin of Lateral Assymetry. In Harnad, S.; Doty, R.; Goldstein, L. (eds.), *Lateralization in the Nervous System*. New York: Academic Press, 1977, pp. 195–209.

41. Levy, J. Psychological Implications of Bilateral Assymetry. In Diamond, S.; Beaumont, J. (eds.), *Hemisphere Function in the Human Brain*. New York: Halstead Press, 1974, pp. 121–83.

42. Seamon, J. G. Coding and Retrieval Processes and the Hemispheres of the Brain. In Diamond, S.; Beaumont, J. (eds.), *Hemisphere Function in the Human Brain*. New York: Halstead Press, 1977, pp. 184–203.

43. Wada, J., Rasmussen, T. Intracarotoid injection of sodium amytal for the lateralization of cerebral speech dominance. *J. Neurosurg. 17:* 266–82, 1960.

44. Beaumont, J. G. Handedness and Hemisphere Function. In Diamond, S.; Beaumont, J. (eds.), *Hemisphere Function in the Human Brain*. New York: Halstead Press, 1974, pp. 89–120.

45. Geschwind, N. Disconnection syndromes in animals and man. P 1, *Brain 88:* 237–94, 1965, P 2, *Brain 88:* 585–644, 1965.

46. Heilman, K. M.; Valenstein, E. (eds.). *Clinical Neuropsychology*. New York: Oxford University Press, 1979.

47. Fisher, M. Left hemiplegia and motor impersistence. *J. Nerv. Ment. Dis. 123:* 201–18, 1956.

48. Ben-Yishay, Y.; Diller, L.; Gerstmann, L.; *et al.* The relationship between impersistence, intellectual function and outcome of rehabilitation in patients with left hemiplegia. *Neurology 18:* 852–61, 1968.

49. Critchley, M. *The Parietal Lobes*. New York: Hafner Press, 1953.

50. Taylor, M. A. *The Neuropsychiatric Mental Status Examination*. New York: SP Medical and Scientific Books, 1981.

51. Quitkin, F.; Rifkin, A.; Klein, D. F. Neurologic soft signs in schizophrenia, organicity in schizophrenia with premorbid asociality and emotionally unstable character disorders. *Arch. Gen. Psychiat. 33:* 845–53, 1979.

52. Taylor, M. A.; Abrams, R.; Faber, R; *et al.* Cognitive tasks in the mental status examination. *J. Nerv. Ment. Dis. 168:* 167–70, 1980.

53. Paulson, G.; Gottlieb, G. Development reflexes: The reappearance of foetal and neonatal reflexes in aged patients. *Brain 91:* 37–52, 1968.

54. Geschwind, N. *Selected Papers on Language and the Brain*. Boston: D. Reidel, 1974.

55. LeDoux, J. E.; Wilson, D. H.; Gazzaniga, M. S. Block design performance following callosal sectioning: Observations on functional recovery. *Arch. Neurol. 35:* 506–8, 1978.

56. Sherwin, I.; Geschwind, N. Neural Substrates of Behavior. In Nicholi, A. M., Jr. (ed.), *The Harvard Guide to Modern Psychiatry*. Cambridge, Mass.: Belknap/Harvard, 1978, p. 78.

57. Monrad-Krohn, G. H. Dysprosody or altered "melody of language." *Brain 70:* 405-15, 1947.

58. Ross, E. D.; Mesulam, M. M. Dominant language functions of the right hemisphere? Prosody and emotional gesturing. *Arch. Neurol. 36:* 144-48, 1979.

59. Weintraub, S.; Mesulam, M. M.; Kramer, L. Disturbances in prosody: A right-hemisphere contribution to language. *Arch. Neurol. 38:* 742-44, 1981.

60. Ross, E. D.; Harney, J. H.; deLacoste-Utamsing, C.; *et al.* How the brain integrates affective and propositional language into a unified behavioral function: Hypothesis based on clinico-anatomic evidence. *Arch. Neurol. 38:* 745-48, 1981.

61. Ross, E. D. The aprosodias: Functional anatomic organization of the affective components of language in the right hemisphere. *Arch. Neurol. 38:* 561-69, 1981.

62. Brown, J. W. *Aphasia, Apraxia and Agnosia: Clinical and Theoretical Aspects.* Springfield: Ill.: C. C. Thomas, 1972.

63. Benson, D. F. *Aphasia, Alexia and Agraphia: Clinical Neurology and Neurosurgery Monographs.* Edinburgh: Churchill Livingstone, 1979.

64. Reich, J. H. Proverbs and the modern mental status exam. *Comp. Psychiat. 22:* 528-31, 1981.

65. Andreasen, N. C. Reliability and validity of proverb interpretation to assess mental status. *Comp. Psychiat. 18:* 465-72, 1977.

66. Reed, J. L. The proverbs test in schizophrenia. *Br. J. Psychiat. 114:* 317-21, 1968.

67. Luria, R. E.; McHugh, P. R. Reliability and clinical utility of the "Wing" present state examination. *Arch. Gen. Psychiat. 30:* 866-71, 1974.

68. Damasio, A. R.; Damasio, H.; Chui, H. C. Neglect following damage to frontal lobe or basal ganglia. *Neuropsychologia 18:* 123-32, 1980.

69. Estes, W. K. (ed.). *Handbook of Learning and Cognitive Processes* vol. 4, *Attention and Memory.* Hillsdale, N.J.: Lawrence Earlbaum Associates, 1976.

70. Cox, S. M.; Ludwig, A. M. Neurological soft signs and psychopathology: I. Findings in schizophrenia. *J. Nerv. Ment. Dis. 167:* 161-65, 1979.

71. Strub, R.; Geschwind, N. Gerstmann syndrome without aphasia. *Cortex 10:* 378-87, 1974.

72. Gerstmann, J. Some notes on the Gerstmann syndrome. *Neurology 7:* 866-69, 1957.

73. Kinsbourne, M.; Warrington, E. A study of finger agnosia. *Brain 85:* 47-66, 1962.

74. Neilsen, J. Gerstmann's syndrome: Finger agnosia, agraphia, comparison of right and left, and acalculia. *Arch. Neurol. Psychiat. 39:* 536-60, 1938.

75. Hecaen, H.; De Ajuriaguerra, J. *Meconnaissances et Hallucinations Corporelles.* Paris: Masson, 1952.

76. Weinstein, E. A.; Kahn, R. L. *Denial of Illness: Symbolic and Physiological Aspects.* Springfield, Ill.: C C. Thomas, 1955.

77. Benton, A.; Van Allen, M. Prosopagnosia and facial discrimination. *J. Neurol. Sci. 15*: 167–72, 1972.

78. Meadows, J. The anatomic basis of prosopagnosia. *J. Neurol. Neurosurg. Psychiat. 37*: 489–501, 1974.

79. Alexander, M. P.; Stuss, D. T.; Benson, D. F. Capgras syndrome: A reduplicative phenomenon. *Neurol. 29*: 334–39, 1979.

80. Christodoulou, G. N. Delusional hyper-identifications of the Fregoli type: Organic pathogenetic contributors. *Acta Psychiat. Scand. 54*: 305–14, 1975.

81. Welton, J. N. *Essentials of Neurology.* 3d ed. Philadelphia: J. B. Lippincott, 1971.

82. Scheinberg, P. *Modern Practical Neurology: An Introduction to Diagnosis and Management of Common Neurologic Disorders.* 2d ed. New York: Raven Press, 1981.

83. Abrams, R.; Taylor, M. A. Differential EEG patterns in affective disorder and schizophrenia. *Arch. Gen. Psychiat. 36*: 1355–58, 1979.

84. Vianna, U. The Electroencephalogram in Schizophrenia. In Lader, M. H. (ed.), *Studies of Schizophrenia: Br. J. Psychiat.* Special pub., ser. no. 10. Kent, England: Headley Bros., 1975, pp. 54–58.

85. Tucker, G. J.; Detre, T.; Harrow, M.; *et al.* Behavior and symptoms of psychiatric patients and the electroencephalogram. *Arch. Gen. Psychiat. 12*: 278–86, 1965.

86. Strub, R. L.; Black, F. W. *Organic Brain Syndromes: An Introduction to Neurobehavioral Disorders.* Philadelphia: F. A. Davis, 1981.

87. Luria, A. R. Frontal Lobe Syndromes. In Vinken, P. J.; Bruyn, G. W. (eds.), *Handbook of Clinical Neurology*, vol. 2, *Localization in Clinical Neurology.* New York: Elsevier/North Holland, 1969, pp. 725–75.

88. Levin, H. S.; Grossman, R. G. Behavioral sequelae of closed head injury: A qualitative study. *Arch. Neurol. 35*: 720–27, 1978.

89. Lishman, W. A. The psychiatric sequelae of head injury: A review. *Psychol. Med. 3*: 304–18, 1973.

90. Miller, E. The long-term consequences of head injury: A discussion of the evidence with special reference to the preparation of legal reports. *Br. J. Soc. Clin. Psychol. 18*: 87–98, 1979.

91. Sisler, G. C. Psychiatric Disorder Associated with Head Injury. In Hendrie, H. C. (ed.), *Psychiatric Clinics of North America*, vol. 1. *Brain Disorders, Clinical Diagnosis and Management.* Philadelphia: W. B. Saunders Co., 1978, pp. 137–52.

92. Alexander, M. P. Traumatic Brain Injury. In Benson, D. F.; Blumer, D. (eds.), *Psychiatric Aspects of Neurologic Disease*, vol. 2. New York: Grune & Stratton, 1982, pp. 219–48.

93. Mershey, H.; Woodforde, J. M. Psychiatric sequelae of minor head injury. *Brain 95*: 521–28, 1972.

94. Harrison, M. S. Notes on the clinical features and pathology of post-

concussional vertigo with special reference to positional nystagmus. *Brain 79:* 474–82, 1956.

95. Rowe, M. J.; Carlson, C. Brain stem auditory evoked potentials in post-concussional dizziness. *Arch. Neurol. 37:* 679–83, 1980.

96. Hall, R. C. W. (ed.). *Psychiatric Presentations of Medical Illness: Somato-psychic Disorders.* New York: SP Medical and Scientific Books, 1980.

97. Speidel, H.; Rodewald, G. *Psychic and Neurological Dysfunctions After Open-Heart Surgery.* First International Symposium, Hamburg, Band 19, Intensivmedizin Notfallmedizin Anasthesiologic. Stuttgart: Georg Thieme Verlag, 1980.

98. Toone, B. Psychoses of Epilepsy. In Reynolds, E. H.; Trimble, M. R. (eds.), *Epilepsy and Psychiatry.* Edinburgh: Churchill Livingstone, 1981, pp. 113–37.

99. Davidson, K.; Bagley, C. R. Schizophrenia-like Psychoses Associated with Organic Disorders of the Central Nervous System: A Review of the Literature. In *Current Problems in Neuropsychiatry. Br. J. Psychiat.* Special pub., no. 4, 1969, pp. 113–84.

100. Trimble, M. R. The Interictal Psychoses of Epilepsy. In Benson, D. F.; Blumer, D. (eds.), *Psychiatric Aspects of Neurologic Disease,* vol. 2. New York: Grune & Stratton, 1982, pp. 75–88.

101. Koella, W. P.; Trimble, M. R. (eds.). *Temporal Lobe Epilepsy, Mania and Schizophrenia and the Limbic System,* vol. 8, *Advances in Biological Psychiatry.* Basel: S. Kruger, 1982.

102. Torack, R. M. *The Pathologic Physiology and Dementia With Indications for Diagnosis and Treatment.* Berlin: Springer-Verlag, 1978.

103. Benson, D. F. The Treatable Dementias. In Benson, D. F.; Blumer, D. (eds.), *Psychiatric Aspects of Neurologic Disease.* vol. 2. New York: Grune & Stratton, 1982, pp. 123–48.

104. Nasrallah, H. A.; Tippin, J.; McCalley-Whitters, M. Neuropsychological soft signs in manic patients: A comparison with schizophrenics and control groups. *J. Aff. Dis. 5:* 45–50, 1983.

105. Nasrallah, H. A.; Jacoby, C. G.; McCalley-Whitters, M.; *et al.* Cerebral ventricular enlargement in subtypes of chronic schizophrenia. *Arch. Gen. Psychiat. 39:* 774–77, 1982.

106. Nyback, H.; Wiesel, F. A.; Berggren, B. M.; *et al.* Computed tomography of the brain in patients with acute psychosis and in healthy volunteers. *Acta Psychiat. Scand. 65:* 403–14, 1982.

107. Frangos, E.; Athanassenas, G. Differences in lateral brain ventricular size among various types of chronic schizophrenics. Evidence based on a CT study. *Acta Psychiat. Scand. 66:* 459–63, 1982.

108. Weinberger, D. R.; DeLisi, L. E.; Perman, G. P.; *et al.* Computed tomography in schizophreniform disorder and other acute psychiatric disorders. *Arch. Gen. Psychiat. 39:* 778–83, 1982.

109. Tenaka, Y.; Hazama, H.; Kawahara, R.; *et al.* Computerized tomography of

the brain in schizophrenic patients: A controlled study. *Acta Psychiat. Scand.* 63: 191-97, 1981.

110. Golden, C. J.; Graber, B.; Coffman, J.; *et al.* Structural brain deficits in schizophrenia: Identification by computed tomographic scan density measurements. *Arch. Gen. Psychiat.* 38: 1014-17, 1981.

111. Tenaka, Y.; Hazama, H.; Fukuhara, T.; *et al.* Computerized tomography of the brain in manic-depressive patients: A controlled study. *Folia Psychiatrica et Neurologica Japanica* 36: 137-43, 1982.

112. Nasrallah, H. A.; McCalley-Whitters, M.; Jacoby, C. G. Cerebral ventricular enlargement in young manic males: A controlled CT study. *J. Aff. Dis.* 4: 15-19, 1982.

113. Reiss, D.; Feinstein, C.; Weinberger, D. R.; *et al.* Ventricular enlargement in child psychiatric patients: A controlled study with planimetric measurements. *Am. J. Psychiat.* 140: 453-56, 1983.

114. Benes, F.; Sunderland, P.; Jones, B. D.; *et al.* Normal ventricles in young schizophrenics. *Br. J. Psychiat.* 141: 90-93, 1982.

115. Jernigan, T. L.; Zatz, L. M.; Moses, J. A., Jr.; *et al.* Computed tomography in schizophrenics and normal volunteers: 1. Fluid volume. *Arch. Gen. Psychiat.* 39: 765-70, 1982.

116. Jernigan, T. L.; Zatz, L. M.; Moses, J. A., Jr.; *et al.* Computed tomography in schizophrenics and normal volunteers: 2. Cranial asymmetry. *Arch. Gen. Psychiat.* 39: 771-73, 1982.

117. Andreasen, N. C.; Smith, M. R.; Jacoby, C. G.; *et al.* Ventricular enlargement in schizophrenia: Definition and prevalence. *Am. J. Psychiat.* 139: 292-96, 1982.

118. Kadrmas, A.; Winokur, G. Manic-depressive illness and EEG abnormalities. *J. Clin. Psychiat.* 40: 306-7, 1979.

119. Kiloh, L. G.; McComas, A. J.; Osselton, J. W. *Clinical Electroencephalography.* 2d ed. London: Butterworth, 1974, pp. 168-200.

120. Itil, T. M.; Saletu, B.; Davis, S. EEG findings in chronic schizophrenics based on digital computer period analysis and analog power spectra. *Biol. Psychiat.* 5: 1-13, 1972.

121. Flor-Henry, P. Lateralized temporal-limbic dysfunction and pathology. *Ann. N.Y. Acad. Sci.* 280: 777-97, 1976.

122. Volavka, J.; Abrams, R.; Taylor, M. A.; *et al.* Hemispheric Lateralization of Fast EEG Activity in Schizophrenia and Endogenous Depression. In Mendlewicz, J.; Van Praag, H. M. (series eds.); Perris, C.; Kemali, D.; Vacca, L. (eds.), *Electroneurophysiology and Psychopathology,* vol. 6, *Advances in Biological Psychiatry.* Basel: Karger, 1981, pp. 72-75.

123. Rockstroh, B.; Elbert, T.; Berbaumer, N.; *et al. Slow Brain Potentials and Behavior.* Baltimore: Williams & Wilkins, 1982, pp. 199-210.

124. Green, J. B.; Walcoff, M. R. Evoked potentials in multiple sclerosis. *Arch. Neurol.* 39: 696-97, 1982.

125. Haldeman, S.; Glick, M.; Bhatia, N. N.; *et al.* Colonometry, cystometry, and evoked potentials in multiple sclerosis. *Arch. Neurol. 39:* 698–701, 1982.

126. Taylor, M. A.; Abrams, R. Cognitive impairment in schizophrenia. *Am. J. Psychiat. 141:* 196–201, 1984.

127. Silverstein, M. Neuropsychological Dysfunction in the Major Psychoses. In Flor–Henry, F.; Gruzelier, J. (eds.), *Laterality and Psychopathology.* Amsterdam: Elsevier–North Holland, 1983, pp. 143–62.

128. Marin, R. S.; Tucker, G. J. Psychopathology and hemispheric dysfunction: A review. *J. Nerv. Ment. Dis. 169:* 546–57, 1981.

129. Morihisa, J. M.; Duffy, F. H.; Wyatt, R. J. Brain electrical activity mapping (BEAM) in schizophrenic patients. *Arch. Gen. Psychiat. 40:* 719–28, 1983.

130. Uytdenhoef, P.; Portelange, P.; Jacquy, J.; *et al.* Regional cerebral blood flow and lateralized hemispheric dysfunction in depression. *Br. J. Psychiat. 143:* 128–32, 1983.

131. Ariel, R. N.; Golden, C. J.; Berg, R. A.; *et al.* Regional cerebral blood flow in schizophrenics. *Arch. Gen. Psychiat. 40:* 258–63, 1983.

132. Mathew, R. J.; Duncan, G. C.; Weinman, M. L.; *et al.* Regional cerebral blood flow in schizophrenia. *Arch. Gen. Psychiat. 39:* 1121–24, 1982.

PART II

PATIENT MANAGEMENT

CHAPTER 4

Principles of
Psychopharmacology

The principles of pharmacology are the same in psychiatry as in other medical specialties. The psychiatrist must consider choice of drug, dosage, preparation, route and schedule of administration, side effects, and duration of treatment. This should be based on a knowledge of pharmacokinetics, metabolism and excretion patterns, and other factors affecting the bioavailability of psychopharmacologic agents. There are fewer classes of drugs to master in psychiatry than in almost any other specialty, and every psychiatrist who prescribes them should make it his business to become a competent psychopharmacologist.

However, the desire to order medications should always be tempered by the need to observe the patient and, at least, "do no harm." A drug-free observation period may be extremely beneficial for the following reasons:

1. *To allow for spontaneous remission of psychopathology of recent, acute onset.* It is surprising how many patients admitted in acutely excited or psychotic states of recent, sudden onset enjoy a full remission without medication after only twenty-four to forty-eight hours of closed-ward observation. Included in this group are doubtless some individuals with reactive or hysterical psychoses and more than a few with drug-induced syndromes, but short-lived attacks of mania or hypomania can also occur. The following case illustrates the value of a pretreatment observation period:

A forty-eight-year-old woman with a fifteen-year history of bipolar affective disorder was admitted to a closed university psychiatric service because she had been turning the light switches on and off in her home. She incorrectly believed her house was on fire, thought her mother was dying, and was convinced she was in Italy "trying to kiss the Pope's ring." These symptoms began two days prior to admission, following a day of feeling "slowed-down," and were ushered in by feelings of euphoria. The day following admission, without any medication, all symptoms remitted with the exception of a very slight residual euphoria. She was discharged in her own care, recovered, on the third day.

The advantages to the patient of being allowed to recover without specific intervention are several. Important prognostic information is gathered concerning the natural course of illness. Such information may be important for the management of future episodes. The patient avoids short-term exposure to the potentially toxic effects of psychoactive medications. Long-term side effects (e.g. tardive dyskinesia) are also avoided: As the observed clinical improvement is not attributed to any drug that was administered, the physician does not then conclude that long-term therapy with such an "effective" agent is indicated.

2. *To allow for observation of symptoms.* Except for an acute emergency requiring immediate symptom control, it is diagnostically critical to observe the patient's psychopathology in its unmodified state. Time is required to observe and record behavior, and in a hospital setting (preferably a closed unit) there is rarely a risk to the patient in allowing his symptoms full manifestation over a twenty-four-to forty-eight-hour period. Not only may treatment modify or remove symptoms before a correct diagnosis can be made, but new symptoms may be added, masking or distorting the correct diagnosis. Neuroleptic drugs may produce motor symptoms of inhibition, rigidity, even stupor, converting an acute manic patient into a catatonic overnight. Akathisia may mimic an agitated state, and the fixed, expressionless facies of drug-induced parkinsonism may lead to an incorrect diagnosis of schizophrenia with emotional blunting.

Psychiatry is no different from other medical specialties in this regard. The neurologist does not rush to administer codeine to a patient with headache, vomiting, and papilledema, even though the patient may complain of agonizing pain. The neurologist needs to observe for pupillary changes characteristic of space-occupying lesions and knows that opiates may alter such pupillary signs.

For patients who require sedation because of agitation, excitement, or hyperactivity, a single dose of sodium amobarbital (250 to 500 mg.) may be given intramuscularly without causing a sustained change in the clinical picture.

3. *To allow for uncontaminated laboratory investigations.* An electroencephalogram and neuropsychological testing are integral parts of a

modern neuropsychiatric evaluation. Both tests may be distorted or even rendered uninterpretable by psychoactive drugs. It is clearly in the patient's best interest to record the results of such evaluations in the drug-free state. Sodium amobarbital may also temporarily obscure interpretation of these tests, but the effects of this compound, unlike the neuroleptics, are gone six to eight hours after administration of a single dose.

Choice of Drug

The decision to select a particular class of drug (e.g. neuroleptic, antidepressant) is always a clinical one and should be based on meticulous and detailed diagnostic considerations. Within classes of drugs, however, there is scant evidence that one or another compound is therapeutically more effective. Among the tricyclic antidepressants, for example, although a number of molecular modifications of the original have been developed and marketed, none has been demonstrated to be more effective than the parent compound (1). For this reason choice of drugs within classes will be based on differences in preparation, routes of administration, and side effects. If a neuroleptic concentrate is required that is colorless, odorless, and tasteless, only haloperidol will suffice. If a long-acting injectable neuroleptic must be given, only fluphenazine is marketed in such a form. And if a neuroleptic is needed for a cardiac patient, thioridazine will be a poor choice in view of its pronounced electrocardiographic effects (2).

Drug Dosage

Next in importance to selecting the appropriate psychotropic agent is the prescription of the appropriate dose of drug. If the drug selected is the correct one, failure to administer an adequate dose is probably the most frequent cause of unsuccessful drug therapy.

In general, as most psychoactive drugs are more effective when administered at the upper, rather than the lower, end of the dosage range, the appropriate dose is the maximum that can be tolerated without undue side effects. It is unusual to achieve a full therapeutic effect without incurring side effects, and the expectation that this can be achieved is probably unrealistic. This is not to say that side effects are prerequisite for therapeutic effects, but simply that side effects are often an indicator of adequate delivery of the drug to the target organ. Dopamine blockade in the mesolimbic system may be related to the antipsychotic activity of neuroleptic drugs, but such blockade may also be expected to occur in the nigrostriatal dopamine system, producing extrapyramidal side effects.

Preparation and Route of Administration

Intramuscular injection of a soluble salt produces the fastest onset of action with drugs of the neuroleptic class. Anxiolytics (e.g. benzodiazepines), on the other hand, are not well absorbed after the usual intramuscular injection (3) and should be given orally (or intravenously, if a rapid effect is required). Tricyclic antidepressants are available in parenteral form, but because of their invariant slow onset of action (one to two weeks) the oral route is always used. There is no parenteral preparation for lithium carbonate, so it must always be given orally.

There are no hard and fast rules, then, that apply to all classes of psychoactive drugs. Within individual drug classes, however, certain factors may be relatively constant. For neuroleptics, intramuscular injection provides the highest blood levels in the shortest time, followed in descending order by oral concentrates, tablets, and multipellet timed-release capsules (4). The management of acute psychotic excitement states invariably requires parenteral therapy, often in very substantial dosages (5). For less severely ill patients oral concentrates are well absorbed and have the added advantage of being difficult to sequester. As many hospitalized psychotic patients are known to "cheek" or otherwise hide their medication for later surreptitious disposal, concentrates are the oral preparation of choice on the inpatient unit.

Dosage Schedules

For neuroleptics and tricyclic antidepressants there is abundant evidence that once-a-day dosing is both safe and clinically effective, in part because of the long half-lives of these drugs. There are several advantages of single daily dosing:

1. If the dose is given at bedtime, many of the side effects may dissipate during sleep, and the quality of sleep may itself be improved by the sedative effects of the drug.
2. Nurses have to prepare and distribute medications only once a day, rather than two to four times, thus freeing their time for other patient-care activities.
3. Patients who are at home find it easier to remember to take a single nighttime dose of medication than multiple doses throughout the day, thus missing fewer doses.
4. Taking medication at bedtime is socially acceptable and avoids the potential embarassment of having to take pills at work or in other public places.

5. For patients taking tablets the cost of a single 100 mg. tablet, for example, is considerably less than four 25 mg. tablets.

In any case, whether given once a day, or in multiple doses, most psychoactive medications are poorly absorbed on a full stomach, and the schedule of administration should be arranged so as not to coincide with mealtimes. A clear exception to this rule is lithium carbonate, which is well absorbed in the presence of food.

Duration of Treatment

For many patients, particularly those suffering from an affective disorder, it is necessary to continue pharmacotherapy for a considerable period of time after satisfactory improvement or remission has been achieved, or else risk a rapid relapse of symptoms. A typical routine for administering a tricyclic antidepressant, for example, is to continue treatment at full therapeutic plasma levels for three or four months after successful completion of the acute phase of treatment. The purpose of such therapy is to maintain symptom suppression for a period of time equivalent to that of an average depressive episode. There is little evidence that prolonging tricyclic therapy beyond this point prevents future bouts of illness; only lithium for affective disorder and anticonvulsants for psychomotor states play such a prophylactic role.

Neuroleptics, on the other hand, because of the risk they present of long-term, irreversible brain damage, should be discontinued at regular intervals, even in chronically ill schizophrenic patients, in order to assess the continued need for such symptom suppression.

Drug Combinations

There is no hard evidence for the existence of true synergism for any two psychopharmacologic agents, although additive effects may certainly occur. Fixed-dose drug combinations of a tricyclic antidepressant and a neuroleptic (e.g. perphenazine–amitriptyline) are to be avoided on two counts. First, the administration of an adequate antidepressant dose invariably yields an excessive dose of the neuroleptic component (and vice versa); and second, the rationale for prescribing such combined therapy is spurious. The manufacturers who market such combinations recommend them in "psychotic" depression, where the antidepressant will alleviate the mood disorder, and the neuroleptic will treat the delusions. But this is nonsense as well as potentially damaging. Depressive delusions do not exist as separate entities but arise from the matrix of the melancholic state as but one of the more severe manifestations. When the melancholia is resolved, with or without treatment, the depressive delusions remit as well. There is no justification for exposing severely depressed patients to neuroleptic-induced sedation, motor slowing, pseudoparkinsonism, and tardive dyskinesia when a safe and effective therapy, ECT, is readily available.

Pharmacokinetics

The pharmacokinetics of specific drugs will be discussed in their individual sections, but some general principles will be covered here.

DRUG METABOLISM

It is important for the physician to be aware of the metabolic and excretion patterns of the drugs he prescribes, for these apparently technical details may have considerable practical clinical relevance. Orally administered neuroleptic and antidepressant drugs, for example, undergo modification first in the intestinal mucosa, and then in the liver via the portal circulation (6). This "first-pass" effect ensures that virtually no orally administered drug enters the systemic circulation or the brain in pristine, unmetabolized form, and although the metabolites are active they may be less effective than unmetabolized drug entering the circulation directly from an intramuscular site. This is reflected clinically by the repeatedly made observation that a patient who becomes excited or aggressive despite substantial oral doses of a neuroleptic will frequently be rapidly controlled by an intramuscular injection of the same drug at a considerably lower dose.

Once in the systemic circulation, these drugs undergo extensive biotransformation in the liver, followed by excretion into the bile, partial reabsorption via the enterohepatic cycle, and further metabolism. This prolonged process, coupled with the fact that these drugs are fat-soluble and extensively protein-bound, results in long half-lives for the neuroleptic and antidepressant compounds, permitting the once-a-day dosage regimen described above (7).

BIOAVAILABILITY

There is an enormous variability among patients' blood levels achieved after single oral doses of medication, and large differences are not uncommon (8). For this reason the most rational method of monitoring drug therapy is by serial blood levels, and such procedures are routinely available for three classes of psychoactive drugs: lithium, the tricyclic antidepressants, and the anticonvulsants. The variability in serum lithium levels after single oral doses is trivial if the patient is in normal health. Lithium excretion is almost entirely a function of renal plasma flow, which varies little from patient to patient. The tricyclic antidepressants, however, for reasons described above, produce extremely variable blood levels after oral doses, and optimal therapy requires serial plasma level determinations.

Two different types of dose-response curves have been obtained for the tricyclic antidepressants (9–10). One is a linear (or sigmoid) curve in which increasing blood levels yield increasing therapeutic effects until a plateau is reached beyond which no further improvement occurs regardless of blood level. A drug of this type (e.g. imipramine) can be pushed to its upper dosage range, limited only by its toxic side effects. The second is a nonlinear (or inverted U) dose-response curve (e.g. nortryptyline) in which clinical improvement falls off at higher blood levels, even in the absence of disabling side effects. Thus, if a patient is unimproved on this type of drug the dose may be either too low or too high, and proper treatment cannot be provided in the absence of blood level monitoring.

DRUG INTERACTIONS

A number of drugs are known inhibitors or inducers of the hepatic enzyme systems for which some of the psychopharmacological agents are substrates and will raise or lower blood levels of these drugs accordingly. Barbiturates, for example, are enzyme-inducers and may lower tricyclic antidepressant blood levels when given for nighttime sedation. For this reason anxiolytic sedatives of the benzodiazepine class, which exhibit little or no enzyme induction, are a more appropriate choice for sedation/hypnosis in depressed patients receiving tricyclics. Methylphenidate, an enzyme-inhibiting compound, has been administered successfully to raise blood levels of tricyclic antidepressants by reducing their rate of metabolism in the liver (11).

In summary, the psychiatrist who prescribes psychoactive drugs is employing potent compounds with potentially toxic short-term and long-term side effects and complex patterns of metabolism and interaction. He must therefore have as thorough a knowledge of the drugs in his field as the internist prescribing beta-blockers or antihypertensives.

References

1. Morris, J. B.; Beck, A. T. The efficacy of antidepressant drugs: A review of research from 1958 to 1972. *Arch. Gen. Psychiat. 30:* 667–74, 1974.
2. Rosenquist, R. J.; Brauer, W. W.; Mork, J. N. Recurrent major ventricular arrhythmias associated with thioridazine therapy. *Minnesota Med. 54:* 877–81, 1971.

3. Gottschalk, L. Pharmacokinetics of the Minor Tranquilizers and Clinical Response. In Lipton, M. A.; DiMascio, A.; Killam, K. F. (eds.), *Psychopharmacology: A Generation of Progress.* New York: Raven Press, 1978, p. 979.

4. Fink, M.; Abrams, R. Selective Drug Therapies in Clinical Psychiatry: Neuroleptic, Anxiolytic and Antimanic Agents. In Freedman, A. M.; Kaplan, H. I. (eds.), *Treating Mental Illness.* New York: Athaneum, 1972, pp. 287–309.

5. SanGiovanni, F.; Taylor, M. A.; Abrams, R.; *et al.* Rapid control of psychotic excitement states with intramuscular haloperidol. *Am. J. Psychiat. 130:* 1155–56, 1973.

6. Davis, J. M.; Erickson, S.; Dekirmenjian, H. Plasma Levels of Antipsychotic Drugs and Clinical Response. In Lipton, M. A.; DiMascio, A; Killam, K. F. (eds.), *Psychopharmacology: A Generation of Progress.* New York: Raven Press, 1978, pp. 905–15.

7. Baldessarini, R. Drugs and the Treatment of Psychiatric Disorders. In Gilman, A. G.; Goodman, L. S.; Gilman, A. (eds.), *The Pharmacological Basis of Therapeutics.* New York: Macmillan, 1980, pp. 404–5.

8. Curry, S. H.; Davis, J. M.; Janowsky, D. S.; *et al.* Factors affecting chlorpromazine plasma levels in psychiatric patients. *Arch. Gen. Psychiat. 22:* 209–15, 1970.

9. Asberg, M.; Cronholm, B.; Sjoqvist, F.; *et al.* Relation between plasma level and therapeutic effect of nortriptyline. *Br. Med. J. 3:* 331–34, 1971.

10. Glassman, A. H.; Perel, J. M.; Shostak, J.; *et al.* Clinical implications of imipramine plasma levels for depressive illness. *Arch. Gen. Psychiat. 34:* 197–204, 1977.

11. Wharton, R. N.; Perel, J. M.; Dayton, P. G.; *et al.* A potential clinical use for methylphenidate with tricyclic antidepressants. *Am. J. Psychiat. 127:* 1619–25, 1971.

CHAPTER 5

Psychopharmacology

Introduction

Psychiatrists have precious few psychoactive agents at their command for the treatment of psychiatric disorders. Four major classes of drugs (neuroleptics, antidepressants, anxiolytics, anticonvulsants) and lithium carbonate basically complete the inventory. The artful practitioner must therefore make up in depth of knowledge what he or she lacks in breadth and must master the intricacies of this limited pharmacopoeia. No matter that more than forty different neuroleptics are marketed worldwide, all having the same therapeutic effects. The psychiatrist's mastery of this class of drugs is demonstrated not by the number of different agents he prescribes but by his intimate and extensive knowledge of the varied and specific characteristics of this class of drugs.

For reasons peculiar to the specialty, few of its members have achieved such mastery. Unlike internal medicine, for example, psychiatry lacks a pharmacological tradition. It is scarcely over thirty years since lithium, the first specifically psychopharmacologic (rather than merely sedative) agent, was introduced to a world of psychiatrists who had only opiates and barbiturates at their command (1). Moreover, those who prescribed lithium —and the subsequently introduced psychoactive agents—were chided by their psychoanalytic colleagues for indulging in mere symptom suppression and failing to deal with "underlying psychodynamic issues." Such treatment was viewed as palliative at best, a "temporary adjunct" to the "more definitive" talking therapies. As recently as 1970 few psychiatric residency training programs offered specific instruction in psychopharmacology (2). Among these, one at a prominent New York institute was billed as "Psychopharmacology and Brief Psychotherapy."

However, this situation has changed dramatically. A vigorous expansion of neuropharmacological and clinical research during the 1970s was accompanied by a profusion of new textbooks on psychopharmacology. The present-day psychiatrist has a wealth of readily available information on the neuropharmacological, behavioral pharmacological, pharmacodynamic, pharmakokinetic, and neurophysiological characteristics of any psychoactive compound he prescribes.

Neuroleptics

The French researchers Delay and Deniker, who in 1952 introduced the first neuroleptic, chlorpromazine, described it primarily as producing emotional quieting, affective indifference, and sedation without sleep (3). Subsequently, beneficial effects also were observed in the treatment of patients with hallucinations, delusions, and formal thought disorder. In the ensuing years dozens of neuroleptics, of several chemical classes, have been introduced, all having approximately the same therapeutic indications and efficacy (4).

Although all neuroleptics are sedating to some degree, they are not truly hypnotic. Unlike barbiturates, neuroleptics do not directly suppress conduction in the reticular activating system. Instead, they increase the central arousal threshold by suppressing afferent sensory transmission from the periphery (5, 6) and filter out incoming stimuli without decreasing alertness. Hence they produce "sedation without sleep."

The most important neuropharmacological effect of neuroleptics is believed to be the blockade of dopaminergic transmission in the central nervous system (7). This is a postsynaptic receptor blockade and occurs (at least in animals) in varying degrees in each of the dopaminergic pathways: nigrostriatal, tuberoinfundibular, mesolimbic, and mesocortical. Blockade of the nigrostriatal system is responsible for the well-known extrapyramidal syndrome seen with the neuroleptics, and is causally unrelated to their antipsychotic activity. Blockade in the tuberoinfundibular system produces a variety of hormonal effects, of which the most prominent are hyperprolactinemia (pseudopregnancy, gynecomastia, lactation) and inhibition of pituitary gonadotrophins. There is no specific evidence for a causal relationship between such endocrine changes and antipsychotic efficacy, although the possibility of such a connection has not been entirely discarded.

Dopamine blockade of the chemoreceptor trigger zone in the hypothalamus is responsible for the well-known antiemetic effects of the neuroleptics (8). Blockade in the mesolimbic and mesocortical dopamine systems remains the most difficult to measure. There is a presumed relationship between such blockade and inhibition of aggressive behavior in animals (and humans), but specific evidence is lacking. For man, the data is entirely hypothetical and circumstantial. Nonetheless, it seems reasonable to posit that the antipsychotic properties of the neuroleptics reside in their ability to block dopaminergic transmission in the limbic structures and related cortex. No practical clinical correlations yet derive from this hypothesis.

Alpha-adrenergic blockade is seen most prominently with the aliphatic tricyclic neuroleptics (e.g. chlorpromazine) and is responsible for the frequent hypotensive effects of this group of compounds (8). The neuroleptics, especially the piperidine tricyclics (e.g. thioridazine), also display anticholinergic effects, which in the case of thioridazine are equipotent with those of the tricyclic antidepressant amitriptyline.

In addition, the neuroleptics exhibit antihistaminic (9) and antiserotonin effects (10), induce hypothermia (10), and potentiate the CNS depressant effects of alcohol, barbiturates, and opiates (11).

Studies in normal humans have demonstrated significant cognitive and electroencephalographic effects of neuroleptics. Single-dose trials generally produce impaired performance on tests of speed, reaction time, and accuracy on timed tasks (12). However, if subjects are allowed to proceed at their own pace, the error rate is not different from that with placebo. The computer-analyzed resting EEG exhibits a characteristic pattern of increased theta and delta abundance with a reduced mean alpha frequency (13).

Clinical Indications and Treatment Techniques

The therapeutic spectrum of neuroleptics is diagnostically nonspecific and is effective against a variety of target syndromes regardless of their etiology. The target syndrome approach defines certain groups of symptoms (and occasionally even individual symptoms) as responsive to neuroleptic drugs regardless of etiology. Thus, psychotic excitement is an indication for neuroleptic therapy whether exhibited by manic, schizophrenic, or epileptic patients. This approach, however, is not to be construed as implying that symptoms exist or can be treated in isolation from the underlying disorder that produces them. One does not use one drug for excitement, a second for hallucinations, and a third for euphoria in a manic patient. Lithium, the drug of choice for such patients, will treat *all* manic symptoms regardless of their form or combination. Psychotic excitement states and delusional-hallucinatory syndromes are particularly responsive to neuroleptics.

Table 5-1 presents a simple classification of neuroleptic drugs with one representative drug given for each class or subclass. The usual list of "equivalent dosages" has been omitted, as no definitive data (e.g. comparative dose-response curves) exist from which to prepare such a list. Instead, for comparison of potencies we have indicated the dose of the greatest-strength individual tablet or capsule provided by the manufacturer. As a rule, as neuroleptic potency increases, the sedative and hypotensive effects decrease and the acute extrapyramidal side effects increase. Neuroleptic potency is also highly correlated with dopaminergic blockade.

We can think of no reason to master more than one drug in each class, and even then there would be great redundancy. Complete familiarity with one low- and one high-potency compound would suffice for all but the most unusual circumstances, and the expertise developed through the intensive use of one or two such drugs would provide the most effective clinical practice.

Psychotic Excitement States

Neuroleptics are most effective in patients with overactive, restless, or agitated behavior. Physiological concomitants of such excitation are dilated pupils, rapid pulse, reduced total sleep time, and a desynchronized EEG. These patients have markedly impaired judgment, are unable to control their excited behavior, and almost always are delusional and hallucinating. It is quite common for such patients to become threatening and physically assaultive. All psychotic excitement states, therefore, require immediate

TABLE 5-1 Neuroleptic Drugs

CLASS (SUBCLASS)	GENERIC	BRAND	TABLET STRENGTH (MG.)
TRICYCLIC			
PHENOTHIAZINE			
ALIPHATIC	CHLORPROMAZINE	(THORAZINE)	200
PIPERIDINE	THIORIDAZINE	(MELLARIL)	200
PIPERAZINE	FLUPHENAZINE	(PROLIXIN)	10
THIOXANTHENE			
ALIPHATIC	CHLORPROTHIXENE	(TARACTAN)	100
PIPERAZINE	THIOTHIXENE	(NAVANE)	20
DIBENZOXAZEPINE	LOXAPINE	(LOXITANE)	50
BUTYROPHENONE	HALOPERIDOL	(HALDOL)	10
DIHYDROINDOLONE	MOLINDONE	(MOBAN)	25

treatment. Mania is the most frequent primary syndrome in this group of patients, although coarse brain disease (e.g. temporal lobe epilepsy) and schizophrenia also may produce excitement states. Psychotic depression with agitation also constitutes an example of a psychotic excitement state, but for reasons described below we do not recommend neuroleptics for patients in this group.

Once the decision has been made to initiate neuroleptic treatment, the drug should always be given parenterally. A neuroleptic with minimal alpha-adrenergic blocking properties should be chosen in order to avoid hypotensive cardiovascular collapse. We have found haloperidol to be the drug of choice. A deep intramuscular injection of 20 mg. (range 10–30 mg.) is given immediately and two to three times daily for a minimum of forty-eight hours before switching to an oral preparation (see below for additional treatment details). There are three rules to follow when changing from parenteral to oral dosing: (1) The oral dose needs to be given only once a day, at bedtime; (2) the daily oral dose should be about 30 percent larger than the parenteral dose; and (3) parenteral administration should not be discontinued until the oral dose has taken effect. This requires administering the first oral dose concomitantly with the evening parenteral one on the day before the switch is made.

DELUSIONAL–HALLUCINATORY SYNDROMES

Patients exhibiting delusional–hallucinatory syndromes are typically guarded and suspicious, with ideas of reference, persecutory delusions, and auditory hallucinations. When severe, such symptoms may require parenteral neuroleptics, particularly if the patient is menacing or becoming increasingly angry. However, most such patients can be managed with oral therapy so long as parenteral medication is immediately available. A typical regimen using haloperidol (another neuroleptic might be used) begins with 20 to 30 mg. twice daily for two to three days, taking advantage of an initial daytime sedating effect and changes to a single nighttime dose of 60 to 80 mg. for the remainder of the treatment course. Some patients may require as much as 120 mg./day of haloperidol for maximum improvement, but doses exceeding this amount rarely augment the clinical response.

OTHER PSYCHOPATHOLOGICAL TARGET SYMPTOMS

The following clinical phenomena, occurring alone or in combinations, are responsive to neuroleptic therapy:

Hallucinations (all modalities)
Delusions (any type)

First-rank symptoms
Formal thought disorder

A reduction in the patient's emotional response to the particular psychotic sign is the first clinical change to be observed, followed by a gradual diminution and eventual disappearance of the sign itself. Thus a patient who is initially tormented by derogatory auditory hallucinations may, after a day or so on neuroleptics, report that he still hears the voices but that he no longer pays attention to them. As the days pass, the voices diminish in frequency and intensity and usually disappear after one or two weeks of treatment. Delusions follow a similar course: The patient initially loses the affective loading of the delusional idea, then claims that the delusional idea occurred only in the past, and eventually (if treatment is fully successful) realizes that the event never occurred.

The response of catatonic motor features to neuroleptic treatment is variable. When mannerisms and stereotypies occur as part of a manic state, for example, these features remit along with the other elements of the syndrome. Mutism, rigidity, catalepsy, and stupor, however, rarely respond to neuroleptics and are frequently aggravated by them. This is consistent with the clinical observation that neuroleptics occasionally induce the syndrome of negativistic stupor in patients previously free from catatonic signs.

Emotional blunting is another phenomenon of the major psychoses that is unresponsive to neuroleptics. Indeed, as neuroleptics are themselves capable of inducing most of the elements of blunting (e.g. expressionless face, monotonous voice, affective indifference), the syndrome may be intensified by their use.

Because of the potential for long-term side effects (tardive dyskinesia) with neuroleptic therapy, conditions that are not known to be specifically responsive to this class of drugs must be considered contraindications to their use. Included here are a variety of neurotic disorders (e.g. anxiety neurosis, panic attacks, phobic disorders, depressive neurosis, dysthymic disorder), personality disorders, and situational reactions. Of course, neuroleptics should never be used solely for their hypnotic/sedative effects.

For patients with psychotic depression, the use of neuroleptics is controversial. Some authors recommend their use in combination with a tricyclic antidepressant, and there is some evidence in the literature that such treatment may be effective (14). It is our practice, however, never to prescribe neuroleptics for any patient with depression, regardless of the presence of psychotic symptoms, so long as the option remains for administering ECT. This latter method is safe, rapid, and highly effective in patients with psychotic (delusional) depression, and we can see no rationale for exposing such patients to the risk of tardive dyskinesia when a course of six to ten bilateral ECT usually induces a full remission of symptoms. The cnly exception to this general rule of practice is for patients who refuse to accept ECT and where it is not possible to administer such treatment involuntarily. In these circumstances a neuroleptic–antidepressant combination is justified, but only after failure of a tricyclic antidepressant given alone, at full therapeutic dosage (e.g. 300 mg./day of imipramine) and with plasma level monitoring. Even then, we would first attempt to enhance the antidepressant effect of the tricyclic with lyothyronine (15) rather than risk the potentially permanent effects of tardive dyskinesia.

Duration of Treatment

The duration of treatment naturally depends on the clinical diagnosis. The details of managing patients with psychoses are presented in the individual chapters devoted to these disorders. In general, where long-term treatment is contemplated, as for patients with schizophrenia or chronic mania that cannot be managed on lithium alone, a maintenance dose about one-third that required for suppression of the acute syndrome will suffice. For example, after a patient with a delusional-hallucinatory syndrome has achieved maximum benefit from acute neuroleptic treatment (generally after four to six weeks at full dosage), the dose should be gradually tapered while the patient is still hospitalized, with the goal of discharging him on about one-third of the acute dose. If symptoms reemerge before this level is reached, the dose will have to be rapidly but briefly returned to the initial level and subsequently reduced to a point about 10 percent above that at which symptoms returned.

The duration of neuroleptic maintenance will depend on the nature and severity of the underlying disorder, the age of the patient, and the number and frequency of illness episodes. In no case is permanent, uninterrupted neuroleptic administration justified. Drug discontinuation studies have amply demonstrated that a substantial portion (up to 60 percent) of patients on maintenance neuroleptics can have their treatment interrupted for many months without experiencing a return of symptoms (16), although as time passes a fairly constant proportion of this drug-free group experiences relapse (17). Considering that the complications of long-term neuroleptic treatment include not only tardive dyskinesia but obesity, parkinsonism, and akathisia, we recommend discontinuation of maintenance neuroleptic therapy after eight to twelve months in every patient who has not had such a drug-free trial. Even in those who relapse and require reinstitution of neuroleptics, such a drug-free trial should be instituted every year or two to determine whether in fact such treatment is still required.

Neuroleptic Side Effects and Their Management

CENTRAL NERVOUS SYSTEM (CNS)

Inhibition of dopaminergic transmission in the nigrostriatal system is responsible for the acute extrapyramidal symptoms, *parkinsonism, akathisia, and dystonia,* seen with the neuroleptics. The parkinsonian triad of tremor, rigidity, and bradykinesia is easy to recognize and may be accompanied by greasy skin, a fixed, unblinking stare, and sialorrhea. This syndrome (and all other extrapyramidal side effects) occurs most frequently with the high-potency neuroleptics (e.g. piperazine phenothiazines, haloperidol) and is readily managed by administration of one of the antiparkinson agents. There is also a reported inverse correlation between neuroleptic drug dosage and the occurrence of extrapyramidal symptoms (18, 19). It is best to try one of the less toxic agents first (e.g. the antihistaminic diphenhydramine or the dopaminergic amantidine) and reserve the more toxic anticholinergics, such as benztropine, for nonresponders to the safer agents. Antiparkinson agents may be discontinued in most instances after three months without a return of parkinsonian symptoms (20). In no instance is "prophylactic" use of these compounds indicated. Akathisia is a particularly troublesome symptom, which presents as a relentless motor restlessness and inability to sit still, and may masquerade as agitation. Dose reduction is the only truly satisfactory management of akathisia.

Acute dystonia is a dramatic and sometimes alarming occurrence, but it carries no permanent morbid risk and responds rapidly to IV or IM benztropine, 1 to 2 mg., or IV or IM diphenhydramine, 25 to 50 mg. Convulsions in patients without prior seizures may occur with very large doses of neuroleptic drugs (e.g. chlorpromazine in doses over 2,000 mg./day), but they are quite rare and respond to dose reduction. A seizure "workup" is always indicated in such patients.

A substantial number of patients receiving long-term (> six months) neuroleptic drug treatment develop tardive dyskinesia, a syndrome of involuntary choreiform movements that persists after the drug is discontinued (21). The symptoms differ from those of the acute extrapyramidal triad and include periodic tongue-protrusion and lip-smacking, puffing and chewing movements of the mouth, athetoid hyperextension of the fingers, and a restless shifting of weight from leg to leg. A comparative study of autopsy material from patients with the syndrome of tardive dyskinesia demonstrated histopathological changes in midbrain structures (22). The biochemical alterations are believed to be either excessive dopamine accumulation in the basal ganglia or an increased dopamine receptor sensitivity (23). One study has reported cognitive deficits as well (24).

The treatment of tardive dyskinesia is unsatisfactory; antiparkinson agents aggravate the syndrome (25) and should not be used to treat it. They apparently do not constitute a risk factor, however (26). Cerebral amine-depleting agents (reserpine), cholinergic agents (diethylaminoethanol, physostigmine, choline, lecithin), and GABA-ergic agents (sodium valproate, baclofen) have all been reported effective in scattered, small clinical trials, but no methodologically adequate studies have shown any of them to be unequivocally and substantially more effective than placebo.

Reinstitution of another neuroleptic, particularly a potent dopamine-blocker, such as haloperidol, also reduces the syndrome, but such treatment is clearly unsatisfactory in the long view.

Tardive dyskinesia has now been reported to occur after only brief (less than six-month) courses of neuroleptic treatment, and for this reason such drugs should be reserved exclusively for the treatment of severely ill or psychotic patients. Their use in depressed or neurotic patients cannot be justified and their use in children and pregnant women should be avoided whenever possible.

Cardiovascular System

Neuroleptics, especially chlorpromazine, thioridiazine, and chlorpro-thixene, produce orthostatic hypotension, which is dose-related and occurs more frequently in older patients and with parenteral administration. Acap-tation to this phenomenon often occurs over a week or two, and patients should be warned to rise slowly and in stages (e.g. lying to sitting, sitting to standing) from lying or sitting positions. For high-dose parenteral neuroleptic treatment, the more potent neuroleptics (e.g. haloperidol, fluphenazine, thiothixene) are best, as they have little hypotensive effect.

Repolarization abnormalities of the electrocardiogram (EKG) frequently are seen with neuroleptics, particularly thioridazine and mesoridazine. Flattening, notching, splitting, and inversion of T-waves, prolongation of P–Q and Q–T intervals, and S–T segment depression may all occur. These EKG changes are partly related to drug-induced myocardial potassium depletion and are reversed by oral potassium replacement (e.g. bananas, apricots, commercial supplements). Neuroleptics should be used cautiously in patients with myocardial disease, as there is a possible relation between the EKG abnormalities and the rare instances of autopsy-negative sudden death in patients receiving these drugs.

Hematopoietic System

Agranulocytosis is a rare and dangerous idiosyncratic allergic response to neuroleptic drugs that usually occurs after two and before six weeks of therapy at doses exceeding 150 mg./day of chlorpromazine (or the equivalent). (This is not to be confused with a relative leukopenia, which is quite common.) Frequent white cell counts are ineffective in the early detection of this syndrome, as the onset can be sudden and precipitous. Painful oropharyngeal infections and fever are the usual presenting complaint, and these may occur within twenty-four hours of a normal white count. The complaint of sore throat or mouth or the occurrence of fever in a patient receiving neuroleptics requires that medication be withheld until a white blood cell count is obtained. If there are less than 2,000 neutrophiles per cubic millimeter (40 percent of a 5,000 total white count), the patient must be seen by a medical consultant without delay. If the white count is adequate, drug therapy may be continued. Once agranulocytosis occurs with a neuroleptic it will always occur with subsequent exposure and is also likely to occur with other neuroleptics of the same class.

AUTONOMIC NERVOUS SYSTEM

The anticholinergic properties of neuroleptics are responsible for their most commonly described side effects. Dry mouth, stuffed nose, impaired taste, blurred vision, constipation, paralytic ileus, and urinary retention are all dose-related, and if severe or persistent respond only to dose reduction. Antiparkinson agents with their own anticholinergic effects merely aggravate these symptoms. Inhibition of ejaculation is a phenomenon seen most frequently with thioridazine and mesoridazine.

SKIN AND EYE

Photosensitivity is reported by patients receiving neuroleptics, and painful sunburn may result from only brief exposure. Patients should be warned of this possibility and should be advised to use a sunscreen preparation to prevent it. Ocular photosensitivity also occurs and can be prevented with sunglasses. A maculopapular erythematous eruption may also be seen with neuroleptics.

Long-term effects of phenothiazine neuroleptics include a characteristic blue-gray pigmentation of the skin, resulting from formation of a neuroleptic–melanin complex, and the development of stellate lenticular and corneal opacities visible only on slit-lamp examination. These changes have no known clinical sequelae but seem to be permanent. They are a function of the total lifetime dose of medication received and have been reported most often after chlorpromazine therapy.

Pigmentary retinopathy leading to blindness has occurred in patients receiving more than 1,200 mg./day of thioridazine, and no more than 800 mg./day of this drug should be given. For this reason, if high-dose neuroleptic treatment is anticipated, thioridazine is a poor initial choice.

LIVER

Benign intrahepatic cholestatic jaundice occurred during the early years of chlorpromazine use but is now a rare complication of neuroleptic treatment. Mildly abnormal liver function tests often occur in patients receiving neuroleptics, but their significance is obscure and no untoward results occur if treatment is continued.

HORMONAL CHANGES

Impaired glucose tolerance with elevated fasting blood sugars may occur with neuroleptics and is observed more commonly in women than in men. This has no known clinical significance, and no treatment is recommended. A temporary pseudopregnancy syndrome (due, in part, to increased prolactin secretion) may also occur in women, with amenorrhea, lactation, breast swelling, and false-positive pregnancy tests. Also, gynecomastia has been reported in men receiving neuroleptics.

FATALITIES

Sudden death in patients receiving neuroleptics has various causes. Autopsy-negative deaths in psychiatric patients were reported before the introduction of neuroleptic drugs, and patients who died in febrile/dehydrated states were described as having lethal catatonia, "Bell's mania," or manic exhaustion. Altered temperature regulation secondary to the anticholinergic effects of neuroleptics and the oft-prescribed antiparkinson agents has produced hyperpyrexic deaths during the hot summer months. Asphyxiation by food bolus has been discovered at autopsy in some patients. Hypotensive deaths also have been reported, and some deaths have been ascribed to drug-induced cardiac arrhythmias. A neuroleptic "malignant syndrome" has also been reported, characterized by fever and rigidity and resembling the malignant hyperpyrexia occasionally seen with anesthetic agents (27). Treatment is generally supportive with the addition of anticholinergic antiparkinson agents, although amantidine (28) and dantrolene sodium (29) have recently been used with some success.

Psychiatric Complications

Symptoms of depression may be observed during or after neuroleptic treatment. Most commonly this occurs when the acute phase of the illness is over. Antidepressant drug therapy or ECT may be required, as there is a risk of suicide in such cases. This is most often seen in acute manics, and it is unclear whether the depressive state is drug-related or simply that which frequently precedes or follows a manic attack even without drug treatment (mislabeled "post-schizophrenic depression").

Contraindications

Absolute contraindications to neuroleptic drugs are rare. Narrow-angle glaucoma is one, and pronounced prostatic hypertrophy another. Naturally, prior idiosyncratic reactions (e.g. agranulocytosis) preclude their further use. These drugs should not be prescribed for pregnant women; neuroleptics cross the placental barrier and enter the fetal brain with unknown (but presumed undesirable) consequences. They also are excreted in mothers' milk.

Antidepressants

The terminology for the antidepressant group of drugs is at present in a state of flux. When originally introduced in the late 1950s as tricyclic antidepressants (TCAs) or monoamine oxidase inhibitors (MAOIs), the two members of this class seemed to have straightforward antidepressant properties and no more. It is now clear that not only are they effective in quite different types of depressive syndromes, but they also have major effects in a variety of anxiety-related disorders such as panic attacks and agoraphobia (29, 30). For this reason the term "mood-stabilizing" drugs was introduced in order to stress their effects on anxiety as well as depressive disorders. This term is not satisfactory either, however, as it implies far more than is known about the mechanism of action of these drugs and ignores other major effects of the TCAs in the management of chronic pain and nocturnal enuresis. Thus, awaiting a better terminology, we have continued to classify these compounds as antidepressants, fully recognizing the limited accuracy of this designation.

CYCLIC ANTIDEPRESSANTS (CAs)

The cyclic group now contains tricyclic and tetracyclic compounds, as listed in Table 5-2. Monocyclic and bicyclic compounds are also under study. The original CA, imipramine, was a minor chemical modification of the neuroleptic chlorpromazine and was introduced to compete in the antipsychotic drug market. It was quickly determined, however, that removal of the sulfur atom in the middle ring had robbed chlorpromazine of its neuroleptic properties and transformed it instead into a moderately effective antidepressant. (It was later determined that as a result of this "minor" structural alteration chlorpromazine lost all dopaminergic blocking activity and gained the ability to block presynaptic re-uptake of norepinephrine.) Subsequent chemical modifications of imipramine yielded amitriptyline and the desmethylated derivatives of both of these parent compounds, without any detectable improvement in antidepressant efficacy.

Unipolar endogenous depression is the primary indication for the CAs. Treatment of these patients is detailed in Chapter 11. The efficacy of CAs for this purpose is only moderate in the majority of studies published. Indeed, about a third of double-blind placebo-controlled comparisons reveal no CA effect at all (31). It is possible that drug dosages have been too low, however, and that plasma-level monitoring might significantly improve the usually reported rate of two-thirds much improved or recovered with CAs.

Plasma-level Monitoring

Several studies have demonstrated a linear relationship between plasma levels of imipramine and clinical response in depressed patients (32). In

TABLE 5-2   Cyclic Antidepressants

| | | | USUAL 24-HOUR DOSAGE RANGE (IN MG.) | |
CLASS/SUBCLASS	GENERIC	BRAND	ACUTE	MAINTENANCE
Tricyclic				
	Imipramine	Tofranil	200–300 oral	150–200 oral
	Amitriptyline	Elavil	200–300 oral	150–200 oral
	Desipramine	Norpramin Pertofrane	150–300 oral	100–150 oral
	Nortriptyline	Aventyl	75–125 oral	50–100 oral
	Protriptyline	Vivactil	30–60 oral	15–30 oral
	Doxepin	Sinequan Adapin	200–300 oral	150–200 oral
	Amoxapine	Asendin	200–300 oral	150–200 oral
Tetracyclic				
	Maprotiline	Ludiomil	200–300 oral	150–200 oral

general the therapeutic effects of imipramine first make their appearance at plasma levels around 150 ng./ml., and increase progressively from that point to around 225 ng./ml., above which level little augmentation of therapeutic response is observed. One study, for example, reported that 73 percent of depressed patients with levels of 180 ng./ml. responded after four weeks, as against only 43 percent who responded at blood levels <180 ng./ml. (33). There is an enormous variability among patients in blood levels achieved by the same drug dose, and without plasma-level monitoring there is no way to determine whether nonresponse is primary or due to inadequate dosage. In the study cited above, although the mean daily dose of imipramine was 225 mg. 40 percent of subjects exhibited subtherapeutic blood levels.

Nortriptyline is another CA for which valid and reliable plasma level determinations have been developed. With this drug, clinical response begins around 50 ng./ml., is maximal between 90 and 120 ng./ml. , and actually falls off at levels exceeding 170 ng./ml. (34). Therefore, in order to achieve maximum therapeutic benefit, some nonresponders will require dose reduction and others an increase in dosage.

Clearly, plasma-level monitoring is less critical in patients who respond as expected to CA therapy, although it will significantly shorten their treatment course by promptly ensuring that adequate dosage has been achieved.

It is in nonresponders that plasma levels are required to provide optimal therapy. Blindly increasing or decreasing dosages and noting the changes in therapeutic and side effects unnecessarily prolongs treatment. Plasma-level monitoring represents the state of the art in prescribing CAs and should be employed in every case. The resultant limitation of drug choice to imipramine and nortriptyline provides no clinical problem, as no CA has been found to have greater efficacy than imipramine, or fewer side effects than nortriptyline.

Treatment of Anxiety

Anxiety disorders provide a second major indication for CAs, although the data are still scanty and conflicting. Imipramine is the CA used in almost all controlled trials of panic and phobic disorders and is reported to be effective in the majority of studies. A reasonable working hypothesis, yet to be proved, is that imipramine is effective in "endogenous" but not "exogenous" anxiety states (e.g. in panic, but not in social or anticipatory anxiety). Thus the recommendation for behavior therapy to reduce anticipatory anxiety in agoraphobic patients whose core panic attacks have been blocked by imipramine (35).

Obsessional disorders may also respond to CAs, although the compound most widely studied for this purpose, chlorimipramine, is not available at this time for general use in the United States.

Side Effects

The cyclic antidepressants share many side effects of the tricyclic neuroleptic parent drugs but have more pronounced anticholinergic properties. Thus postural hypotension, EKG changes, dry mouth, blurred vision, heartburn, constipation, adynamic ileus, and urinary hesitancy and retention all occur. Tetracyclics are reported to induce fewer anticholinergic side effects than tricyclics, but the data are unimpressive. However, extrapyramidal syndromes do not occur, and there are no reports of tardive dyskinesia. A troublesome, persistent fine tremor does occur, similar to that in thyrotoxicosis. It is resistant to antiparkinson agents and does not diminish over time. Dose reduction may be required, but when this is not advisable, the beta-adrenergic blocking agent propranolol may be used concurrently with some success in doses of 10–30 mg./day.

EKG alterations are more frequent with the CAs (36) than their parent neuroleptic compounds, and there is a significant incidence of unexplained sudden death in cardiac patients receiving these drugs for the treatment of depression (37). For this reason, we believe ECT is a more conservative method than tricyclic antidepressants for the treatment of depressed patients with myocardial disease.

Hematologic abnormalities also occur with the CAs, and one of us treated a patient who developed a near-fatal total aplastic anemia with imipramine. Treatment is the same as for agranulocytosis, noted above. Intrahepatic cholestatic jaundice is also reported as a rare idiosyncratic response to amitriptyline and requires stopping the drug. Profuse sweating frequently occurs with the tricyclics, particularly imipramine, a phenomenon not observed with the neuroleptics.

The CAs may induce mania in bipolar patients receiving these drugs for depression, a response also observed with ECT. It is unclear whether this occurs with greater frequency than in patients not so treated, however. The occurrence of mania or hypomania in a depressed patient without prior history of such suggests that he suffers from bipolar disorder.

Overdosage with CAs can induce a toxic psychosis. This anticholinergic delirium is characterized by confusion, disorientation, clouding of consciousness, dilated pupils, dry skin, and a history of tricyclic drug ingestion. It is responsive to the cholinesterase-inhibitor physostigmine, 2 mg. intravenously, which may be repeated in twenty minutes and again in a half-hour (38).

Narrow-angle glaucoma and severe prostatic hypertrophy are absolute contraindications to CAs, a subject discussed more fully below.

MAOIs

Although MAOIs were initially introduced for the treatment of endogenous depression, two major controlled trials have amply demonstrated the inefficacy of these drugs in this diagnostic group (39, 40). Instead, studies over the past decade have shown the MAOIs to be effective in neurotic, reactive, or atypical depressives, those invariably classified as TCA nonresponders (41, 42). It is important to note that dosages were too low in earlier studies. Phenelzine, the most widely-used MAOI, should be given in a starting dose of 15 mg./day, increasing by 15 mg. each day to a total of 90 mg./day for the average patient, rather than the previous recommended maximum of 60 mg./day (43). Twice-a-day dosage is satisfactory, and the second dose should be given before 6 P.M. in order not to cause insomnia. As more experience has accumulated with phenelzine, there is little reason to prescribe the two other available MAOIs, isocarboxazide or tranylcypromine, especially as neither exhibits therapeutic benefits greater than those of phenelzine.

Like TCAs, MAOIs have also been demonstrated to be effective in dysthymias (e.g. panic disorders, agoraphobia) (30). This anxiolytic effect occurs at dosages in the same range as used to treat depression and is independent of relief from any accompanying or "underlying" depressive symptoms. Again, almost all of the data refer to phenelzine.

Side Effects

The most important side effect of MAOIs is a hypertensive crisis that may occur in patients who eat foods with high tyramine content (44). This "cheese" reaction (so called because ripened cheeses have been associated with a majority of the severe reactions, although ordinary processed American cheese can precipitate a crisis) may range from a sudden, throbbing headache to a paroxysmal hypertensive crisis with subarachnoid hemorrhage and, rarely, death. It results from failure of the body to metabolize the ingested pressor amine tyramine because of inhibition of monoamine oxidase, for which tyramine is a substrate. Treatment of the hypertensive crisis requires an alpha-adrenergic blocking agent, and parenteral phentolamine (5 mg. intravenously) is the standard. Many physicians provide their patients on MAOIs with one or two tablets of chlorpromazine and instruct the patients to take one immediately for its alpha-adrenergic blocking action should a "slip" occur in dietary observance or should signs of acute hypertension be noticed.

Foods that have been associated with severe headache or paroxysmal hypertension include cheese (except cottage or cream cheese), pickled herring, liver (especially chicken liver), raw yeast or yeast extracts such as

"Bovril" or "Marmite," beer and wine (especially Chianti) and Italian broad beans (fava beans). Despite these caveats, there are data to show that even if the dietary proscriptions are occasionally transgressed, serious or fatal reactions are quite rare (45). Patients also must not take any medications with adrenergic properties, including amphetamines and related compounds, or cocaine. Central nervous system depressants are potentiated by MAOIs, and alcohol, opiates, and barbiturates should be avoided. Patients should be instructed to "clear" any over-the-counter medications with their physician, as many such preparations contain pressor amines for their decongestant action. Phenylephrine and ephedrine, contained in many nosedrop preparations, should be avoided. If dental procedures are contemplated, local anesthetics without epinephrine should be employed.

For many years it was asserted that tricyclics and MAOIs should never be combined, because fatal reactions had ensued from such treatment. However, a detailed review (46) of such cases failed to demonstrate convincingly a negative drug interaction, and a number of reports on the safety of TCA–MAOI combined therapy have appeared in recent years (47). Indeed, one study demonstrated a protective effect of imipramine against tyramine-induced hypertension in patients on MAOIs (48). Unfortunately, there are no data from controlled trials at adequate dosages demonstrating the superiority of TCA–MAOI therapy over either compound given alone.

Autonomic side effects are similar to those of the tricyclics and include postural hypotension, blurred vision, dry mouth, constipation, paralytic ileus, and urinary retention. Increased libido is experienced by some, and transient impotence or delayed ejaculation has also occurred. Some patients with personality disorders abuse tranylcypromine because of its amphetamine-like properties. Initially patients should be instructed not to take MAOIs within four hours of bedtime, as insomnia occasionally results. However, some patients will eventually handle it closer to bedtime, and for some it could be more convenient to take then.

An amphetamine-like psychosis can occur with the MAOIs, especially tranylcypromine. This toxic psychosis occurs in a clear consciousness, unlike the delirium of tricyclic drug overdosage, and responds to neuroleptic drugs or ECT.

Anxiolytics

It should now be obvious that the designation "anxiolytic" should no longer be limited to the benzodiazepines and similar agents, as both TCAs and MAOIs reduce chronic anxiety.

However, standard usage limits the term to the barbiturate and nonbarbiturate sedative/hypnotics, of which the benzodiazepines represent by far the largest group. Other nonbarbiturate sedative/hypnotics (e.g. glutethimide, meprobamate) will not be considered here, as they provide no advantage and a considerably increased risk over the benzodiazepines.

These compounds share with the barbiturates the properties of addiction/habituation, seizure suppression (and withdrawal seizures after prolonged high dosage), and inhibition of spinal interneuronal transmission (muscle relaxation). Compared with barbiturates, however, benzodiazepines have reduced activity in suppressing respiration and rapid-eye-movement sleep and inducing hepatic enzymes.

Most of the benzodiazepines available in the United States at the time of this writing are biotransformed to desmethyldiazepam, an active metabolite with a very long (several days) half-life (49). These compounds include diazepam, chlordiazepoxide, chlorazepate, and halazepam. Flurazepam has a similarly long half-life by virtue of its conversion to the slowly excreted active metabolite desalkylflurazepam. In contrast, lorazepam and oxazepam are excreted unconjugated, or as the glucuronide, and have a half-life of twelve to eighteen hours (50).

The benzodiazepines have three main uses in psychiatry: to treat acute anxiety states, to provide bedtime hypnosis, and to treat delirium tremens.

Acute Anxiety States

Benzodiazepines are the treatment of choice for managing acute anxiety states (panic attacks). Intramuscular administration is never used for this purpose, as these compounds are poorly absorbed from intramuscular sites but rapidly and thoroughly absorbed from the vascular bed or from the G–I tract. When the patient is extremely agitated, intravenous administration is preferable. Substantial dosages may be required to inhibit a panic attack (e.g. 15 to 20 mg. diazepam or 25 to 30 mg. chlordiazepoxide), but these drugs rarely have to be repeated in a single day thanks to their long half-life. For most patients, therefore, one or two days' treatment suffices to abolish the panic attack, after which the drug can abruptly be discontinued. In no case, however, do benzodiazepines provide rational long-term treatment in the prevention of panic attacks or in the management of chronic anxiety. The invariable requirement for increasing the dose as tolerance develops over time eventually leads to habituation and addiction and to the undesirable and potentially dangerous side effects of ataxia and impaired cognition.

Bedtime Sedation/Hypnosis

The benzodiazepines have now almost entirely replaced the older barbiturates for this purpose. Any of the compounds will do—flurazepam is no better as a hypnotic than diazepam—if given in adequate dosage. However, the long half-lives of most of these drugs will eventually lead to significant daytime accumulation of sedative effects, and for this reason the short half-life compounds such as lorazepam and oxazepam are safer choices where daily bedtime sedation is indicated.

Delirium Tremens

The benzodiazepines are also the treatment of choice for this withdrawal syndrome manifested by tremor, restlessness, perceptual disturbances, disorientation, and clouded sensorium. One of the long half-life compounds should be chosen, and as the intravenous route is generally required because of the patients' inability to retain gastric contents, chlordiazepoxide or diazepam are usually employed. A typical regimen with chlordiazepoxide is to give 100 mg. intravenously and to repeat this dose every four to six hours during the first twenty-four hour period. After that time oral medication can usually be tolerated and a dose of 50 mg. QID is given the second day and rapidly tapered off and discontinued by the fourth day of treatment.

Side Effects

The side effects of the benzodiazepines are limited to the CNS and include drowsiness, ataxia, and slurred speech. When administered in high dosage for a long time, there is a substantial risk of addiction, with seizures and delirium manifested after abrupt withdrawal. Thus therapy with these compounds should always be brief and intermittent.

Lithium

Lithium is the only psychopharmacological agent that is not an organic (i.e. cyclical) compound. It is one of the alkali metals and precedes sodium in the periodic table of the elements. It is widely distributed in the earth's crust, where it leaches into the drinking water and is daily ingested in minute amounts by everyone.

Lithium is rapidly and almost completely absorbed from the G-I tract, and peak serum lithium concentrations are reached about two hours after an oral dose. The half-life of a single dose (about thirty-six hours) is significantly longer in manic-depressive patients than matched normal controls, suggesting an illness-related lithium retention in the former group (51).

The above-mentioned retention of a lithium loading dose is also reflected in an increased RBC:plasma lithium concentration ratio in manic-depressives compared to controls (52).

More than 95 percent of ingested lithium is excreted in the urine, and the remainder in the sweat and feces. Lithium diffuses freely into all body compartments, as well as the glomerular filtrate, and has a renal clearance of about 80 ml./minute, substantially less than the glomerular filtration rate of 120 ml./minute. Active reabsorption of lithium takes place in the proximal tubule, utilizing the same transport system as for sodium, with which it competes (53). Thus in the presence of a reduced renal sodium load (e.g. as with a low-salt diet), more lithium will be reabsorbed, leading to toxicity. This is undoubtedly the mechanism for most of the deaths reported when lithium was marketed as a salt substitute in the 1940s.

Lithium diffuses passively across all cell membranes and is actively extruded against a gradient by a variety of mechanisms (54). During the first week or so of lithium therapy there is a sodium diuresis, with polyuria, as lithium replaces a portion of intracellular sodium, followed by several days' lithium diuresis around the time of clinical improvement (55, 56). Following this a "steady state" is achieved in which lithium and sodium (as well as water and potassium) reach a stable balance and maintain equilibrium for the remainder of the treatment course.

The daily dosage required to produce a specified steady-state serum lithium level can be predicted from any two serum lithium levels (57). The same program can be used to determine the time required for the serum lithium levels of a lithium-toxic patient to return to a nontoxic range.

In comparison with neuroleptics and antidepressants, very little is known of the neuropharmacology of lithium, and hence of its mechanism of action. It is an inhibitor of cyclic AMP (cAMP), a substance that, among other things, mediates the transfer of regulatory influences from the external milieu of a cell to its internal metabolic machinery. Two specific actions of cAMP inhibited by lithium involve the effects of vasopressin (antidiuretic hormone) on the kidney and the release of T_3/T_4 from the thyroid gland (58). In the first instance, lithium induces a nephrogenic diabetes insipidus–like syndrome, and in the second, hypothyroidism. The reported increased cellular norepinephrine reuptake induced by lithium in animals may also be related to its effect on cAMP, as this substance is involved in the regulation of tyrosine hydroxylase, the rate-limiting step in norepinephrine synthesis.

Animal and human behavioral pharmacology of lithium has also been little studied. In general, few behavioral effects are observed at nontoxic doses. Animals given lithium exhibit modest decrements in spontaneous motor behavior, and normal human subjects exhibit a modest reduction in "mental efficiency," manifested by impairment on timed cognitive tasks at blood levels around 1.0 mEq/L (59). At doses close to the toxic range lithium induces EEG slowing (60).

Clinical Indications and Treatment Techniques

The primary indication for lithium administration is in the treatment and prevention of affective disorders, both bipolar and unipolar types. The greatest experience with lithium has been garnered in the treatment and prevention of mania, which is clearly the prime indication for this form of therapy.

ACUTE MANIA

Many manic patients are too ill to be managed initially with lithium alone. Even if they are willing to cooperate with oral treatment, as most are not, the five- to seven-day lag in onset of lithium's antimanic effects usually proves too great a burden for the other patients and the staff to bear. If we had to choose but a single drug for the treatment of acute mania it would have to be a neuroleptic (preferably haloperidol). After several days of neuroleptic therapy, however, it is almost always possible to start lithium with the aim of tapering and discontinuing the neuroleptic when steady-state lithium levels are achieved (see pp. 232–237 for more treatment details). For those manic patients initially treated with lithium alone, the rate of marked improvement/recovery is about 80 percent. Attempts to define the specific variables responsible for nonresponsiveness to lithium have thus far been generally unsuccessful (61, 62). Rapid cycling (four or more episodes per year prior to initiation of lithium) and paranoid-destructive attitudes have not been confirmed as predictors of lithium failure, nor have reduced RBC/plasma lithium ratios or a family history negative for affective disorder. Regardless of the cause, however, lithium nonresponders who then receive additional or alternate treatments (e.g. neuroleptics, ECT), ultimately show as much improvement as those who do not, although at the cost of a significantly longer hospital stay (62).

The same 80 percent efficacy rate holds initially for preventive (prophylactic) lithium treatment in mania, and the effectiveness of such treatment increases with each passing year (63). Thus relapse and hospital readmission during a patient's first year on lithium prophylaxis are no reasons to terminate such treatment. Continued lithium prophylaxis significantly decreases the likelihood of such relapse the following year, and even more so the year after.

ACUTE DEPRESSION

The evidence for direct antidepressant effect of lithium is scant, although some data from controlled trials suggest that a proportion of bipolar depressives respond to such treatment (64). Much better evidence exists for a prophylactic effect of lithium in depression, which is about the same in unipolar as bipolar patients and approaches that obtained in the prophylaxis of mania (65, 66). Anecdotally, however, we have occasionally achieved excellent results in the acute treatment of bipolar depression with lithium alone.

Serum-Level Monitoring

Serial serum lithium determinations are used to monitor the course of lithium treatment. Blood levels are obtained in the morning, twelve hours after the last dose, and should be in the range of 1.0 to 1.5 mEq./L. for successful treatment of acute mania. After remission of symptoms has been achieved, the dosage should be reduced to provide a blood level between 0.8 to 1.2 mEq./L. Blood levels are obtained twice weekly until a steady state has been reached, after which time weekly levels will suffice for inpatients and monthly levels for outpatients.

Side Effects, Precautions, and Contraindications

During the initial week or so of treatment patients may experience a fine tremor, mild fatigue or drowsiness, nausea, abdominal fullness, increased thirst, and polyuria. These symptoms do not require reduction of dosage and usually remit when stable blood levels are achieved. Vomiting immediately after ingestion of lithium sometimes occurs and can be avoided by instructing patients to take their lithium with food. Genuine toxicity rarely appears below serum lithium levels of 2.0 mEq./L. and is characterized by profuse vomiting or diarrhea, slurred speech, ataxia, coarse tremor, lethargy, myoclonus, stupor, and coma. Atypical neurologic syndromes may occur, with unilateral focal signs mimicking a stroke. Treatment of moderate lithium toxicity is supportive. The drug is stopped, fluids are forced, and an adequate food (and salt) intake is encouraged. No specific antidote is yet available for lithium toxicity.

Renal dialysis is the only known method for actively removing lithium from the body (67). Although insufficient data have been accumulated for a definitive statement on its efficacy, dialysis should be instituted in the presence of severe lithium toxicity (e.g. patient in coma; renal elimination of lithium inadequate; serum lithium level > 4 mEq./L.). In addition, standard supportive procedures are instituted (parenteral fluids, prophylactic antibiotics, frequent turning in bed, airway maintenance).

Lithium should be used with extreme caution in patients with impaired renal function, employing low doses (e.g. 150 mg. BID or TID) and frequent serum lithium determinations. Caution also should be observed in cardiac patients as EKG repolarization abnormalities occur with lithium. This drug should not be prescribed for patients receiving diuretics or a low-sodium diet, as severe lithium poisoning may rapidly occur in salt-depleted patients. (An exception is the use of chlorothiazide, described below.)

As an inhibitor of cyclic-AMP/adenylcyclase, lithium impairs the function of two major hormones mediated by this system: antidiuretic hormone (ADH) and thyroid hormone (T_3/T_4). The effect on ADH is to prevent its action on the kidney, producing a nephrogenic diabetes insipidus–like syndrome (which is, of course, ADH-resistant), manifested by a large output of dilute urine. With such a large urine volume it becomes difficult to maintain adequate serum lithium levels, and the therapeutic results may suffer. In such cases chlorothiazide is indicated in order to reduce urine volume and increase serum lithium levels (68). There may be long-term effects related to this syndrome as well. Several reports have appeared in the literature of patients with this syndrome who demonstrate glomerular changes on renal biopsy (69, 70). Often in such cases the patients have a prior history of severe lithium toxicity. However, despite the biopsy findings mentioned above, follow-up studies have not shown significant long-term impairment in renal function in patients maintained on lithium (71), and we are aware of no case as yet reported of end-stage renal disease in a patient on maintenance lithium. However, at this stage of our knowledge it would be prudent to reduce or discontinue lithium whenever possible in patients who develop the diabetes insipidus-like syndrome.

Because of the antithyroid effect of lithium, a few patients receiving long-term maintenance lithium treatment develop nontoxic goiters that shrink with discontinuation of lithium or the addition of small doses of thyroid. The patients are usually clinically euthyroid, but signs of hypothyroidism may occur. The T_3/T_4 levels are often reduced, and there is an increased uptake of radioactive iodine. Women are more frequently affected than men.

The safe use of lithium in pregnant women is not established, and sporadic reports of possible teratogenic effects (particularly cardiovascular) continue to accumulate (72). Lithium is excreted in mother's milk (73), and mothers on lithium treatment should bottle-feed their babies. Excessive weight gain and acneiform eruptions are frequent troublesome side effects of lithium that respond to dose reduction. The former phenomenon, is, unfortunately, a frequent occurrence in women and is often the primary reason for inability to maintain female patients on lithium therapy.

There are no specific guidelines on the duration of lithium maintenance treatment. Patients who have remained well on such a regimen for years may relapse in a week's time when lithium is discontinued. The duration of treatment will depend largely on the number, rate, and severity of prior attacks of illness.

As noted in the section on neuroleptic drugs, manic episodes are frequently followed by depression. This pattern also occurs in patients receiving lithium, and it is unclear whether the drug increases the frequency of the pattern. If depression occurs, and is mild, lithium should be continued and the appropriate antidepressant treatment started (e.g. a tricyclic antidepressant). If this fails, or if depression is severe, all drugs should be discontinued and ECT initiated.

References

1. Cade, J. F. J. Lithium salts in the treatment of psychotic excitement. *Med. J. Aust. 2:* 349–52, 1949.

2. Abrams, R.; Fink, M. Unpublished data.

3. Delay, J.; Deniker, P. 38 cas de psychoses traités par la cure prolongée et continuée de 4,568 R. P. *Ann. Med.-Psychol. 110:* 364 ff., 1952.

4. Hollister, L. E.; Overall, J. E.; Kimbell, I.; *et al.* Specific indications for different classes of phenothiazines. *Arch. Gen. Psychiat. 30:* 94–99, 1974.

5. Bradley, P. B. The Central Action of Certain Drugs in Relation to the Reticular Formation of the Brain. In Jasper, H. H., *et al.* (eds.), *Reticular Formation of the Brain.* Boston: Little, Brown, 1958, pp. 123–49.

6. Killam, K. F.; Killam, E. K. Drug Action on Pathways Involving the Reticular Formation. In Jasper, H. H. *et al* (eds.), *Reticular Formation of the Brain.* Boston: Little, Brown, 1958, pp. 111–22.

7. Baldessarini, R. J. Schizophrenia. *New Eng. J. Med. 297:* 988–95, 1977.

8. Baldessarini, R. J. Drugs and the Treatment of Psychiatric Disorders. In Gilman, A. G.; Goodman, L. S.; Gilman, A. (eds.), *The Pharmacological Basis of Therapeutics.* 6th ed. New York: Macmillan, 1980, pp. 391–447.

9. Shepherd, M.; Lader, M.; Rodnight, R. *Clinical Psychopharmacology.* New York: Lea & Feibiger, 1968, p. 91.

10. Domino, E. F. Substituted Phenothiazine Antipsychotics. In Efron, D. H.; Cole, J. O.; Levine, J.; Wittenborn, J. R. (eds.), *Psychopharmacology: A Generation of Progress, 1957–1967.* Washington, D.C.: U.S. Government Printing Office, 1968, pp. 1045–63.

11. Hollister, L. *Clinical Pharmacology of Psychotherapeutic Drugs.* Edinburgh: Churchill Livingstone, 1978, p. 179.

12. Mirsky, A. F.; Kornetsky, C. On the dissimilar effects of drugs on the digit symbol substitution and continuous performance tests. *Psychopharmacologia Berlin 5:* 161–77, 1964.

13. Fink, M. Quantitative EEG in Human Psychopharmacology: Drug Patterns. In Glaser, G. H. (ed.), *EEG and Behavior.* New York: Basic Books, 1963, pp. 177–97.

14. Nelson, J. C.; Bowers, M. B., Jr. Delusional unipolar depression: Description and drug response. *Arch. Gen. Psychiat. 35:* 1321–28, 1978.

15. Wilson, I. C.; Prange, A. J., Jr.; McClure, T. K. Thyroid hormone enhancement

of imipramine in non-retarded depressions. *New Eng. J. Med. 282:* 1063–57, 1970.

16. Prien, R. F.; Cole, J. O.; Belkin, N. J. Relapse in chronic schizophrenics follow ng abrupt withdrawal of tranquillizing medication. *Br. J. Psychiat. 115:* 679–36, 1968.

17. Davis, J. M. Overview: Maintenance therapy in psychiatry: 1. Schizophrenia. *Am. J. Psychiat. 132:* 1237–45, 1975.

18. Rifkin, A.; Quitkin, F.; Carillo, C.; *et al.* Very high dosage fluphenazine for non-chronic treatment-refractory patients. *Arch. Gen. Psychiat. 25:* 398–403, 1971.

19. San Giovanni, F.; Taylor, M. A.; Abrams, R.; *et al.* Rapid control of psychotic excitement states with intramuscular haloperidol. *Am. J. Psychiat. 130:* 1155–60, 1973.

20. Klett, C. J.; Caffey, E. Evaluating the long-term need for antiparkinson drugs by chronic schizophrenics. *Arch. Gen. Psychiat. 26:* 374–79, 1972.

21. Crane, G. E. Tardive dyskinesia in patients treated with major neuroleptics: A review of the literature. *Am. J. Psychiat. 124* (February Supplement): 46–48, 1968.

22. Christensen, E.; Moller, J. E.; Faurbye, A. A neuropathological investigation of 28 brains from patients with dyskinesia. *Acta Psychiat. Scand. 46:* 14–23, 1970.

23. Klawans, H. L., Jr. The pharmacology of tardive dyskinesia. *Am. J. Psychiat. 130:* 82–86, 1973.

24. Struve, F. A.; Willner, A. E. Cognitive dysfunction and tardive dyskinesia. *Br. J. Psychiat. 143:* 597–600, 1983.

25. Baldessarini, R. J.; Tarsy, D. Tardive dyskinesia. In Lipton, M. A.; DiMascio, A.; Killam, K. F. (eds.), *Psychopharmacology: A Generation of Progress.* New York: Raven Press, 1978, p. 997.

26. Gardos, G.; Cole, J. O. Tardive dyskinesia and anticholingeric drugs. *Am. J. Psychiat. 140:* 200–202, 1983.

27. Caroff, S. N. The neuroleptic malignant syndrome. *J. Clin. Psychiat. 43:* 79–83, 1980.

28. McCarron, M. M.; Boettger, M. L; Peck, J. J. A case of neuroleptic malignant syndrome successfully treated with amantidine. *J. Clin. Psychiat. 43:* 381–82, 1982.

29. Klein, D. F. Importance of psychiatric diagnosis in prediction of clinical drug effects. *Arch. Gen. Psychiat. 16:* 118–26, 1967.

30. Sheehan, D. V.; Ballenger, J.; Jacobsen, G. Treatment of endogenous anxiety with phobic, hysterical, and hypochondriacal symptoms. *Arch. Gen. Psychiat. 37:* 51–59, 1980.

31. Klein, D. F.; Davis, J. *Diagnosis and Drug Treatment of Psychiatric Disorders,* Baltimore: Williams & Wilkins, 1969, pp. 187–298.

32. Glassman, A. H.; Perel, J. M. Tricyclic Blood Levels and Clinical Outcome: A Review of the Art. In Lipton, M. A.; DiMascio, A.; Killam, K. F. (eds.), *Psychopharmacology: A Generation of Progress.* New York: Raven Press, 1978, pp. 917–22.

33. Glassman, A. H.; Perel, J. M.; Shostak, J.; *et al.* Clinical implications of imipramine plasma levels for depressive illness. *Arch. Gen. Psychiat. 34:* 197–204, 1977.

34. Asberg, M.; Cronholm, B.; Sjoqvist, F.; *et al.* Relation between plasma level and therapeutic effect of nortriptyline. *Brit. Med. J. 3:* 331–34, 1971.

35. Zitrin, C. M.; Klein, D. F.; Woerner, M. G. Behavior therapy, supportive psychotherapy, imipramine, and phobias. *Arch. Gen. Psychiat. 35:* 307–16, 1978.

36. Burrows, G. D.; Vohra, J.; Hunt, D.; *et al.* Cardiac effects of different tricyclic antidepressant drugs. *Br. J. Psychiat. 129:* 335–41, 1976.

37. Coull, D. C.; Crooks, J.; Dingwall-Fordyce, I.; *et al.* Amitriptyline and cardiac disease: Risk of sudden death identified by monitoring system. *Lancet 2:* 590–91, 1970.

38. Burks, J. S.; Walker, J. E.; Rumack, B. H.; *et al.* Tricyclic antidepressant poisoning: Reversal of coma, choreoathetosis, and myoclonus by physostigmine. *JAMA 230:* 1405–7, 1974.

39. Greenblatt, M.; Grosser, G. H.; Wechsler, H. A comparative study of selected antidepressant medications and EST. *Am. J. Psychiat. 119:* 144–53, 1962.

40. Medical Research Council. Clinical trial in the treatment of depressive illness. *Br. Med. J. 5439:* 881–86, 1965.

41. Robinson, D. S.; Nies, A.; Ravaris, C. L.; *et al.* The monoamine oxidase inhibitor, phenelzine, in the treatment of depressive-anxiety states. *Arch. Gen. Psychiat. 29:* 407–13, 1973.

42. Johnstone, E. C.; Marsh, W. Acetylator status and response to phenelzine in depressed patients. *Lancet 1:* 567–70, 1973.

43. Tyrer, P.; Gardner, M.; Lambourn, J.; Whitford, M. Clinical and pharmacokinetic factors affecting response to phenelzine. *Br. J. Psychiat. 136:* 359–65, 1980.

44. Marley, E.; Blackwell, B. Interactions of monoamine oxidase inhibitors, amines, and foodstuffs. *Adv. Pharmacol. Chemother. 8:* 185–239, 1970.

45. Foulks, D. G. Monoamine oxidase inhibitors: Reappraisal of dietary considerations. *J. Clin. Psychopharm. 4:* 249–52, 1983.

46. Schuckit, M.; Robins, E.; Feighner, J. Tricyclic antidepressants and monoamine oxidase inhibitors: Combination therapy in the treatment of depression. *Arch. Gen. Psychiat. 24:* 509–14, 1971.

47. Ananth, J.; Luchins, D. A review of combined tricyclic and MAOI therapy. *Comp. Psychiat. 18:* 221–30, 1977.

48. Pare, C. M. B.; Kline, N.; Hallstrom, C.; *et al.* Will amitriptyline prevent the "cheese" reaction of monoamine-oxidase inhibitors? *Lancet 2:* 183–86, 1982.

49. Greenblatt, D. J.; Shader, R. I. New anxiolytics: Are they really new? *Psychopharm. Bull. 18:* 58–61, 1982.

50. Harvey, S. C. Hypnotics and Sedatives. In Gilman, A. G.; Goodman, L. S.; Gilman, A. (eds.), *The Pharmacological Basis of Therapeutics.* New York: MacMillan, 1980, pp. 339–75.

51. Almy, G. L.; Taylor, M. A. Lithium retention in mania. *Arch. Gen. Psychiat.* 29: 232–34, 1973.

52. Lyttkens, L.; Soderberg, V.; Wetterberg, L. Increased lithium erythrocyte-plasma ratio in manic depressive illness. *Lancet 1:* 40, 1973.

53. Thomsen, K.; Schou, M. Renal lithium excretion in man. *Am. J. Physiol. 215:* 823–27, 1968.

54. Pandey, G. N.; Ostrow, D. G.; Haas, M., *et al.* Abnormal lithium and sodium transport in erythrocytes of a manic patient and some members of his family. *Proc. Nat. Acad. Sci. 74:* 3607–11, 1977.

55. Trautner, E. M.; Morris, R.; Noack, C. H.; *et al.* The excretion and retention of ingested lithium and its effect on the ionic balance of man. *Med. J. Aust. 2:* 280–91, 1955.

56. Tupin, J. P.; Schlagenhauf, G. K.; Creson, D. L. Lithium effects on electrolyte excretion. *Am. J. Psychiat. 125:* 536–42, 1968.

57. Swartz, C. M. Predicting lithium levels with a microcomputer. *Computers in Psychiatry/Psychology 5:* 13–17, 1983.

58. Forn, J. Lithium and Cyclic AMP. In Johnson, F. N. (ed.), *Lithium Research and Therapy.* New York: Academic Press, 1975, pp. 485–97.

59. Judd, L. L.; Hubbard, B.; Janowsky, D. S.; *et al.* The effect of lithium carbonate on the cognitive functions of normal subjects. *Arch. Gen. Psychiat. 34:* 355–57, 1977.

60. Johnson, G. Lithium and the EEG: An analysis of behavioral, biochemical and electrographic changes. *EEG Clin. Neurophysiol. 27:* 656–57, 1969.

61. Taylor, M. A.; Abrams, R. Acute mania: A clinical and genetic study of responders and nonresponders to somatic treatments. *Arch. Gen. Psychiat. 32:* 863–65, 1975.

62. Krishna, N. R.; Taylor, M. A.; Abrams, R. Response to lithium carbonate. *Biol. Psychiat. 13:* 601–6, 1978.

63. Dunner, D. L.; Fieve, R. R. Clinical factors in lithium carbonate prophylaxis failure. *Arch. Gen. Psychiat. 30:* 229–33, 1974.

64. Mendels, J.; Ramsey, A.; Dyson, W. L.; *et al.* Lithium as an antidepressant. *Arch. Gen. Psychiat. 36:* 845–46, 1979.

65. Baastrup, P. C.; Poulsen, J. C.; Schou, M.; *et al.* Prophylactic lithium: Double-blind discontinuation in manic-depressive and recurrent depressive disorders. *Lancet 1:* 326–30, 1970.

66. Coppen, A.; Noguera, R.; Bailey, J.; *et al.* Prophylactic lithium in affective disorders: Controlled trial. *Lancet 2:* 275–79, 1971.

67. Thomsen, K.; Schou, M. The Treatment of Lithium Poisoning. In Johnson, F. N. (ed.), *Lithium Research and Therapy.* New York: Academic Press, 1975, pp. 227–36.

68. Levy, S. T.; Forrest, J. R.; Heninger, G. R. Lithium-induced diabetes insipidus: Manic symptoms, brain and electrolyte correlates, and chlorothiazide treatment. *Am. J. Psychiat. 130:* 1014–18, 1973.

69. Hestbech, J.; Hansen, H. E.; Amdisen, A.; *et al.* Chronic renal lesions following long-term treatment with lithium. *Kidney Internat.* 12: 205–13, 1977.

70. Burrows, G. D.; Davies, B.; Kincaid-Smith, P. Unique tubular lesion after lithium. *Lancet 1:* 1310, 1978.

71. Gerner, R. H.; Psarras, J.; Kirschenbaum, M. A. Results of clinical renal function tests in lithium patients. *Am. J. Psychiat.* 137: 834–37, 1980.

72. Weinstein, M. R.; Goldfield, M. D. Cardiovascular malformations with lithium use during pregnancy. *Am. J. Psychiat.* 132: 529–31, 1975.

73. Schou, M.; Amdisen, A. Lithium and pregnancy: 2. Lithium ingestion by children breast-fed by women on lithium treatment. *Br. Med. J. 2:* 138, 1973.

CHAPTER 6

Electroconvulsive Therapy

Electroconvulsive therapy (ECT) is a widely used treatment throughout the Western world. For example, in the United States the estimated rate of use was 4.4 per 10,000 population when last surveyed in 1978 (1). About 73,000 patients a year in the United States receive ECT, virtually always in a hospital setting, although not always as inpatients. Despite its wide use and established efficacy, ECT remains controversial in the United States (2). The controversy results in part from the peculiar historical development of American psychiatry, which was for many years dominated by a psycho-analytic movement that characterized all biological forms of treatment, especially ECT, as harmful to the patient's best interests. More recently ECT and other biological treatments in psychiatry have been attacked by a loose coalition of quasi-religious organizations, patient self-help groups, and civil libertarians on grounds that such physical treatments infringe patients' rights, are abused by psychiatrists unwilling or unable to provide "genuine" (e.g. talking) therapy, and cause brain damage. This attack, really only one manifestation of a worldwide general antiscientific, antimedical, and evangelical movement, has unfortunately convinced legislators in several states (most notably California) to pass laws restricting the use of ECT.

Some psychiatrists have contributed to this course of events. A small but significant number of private practitioners have abused ECT for their finan-cial gain, administering the treatment indiscriminately or for excessively long courses. Others, working in public institutions, have given ECT thoughtlessly, mechanically, and in grim surroundings, callously referring to the procedure as "shocking" or "buzzing" their patient and remaining ignorant of advances in knowledge and technique that would improve treatment results, reduce side-effects, and render the method more acceptable to patients and staff alike. Until the early 1950s ECT was administered without anesthesia or muscle-relaxation, and in many hospitals where ECT was given in full view of other patients, the unmodified convulsive seizure was undoubtedly frightening and disturbing. ECT today bears no resemblance to this primitive procedure, but portrayal of these archaic methods in films such as *The Snake Pit* and *One Flew Over the Cuckoo's Nest* continues to have an important negative effect on public opinion and legislators.

Modern ECT, when correctly done, is a medical procedure carried out under general anesthesia in a special suite set aside for the purpose, with a full complement of medical staff in attendance, including a psychiatrist, anesthetist/anesthesiologist, nurse, and nursing assistant. EKG and EEG monitoring are routine, vital signs are measured and recorded at regular intervals, and the patient is observed by trained personnel following treatment in a separate recovery area until fully alert and ambulatory. Patient apprehension has been reduced or eliminated by premedication and fast-acting barbiturates. Muscle relaxants now modify the intensity of the contractions of the induced seizure, and improvements in equipment and technique of seizure-induction permit many patients to be treated with minimal memory loss or confusion.

Most important, the diagnostic indications for ECT have been refined and reduced in scope, ensuring a predictably good treatment response in patients properly selected according to modern criteria and avoiding unnecessary and unsuccessful treatment in those patients now known not to benefit from ECT. As diagnostic indications have become more specific, the average length of a course of ECT has been sharply reduced. One now almost never hears of a patient receiving twenty or thirty ECT, a procedure once considered mandatory in the treatment of schizophrenia but now recognized as inappropriate for patients who satisfy modern diagnostic criteria for this diagnosis.

A legitimate question remains concerning the duration of the cognitive impairment usually induced by bilateral ECT. Although many patients find memory fully restored to normal by thirty days following a course of ECT, some experience a longer-lasting but finite period of dysfunction and a few assert that the treatment has permanently impaired their memory (3). Although recent well-controlled studies have not found evidence for permanent post-ECT memory disturbance as measured by mean memory-test scores in patients versus control groups, there is always the possibility that an individual patient, because of idiosyncratic sensitivity or unusual predisposition, might in fact suffer permanent memory impairment after ECT. Such an occurrence would be rare, as most patients experience no such difficulty. The impairment would have to be very limited in extent; when patients who claim such impairment are tested, they invariably function normally on standard memory test batteries.

In any event ECT is a treatment that, like other medical procedures carried out under general anesthesia, should never be prescribed casually or without regard for its potential undesirable side effects, against which its benefits must be weighed. The severity and potential morbidity and mortality of the illness to be treated, and the efficacy of alternate treatments, must also be weighed in the balance. If a psychotic depressive commits suicide while waiting for his antidepressant drug to take effect, all questions concerning real or imagined side effects of ECT become academic.

Indications for ECT

The primary indication for ECT is in the treatment of patients with major affective disorders, depressed or manic type. The depressive syndrome specifically responsive to ECT is characterized as "endogenous" or "melancholic" (see Chapter 11). Patients with this syndrome often respond dramatically, leading many clinicians to consider ECT the treatment of choice for major depression. Mania is also extremely responsive to ECT (4), although more treatments are often required to induce a remission, and many practitioners would reserve ECT for patients who had failed to respond to lithium or a short course of parenteral neuroleptics.

The catatonic syndrome of negativistic stupor, characterized by mutism, negativism, stupor, and catalepsy, is also extremely ECT-responsive. This motor syndrome is most frequently a manifestation of endogenous depression (5) but can also occur in patients with coarse brain disease, mania, or schizophrenia. Although the syndrome may fully respond to only two or three induced seizures, additional treatments are needed to prevent relapse, and the eventual outcome is determined by the prognosis of the underlying condition.

Finally, a miscellaneous group of organically based psychoses respond to ECT, with etiologies as varied as drug abuse (e.g. LSD, amphetamines), endocrinopathy (myxoedema, Cushing's syndrome), infection (encephalitis), toxicity (bromide psychosis) and epilepsy (6). Most of these conditions will respond to treatment of the primary problem, with co-administration of an appropriate psychoactive agent, but some who remain resistant to these measures will respond to a short course of ECT.

ECT is not of use in treating patients with reactive or neurotic depression (dysthymic disorder) or other anxiety-related disorders (anxiety neurosis, panic attacks, phobic disorder), chronic schizophrenia, or personality disorders. The continued use of ECT in patients with these diagnoses only serves to bring a useful treatment into disrepute and is not worth the very infrequent unexpectedly good result achieved.

Pretreatment Examinations

ECT is inherently a very safe treatment (see below), rendered more so by obtaining routine medical screening information required of all patients about to undergo general anesthesia, including a complete history and physical examination, chest x-ray, EKG, CBC, urinalysis, FBS, and BUN. Patients with a history or symptoms of a specific medical condition should have all additional tests relevant to the organ system potentially involved. The purpose of these screening evaluations is not to detect conditions that contraindicate ECT, for few exist, but to uncover previously unsuspected pathology so that it may be corrected or ameliorated prior to initiating treatment.

The advice of a medical consultant should be sought as needed, but not for the purpose of "clearing" the patient for ECT. The consultant should be asked to provide an assessment of the nature and severity of the patient's medical condition, as well as an opinion as to the appropriate medical intervention required to restore the maximum possible degree of function in the affected system. The final medical decision to administer ECT rests with the psychiatrist, as the only person fully cognizant of the morbid and mortal risks of withholding as well as giving treatment. Moreover, some internists, not fully aware of the brief duration of ECT anesthesia or the generally modest systemic effects of a medically controlled grand mal seizure, seriously overestimate the stress of the procedure on the organism and will reject as inappropriate risks some patients for whom ECT is actually the conservative treatment of choice.

Neither skull x-rays nor an EEG is a useful screening test prior to ECT. The former are insensitive in detecting intracerebral pathology and the latter lacks specificity for all but seizure disorders. As almost one-third of all melancholics will exhibit pretreatment nonspecific EEG abnormalities that do not predict an unfavorable outcome (7), their presence is unhelpful in deciding whether or not to give ECT. If intracerebral lesions are suspected, a CT or NMR scan is the diagnostic procedure of choice.

Prior to the introduction in 1955 of succinylcholine muscle relaxation for ECT, many patients sustained spinal compression fractures during the tonic phase of the induced seizure (8), and x-rays of the dorsolumbar spine were routinely obtained pretreatment for medicolegal documentation. It is now almost thirty years since such documentation became unnecessary, and the archaic requirement in some hospitals for pre-ECT spine films only produces needless expense and radiation exposure.

Some authorities recommend plasma pseudocholinesterase determination prior to ECT (9) in order to detect the rare (1:3,000) individual whose deficient levels of this enzyme predispose him to prolonged post-ECT apnea due to impaired metabolism of succinylcholine, the muscle-relaxant used for the procedure. The fact is that screening for pseudocholinesterase deficiency is of no value for the following reason: When a sensitive (albeit quite specific) test is used to screen for a rare disorder, over 90 percent of the positive results are false, providing no guide to action (10).

Consent for ECT

Ideally ECT should be given only to competent patients who voluntarily provide their written consent after a full and free discussion of its potential benefits and risks, as well as the benefits and risks of alternate treatments or no treatment at all. In practice this ideal is often difficult to achieve. Many endogenously depressed patients who are on voluntary status and fully competent are simply unable to attend to the fine details of the informed consent process because of distractibility or preoccupation with their own thoughts. Or they may have "gone beyond caring," be indifferent to their fate, and perfunctorily sign any document shown to them. Others, who comprehend the elements of the procedure, have no objection to it, and strongly desire relief from symptoms, must be encouraged, coaxed, and pressed into signing, as their indecision or psychomotor retardation prove almost insurmountable obstacles to obtaining consent. Their families are often asked, or may volunteer, to aid in this process. All of the above surely stretch the doctrine of informed consent.

The psychiatrist, like other physicians, is frequently faced with this conflict between the letter and the spirit of the law, between what he believes is best for his patient and what the law says is best for society. Ultimately each physician decides for himself, case by case, the degree of ambiguity he can tolerate in applying these legal doctrines within the context of responsible medical practice.

The law, however, is generally clear. It may vary somewhat from state to state but usually includes the following elements. Voluntary patients may receive ECT only after providing their written, informed consent. In some states an exception to this rule is the patient who suddenly and unexpectedly becomes acutely suicidal and presents a clear and immediate danger of killing himself. Many psychiatrists would give emergency ECT to such a patient after converting his status to involuntary, often (but not always) first obtaining the family's consent and that of the hospital director or service chief. In such instances the emergency must be genuine and clearly documented in writing in the patient's chart.

Many states now also insist that informed consent for ECT be obtained from involuntary patients as well, recognizing that a psychosis does not necessarily rob a patient of the ability to understand the nature of the treatment offered and rationally to refuse it. The empathic clinician, eager to restore his patient to health through a safe, quick, and demonstrably effective method, may well chafe at these legal intrusions into medical practice. However, many patients in the past were treated involuntarily but doubtless also unnecessarily and even inappropriately by otherwise well-meaning and dedicated physicians convinced of the efficacy of ECT in chronic schizophrenia, for example. If ECT is to survive as a treatment method it is probably just as well that patients and staff are spared the disturbing spectacle of an unwilling patient being forcibly restrained in order to receive ECT. If the treating psychiatrist is thoroughly convinced that the potential benefits of ECT justify involuntary treatment, it behooves him to petition the court to direct that ECT be given against the patient's will. If successful, this process not only provides much-needed treatment for the patient, but serves to educate the courts as well.

ECT Orders

Once the decision to give ECT has been made, and a starting date set, standard orders for the procedure are as follows:

1. ECT Mondays, Wednesdays, and Fridays, starting _____
2. Nothing by mouth after midnight before ECT
3. Consent signed and placed in chart
4. Atropine 0.6–1.0 mg. intramuscular forty-five minutes before treatment

Dentures and eyeglasses should be removed and stored in a safe place; they tend to get lost, dropped, or stepped on in the bustle of the treatment and recovery rooms. Patients should urinate before going for treatment as incontinence occasionally occurs during the seizure. Hair oils, creams, and sprays should not be applied on treatment mornings. Patients with oily hair or residues from hair preparations should have a shampoo the night before. These precautions will ensure good electrode-scalp contact.

The ECT Unit

The modern ECT unit includes separate treatment and recovery areas and is similar in many ways to a minor surgery suite. The present description is based on a unit that serves a thirty-bed psychiatric service and assumes that about 15 percent of patients will receive ECT at any time.

Floor Space

The treatment area must comfortably accommodate several pieces of equipment (treatment machine, pacemaker-defibrillator, oxygen tank, "crash cart"), the patient on a stretcher, and four to six personnel (depending on whether residents or medical students are present). A minimum of 225 sq. ft. of space is thus required, and 400 sq. ft. is by no means excessive. The recovery room must accommodate five or six patients on stretchers, oxygen and suction equipment, and two to four personnel; it should be approximately the same size as the treatment room.

Treatment and recovery rooms should be separate but connected by a door. The ideal procedure is for patients to enter the treatment room through one door, be transferred to the recovery room through another door, and leave the recovery room through a third door.

Equipment

Treatment Room
    six rolling stretchers, OR type,
        with IV holders
    ECT apparatus and stand
    pacemaker–defibrillator and stand
    oxygen tank with valve, flow-meter, and
        positive-pressure bag
    tracheal suction apparatus
    refrigerator
    IV pole on wheels
    medication/supplies cabinet
    medication cart on wheels
    emergency medication tray to contain:
        atropine
        diazepam
        diphenhydramine
        epinephrine
        levarterenol
        lidocaine
        methylprednisolone
        propranolol
    laryngoscope with three sizes of blades
    assorted cuffed endotracheal tubes
    assorted plastic airways, rubber
        mouth-bites

Recovery Room
    tracheal suction apparatus
    portable positive-pressure ventilation
        (e.g., Ambu bag)

PATIENT FLOW AND DIVISION OF STAFF RESPONSIBILITY

ECT is a brief procedure, which, if performed efficiently, requires no more than eight to ten minutes' time per patient. Efficiency can be maximized by controlling patient flow as follows:

1. The patient to be treated has emptied his bladder, his vital signs have been recorded, and he is lying on a stretcher outside the treatment room.

2. When the treatment team is ready, the patient is wheeled into the treatment room, and the next patient is prepared and placed on the stretcher outside.

3. While an intravenous infusion is being started, the nursing assistant applies the EKG and EEG electrodes. As soon as a few seconds of baseline recording are obtained, anesthesia is rapidly induced and the anesthetist starts forced oxygenation immediately when the patient loses consciousness. The muscle-relaxant is injected at the same time, and as soon as the fasciculations disappear in the calf muscles the psychiatrist applies the treatment electrodes, the anesthetist inserts the rubber bite block if needed and hyperextends the neck, and the electrical stimulus is given. The anesthetist continues forced ventilation throughout the seizure until the return of spontaneous respirations, at which time the patient is placed on his side, an airway inserted, and the stretcher is rolled into the recovery room.

4. The next patient is then brought into the treatment room.

The ECT Team

ECT is not a trivial or innocuous procedure, to be relegated to a lone psychiatric resident or casually administered, unassisted, in the office. It is a significant medical procedure carried out under general anesthesia, and it entails definite risks, however small, of morbidity and mortality. To maximize safety and efficiency ECT should be given by an experienced team composed of (at a minimum) a psychiatrist, a nurse, an anesthetist or anesthesiologist, and a nursing assistant.

The psychiatrist is the director of the ECT unit and has overall medical responsibility for the procedure, analogous to the surgeon's role in the operating suite. His specific functions are as follows:

1. To determine the clinical appropriateness of ECT for each patient referred for treatment.
2. To evaluate the potential risks and benefits of ECT for each patient
3. To monitor the patient's progress in treatment and determine the point of maximum benefit
4. To monitor treatment side effects and modify the course of treatment accordingly (e.g. reduce frequency of treatment if excessive memory loss occurs)
5. To monitor the treatment itself by
    a. establishing and adjusting the anesthetic dosage
    b. establishing and adjusting the electrical stimulus parameters

The ECT nurse is responsible for the coordination of the unit, a role that carries a large administrative responsibility along with traditional nursing functions, as follows:

1. To ascertain that patients are properly prepared for ECT (e.g. that they have not eaten breakfast) and that the required paperwork and laboratory examinations are completed and in the patient's chart
2. To monitor and maintain medical supplies for the ECT unit (e.g. succinylcholine, intravenous sets, syringes) and to maintain records of any controlled substances (e.g. methohexital) used
3. To monitor patient flow from waiting area to treatment room to recovery room and back to home unit
4. To supervise nursing personnel in treatment room and recovery areas
5. To monitor and record vital signs before, during, and after ECT
6. To prepare intravenous solutions and injectable medications in syringes

The role of the anesthetist or anesthesiologist is:

1. To induce anesthesia
2. To maintain airway and oxygenation
3. To assume charge of any emergency or resuscitative procedures that may be required (e.g. intubation, defibrillation)

The nursing assistant performs the following functions:

1. Ascertains that patients are prepared for treatment (properly attired, bladder empty, jewelry removed, not smoking or chewing gum, dentures and glasses removed and safely stowed), and to assist in transferring the patient to his bed
2. Wheels patients to and from ECT unit
3. Applies EKG and EEG electrodes
4. Prepares ECT unit for next treatment day after ECT is over, assuring the suite's neatness and cleanliness

In addition, two trained nursing assistants should be stationed in the recovery room to assist in transferring patients from stretcher to bed, and to reassure patients as they emerge from anesthesia.

Preanesthesia and Anesthesia

Atropine, 0.6–1.0 mg. intramuscular, is given forty-five minutes prior to anesthesia to attenuate the seizure-induced parasympathetic discharge with its consequent bradycardia and increased tracheobronchial secretions. If a potent vagal-blocking effect is required, as in treating a patient with preexisting heart block, 1.2 mg. of atropine should instead be given intravenously immediately after the barbiturate anesthesia.

The ultra-short-acting barbiturate methohexital is now the anesthetic agent of choice, having entirely replaced the older thiopental sodium with its greater risk of EKG abnormalities (11). An intravenous drip infusion is started with a 250 cc. container of glucose and water, using a 19–21 gauge, thin-walled butterfly needle assembly (alternatively, a 50 cc. syringe filled with glucose and water may be attached to the butterfly). After recording vital signs, 60–80 mg. of methohexital (1 mg./kg.) is rapidly given intravenously by "bolus push" into the IV tubing. The patient is asked to count aloud to fifty. When he ceases counting, 40–50 mg. succinylcholine is injected in the same manner as the methohexital. (Subsequent succinylcholine dosage will be modified according to the strength of the first seizure.) The patient is then closely observed for muscle fasciculations representing the first (depolarization) phase of succinylcholine activity. These start in the face, chest, and upper extremities and progress to lower extremities over ten to twenty seconds. When the fasciculations begin to fade in the calves and small muscles of the feet, the patient is ready to be treated.

Treatment Electrode Application

Bilateral ECT is the original method and is administered through bifrontotemporal electrodes, one on each side of the head, placed an inch above the midpoint of an imaginary line joining the outer canthus of the eye and the external auditory meatus. Unilateral ECT, a modification introduced in 1958 (12), is most frequently administered through electrodes placed temporoparietally over one side of the head only, the nondominant hemisphere. The lower (temporal) electrode is placed as for bilateral ECT, and the upper (parietal) electrode is placed 3 to 4 inches above this, in the direction of the vertex. Right-sided unilateral ECT should initially be given in all patients, as the left hemisphere is dominant for speech in almost all right-handers and many left-handers. If a left-handed patient exhibits verbal memory impairment after the first treatment, he may be assumed to be right hemisphere dominant for speech, and the treatment electrodes should be moved to the left hemisphere for subsequent treatments.

Unilateral ECT was introduced in a successful attempt to reduce the memory loss and confusion so frequently observed after conventional, bilateral ECT. Controversy remains over the relative therapeutic efficacy of unilateral and bilateral ECT in endogenous depression (melancholia), and a recent controlled study from this department demonstrated a significant and important clinical advantage for bilateral ECT (13). The majority of studies, however, find the two methods to be equally efficacious (14).

Where there is no special urgency to achieve symptom relief, patients may be started on unilateral ECT, changing over to bilateral ECT if significant improvement is not observed after four or five treatments. Where a rapid response is required, as in suicidal, psychotic, agitated, or severely retarded depressives, or manics, we prefer to give bilateral ECT directly.

Treatment Devices

Two types of ECT devices are available, which employ either sinusoidal or pulsed currents.

Sinusoidal Current Devices

Sinusoidal (alternating) currents are characterized by a continuous flow of electricity, first in one direction and then in the other, at a frequency of 60 Hz. Such currents were used in 1938 to give the first ECT, and are still employed today in some devices of older design. One such apparatus (Medcraft™) has settings for voltage (70–170 volts) and stimulus duration (0.1–1.0 seconds). A typical initial setting is 140 volts for 0.5 seconds, increasing the dose in a stepwise fashion if a seizure is not obtained, first by increasing the duration to 1.0 second and then by raising the voltage to 170 if the first maneuver fails. This apparatus also has a "glissando" dial which was introduced in the pre-succinylcholine era in an attempt to reduce the incidence of fractures by slowing the rate of application of the treatment stimulus. The "glissando" mode substantially increases the electrical dosage, however, and as the advent of succinylcholine muscle-relaxation has rendered the dial merely decorative, it should be left permanently off.

PULSED CURRENT DEVICES

Sinusoidal currents can be modified electronically to provide a series of brief rectangular pulses which more efficiently stimulate the brain, inducing seizures with substantially less electrical energy and therefore less memory loss (15). One pulsed current device (Mecta™) has dials to control pulsewidth, frequency, and stimulus duration; typical initial settings are pulsewidth = 0.75 ms., frequency = 30 Hz., stimulus duration = 1 sec. If a seizure is not obtained at these settings, the stimulus duration should be increased to 2 sec. and the treatment readministered. If a seizure is still not obtained, the frequency and then the pulsewidth should be raised to the maximum, in that order, in an attempt to pass the convulsive threshold.

Another pulsed current instrument (Thymatron™) has a single dial which directly controls the percent of total available energy delivered. If a seizure is not obtained at an initial setting of 50 percent energy, restimulation should be applied at 75 percent and then 100 percent energy, at which point the seizure threshold should virtually always be passed.

Regressive ECT and Multiple ECT

Regressive ECT was introduced in the 1940s as a technique to induce a transient, profound dementia through a series of 30–40 seizures administered on consecutive days (16). It was based on the belief that this demented state resembled psychoanalytic regression and the hope that patients could be therapeutically reintegrated as they emerged from this severely disorganized condition. The theory was, of course, nonsense, and as the method was never shown to be more effective than conventional ECT it died a natural death.

Multiple ECT is a conceptually unrelated technique introduced in order to shorten the required course of treatment and reduce the number of anesthesia exposures by administering several seizures in a single treatment session (17). The original authors called the procedure multiple monitored ECT, because they recorded the EKG and EEG during treatment. Such monitoring, however, is not an essential aspect of the method.

Like regressive ECT, multiple ECT has never been subjected to a controlled comparison with conventional ECT, and because of its markedly increased side effects multiple ECT has been largely abandoned (18).

The Seizure

Although the relative therapeutic roles of the induced cerebral seizure and the electrical stimulating current remain as yet undefined, there is little doubt that a fully-developed grand mal seizure is a major element in the treatment process (15). The motor manifestation of this seizure is irrelevant, so long as a cerebral seizure has occurred. In most patients this event will be easily recognized, despite the effects of succinylcholine, which rarely entirely obscures the stereotyped tonic–clonic progression of the induced seizure. Missed, abortive, or partial seizures occasionally occur, most often with unilateral ECT, and when this happens the electrical stimulation must be repeated until a full seizure is obtained. Even with extreme degrees of muscle relaxation, a tonic seizure phase can usually be observed, characterized by pronounced plantarflexion lasting for five to ten seconds. In the absence of such a response it is best to repeat the electrical stimulation as quickly as possible in order to take advantage of the temporarily lowered seizure threshold from the initial stimulus. Additional evidence for the occurrence of a seizure may be deduced from the presence of piloerection (gooseflesh), pupillary dilatation, and tachycardia. An EEG monitor is only of modest assistance in this regard, as the passage of the stimulating current overloads the EEG amplifiers, so that it takes at least ten seconds for the recording pens to return to baseline. By then the tonic phase will have passed, along with the optimal period during which a repeat stimulus of the same intensity is likely to induce a seizure. A simple and effective technique for monitoring seizure activity is to inflate a blood pressure cuff over one arm to exceed the systolic blood pressure before the succinylcholine is given. The unmodified seizure can then be observed in the occluded extremity.

EEG monitoring is primarily of value to ensure adequate seizure duration, for unlike the tonic phase the clonic seizure phase may be markedly attenuated and even totally obscured by succinylcholine (although experienced clinicians will recognize the very fine rhythmical twitching movements of the small muscles underlying the skin around the eyes and nose). If total seizure time, as measured by stopwatch or EEG, is less than twenty-five seconds, the electrical stimulation should be repeated at a higher intensity, after waiting at least one minute for the refractory period to pass. It is almost never necessary to give additional succinylcholine in this event, as an adequate degree of muscle relaxation for ECT continues for several minutes after the peak effect has been reached.

Recovery Phase

Termination of the seizure signals the end of the treatment phase. The remaining task is to monitor the patient's emergence from anesthesia and the cognitive disruption of the seizure. Assisted ventilation is continued for several minutes until spontaneous respirations return, at which time the IV is removed, and the patient is turned on his side and wheeled to a nearby recovery area, where he will be observed by trained personnel until he awakens. Maintenance of an airway and adequate exchange of air are the main tasks of the recovery phase, and suction and oxygen equipment, although rarely required, must be maintained for immediate use should the occasion arise.

Medical Physiology of ECT

ECT exerts its most prominent effects on the cardiovascular system, both through a direct initial Valsalva effect and from a subsequent seizure-induced generalized autonomic and motor discharge.

Heart rate and blood pressure increase moderately during the initial Valsalva effect, followed by further marked increases during a period of one to two minutes following the electrical stimulus. Pulse rates typically rise to 130–190/minute with accompanying systolic blood pressure levels of 200–250 mmHg. These levels return to baseline by a minute or so after the seizure ends. Cerebral blood flow increases after an initial brief reduction during the electrical stimulus, and this is accompanied by doubling of cerebral oxygen consumption and glucose utilization during the induced seizure. However, there is no evidence for cerebral anoxia during succinylcholine-modified ECT, probably explained by the very small amounts of oxygen used up peripherally by the paralyzed muscles.

Complications and Side Effects

About 5 to 10 percent of patients develop a state of pronounced restless agitation as they emerge from anesthesia. This is an "emergence delirium," for which patients later display a dense amnesia. No amount of calm reassurance or firm persuasion is of any avail in preventing them from climbing out of bed, over the side rails if raised, and possibly injuring themselves. The patient must be restrained and given intravenous sedation, preferably with diazepam, 10 mg., in order to terminate the episode. Repeat episodes usually occur with each subsequent treatment and may be prevented by giving diazepam, 10 mg., by direct intravenous injection immediately after the induced seizure terminates. The rapid response of this syndrome to intravenous sedatives, as well as its clinical characteristics of automatisms and amnesia, suggest that it may be similar to a psychomotor seizure. Untreated, it rarely lasts longer than fifteen to twenty minutes.

Prolonged apnea is a rare complication of ECT anesthesia and results from a relative deficiency of pseudocholinesterase, the enzyme that degrades succinylcholine. If spontaneous respirations do not return by five minutes after the seizure has ended, preparation should be made for intubation; if assisted respiration is still required after ten minutes, a cuffed endotracheal tube should be inserted and inflated in order to maximize the efficiency of air exchange. Most patients with this complication will breathe spontaneously within a half-hour; those who do not may be given a unit of typed and crossmatched *fresh* whole blood to supply an exogenous source of pseudocholinesterase.

The principal side effect of ECT is the temporary confusion and memory loss seen most clearly after bilateral ECT. These phenomena are directly related to the number and frequency of treatments and may be exaggerated in patients over age sixty. The memory loss consists of two parts: a fully recoverable retrograde amnesia for events preceding the first treatment, exhibiting a gradient of severity more pronounced for recent than remote events, and an anterograde amnesia for events occurring after the patient awakens from treatment, permanent because it results from failure to consolidate new memories during several postictal hours. Once a course of treatments has ended, the retrograde amnesia shrinks gradually over a period of several weeks and generally disappears entirely by thirty to sixty days. Because of anterograde amnesia, however, patients often complain of memory gaps for parts of their hospital stay.

Memory changes following unilateral ECT administered to the nondominant hemisphere are markedly reduced as compared with bilateral ECT (19). Immediately following a seizure, personal orientation returns more rapidly with unilateral than with bilateral ECT, as does recall of items learned prior to the seizure. Both retrograde and anterograde amnesia are reduced, as well as the cumulative memory impairment following a course of treatment.

Induced convulsions are characterized not only by the electrical discharge of the seizure but by EEG changes, which persist into the interseizure period. These changes take the form of slowing, increased amplitude, and increased rhythmicity. They appear all over the head, with the degree of slowing directly related to the number and frequency of seizures and the location of the treatment electrodes (20).

Risks, Precautions, and Contraindications

ECT is among the safest of medical procedures carried out under general anesthesia. The most recent large-scale survey found 4.5 deaths per 100,000 treatments, or a fatality rate of 0.0045 percent (21).

Cardiovascular conditions are responsible for most of the mortality of ECT (11), and special caution is required when treating patients who have arrhythmias, conduction defects, ischemia, heart failure or other significant pathology. Appropriate medical therapy should be instituted to maximize cardiac function and efficiency (e.g. digitalization for congestive heart failure, quinidinization for atrial fibrillation). The decision whether to give ECT will then be based on the relative risk of giving or withholding such treatment. In the severely depressed melancholic, the decision will frequently be in favor of giving ECT in view of the lack of effective alternate treatments and the deleterious effect of the melancholia upon cardiac status.

Reserpine and its congeners should not be given with ECT, as fatal hypotension may ensue (22). Caution should be observed when combining ECT with phenothiazines, as cardiovascular collapse has occurred following such a combination. There are no reported fatalities or complications arising from the combination of ECT with either tricyclic or MAOI antidepressant drugs. Lithium should be avoided in patients receiving ECT, because it may increase the succinylcholine-induced neuromuscular blockade (23) and may also magnify the cognitive side effects (1).

The principal contraindication to convulsive therapy is a space-occupying lesion of the brain with increased intracranial pressure.

Age in itself is no contraindication to treatment. Some of the most rewarding results with convulsive therapy are obtained in elderly, debilitated patients whose primary affective or delusional disorder masquerades as senile dementia.

When considering indications and contraindications the suicidal potential of the patient must be carefully evaluated; this will occasionally take precedence irrespective of the physical condition. A determined patient may successfully commit suicide despite stringent precautions and constant individual surveillance. Once ECT is started, however, suicide attempts are rare.

Maintenance ECT

For patients who relapse despite continuation therapy with tricyclics or lithium, maintenance ECT has been used successfully, although few objective data have yet been provided in support of this technique. With maintenance ECT, patients return at regular intervals for additional treatments even in the absence of any recurrence of symptoms. A typical schedule for a patient who has fully recovered with a course of six ECT might have the patient return for 4–6 additional treatments at biweekly intervals for the first 2–3, and monthly thereafter. There is no rationale for continued maintenance ECT for prolonged periods (e.g., over six months), except in unusual circumstances. The continued use of prolonged maintenance ECT has no clinical justification and may result in continuous cognitive dysfunction.

References

1. Fink, M. *Convulsive Therapy: Theory and Practice.* New York: Raven Press, 1979, p. 75.

2. Abrams, R. The ECT controversy: Some observations and a suggestion. *Psychiatric Opinion 16:* 11–15, 1979.

3. Taylor, J. R.; Tompkins, R.; Demers, R.; *et al.* Electroconvulsive therapy and memory dysfunction: Is there evidence for prolonged defects? *Biol. Psychiat. 17:* 1169–93, 1982.

4. McCabe, M. S. ECT in the treatment of mania: A controlled study. *Am. J. Psychiat. 133:* 688–91, 1976.

5. Abrams, R.; Taylor, M. A. Catatonia: A prospective study. *Arch. Gen. Psychiat. 33:* 579–81, 1976.

6. Taylor, M. A. Indications for Electroconvulsive Treatment. In Abrams, R.; Essman, W. B. (eds.), *Electroconvulsive Therapy: Biological Foundations and Clinical Applications.* New York: Spectrum, 1982, pp. 7–30.

7. Abrams, R.; Volavka, J.; Dornbush, R.; *et al.* Lateralized EEG changes after unilateral and bilateral electroconvulsive therapy. *Dis. Nerv. Syst. GWAN Supplement 31:* 28–33, 1970.

8. Kalinowsky, L. B.; Hippins, H. (eds.). *Pharmacological, Convulsive and Other Somatic Treatments in Psychiatry.* New York: Grune & Stratton, 1969, p. 213.

9. A.M.A. *Task Force Report 14: Electroconvulsive Therapy.* Washington, D.C.: American Psychiatric Association, 1978, p. 107.

10. Galen, R. S.; Gambino, S. R. *Beyond Normality: The Predictive Value and Efficiency of Medical Diagnoses.* New York: John Wiley, 1975, p. 17.

11. Pitts, F. Medical Physiology of ECT. In Abrams, R.; Essman, W. B. (eds.), *Electroconvulsive Therapy: Biological Foundations and Clinical Applications.* New York: Spectrum, 1982, pp. 57–89.

12. Lancaster, N. P.; Steinert, R. R.; Frost, I. Unilateral electro-convulsive therapy. *J. Ment. Sci. 104:* 221–27, 1958.

13. Abrams, R.; Taylor, M. A.; Faber, R.; *et al.* Bilateral versus unilateral ECT: Efficacy in melancholia. *Am. J. Psychiat. 140:* 463–56, 1983.

14. D'Elia, G.; Raotma, H. Is unilateral ECT less effective than bilateral ECT? *Br. J. Psychiat. 126:* 83–89, 1975.

15. Weiner, R. D.; Rogers, H. C.; Welch, C. A., Jr.; *et al.* ECT Stimulus Parameters and Electrode Placement: Relevance to Therapeutic and Adverse Effects. In Lerer, B., Weiner, R. D., and Belmaker, R. H. (eds.), *ECT: Basic Mechanisms.* London: John Libbey, 1983, pp. 139–147.

16. Glueck, B. J., Jr.; Reiss, H.; Bernard, L. E. Regressive electric shock therapy. *Psychiat. Quart. 31:* 117–36, 1957.

17. Blachly, P.; Gowing, D. Multiple monitored electroconvulsive treatment. *Comp. Psychiat. 7:* 100–109, 1966.

18. Abrams, R. Multiple ECT: What Have We Learned? In Fink, M.; Kety, S.;

McGaugh, J.; *et al.* (eds.), *Psychobiology of Convulsive Therapy.* New York: John Wiley & Sons, 1974, pp. 79–84.

19. Squire, L. Neuropsychological Effects of ECT. In Abrams, R.; Essman, W. B. (eds.), *Electroconvulsive Therapy: Biological Foundations and Clinical Applications.* New York: Spectrum, 1982, pp. 169–85.

20. Abrams, R.; Volavka, J. Electroencephalographic Effects of ECT. In Abrams, R.; Essman, W. B. (eds.), *Electroconvulsive Therapy: Biological Foundations and Clinical Applications.* New York: Spectrum, 1982, pp. 157–67.

21. Heshe, J.; Roeder, E. Electroconvulsive therapy in Denmark. *Br. J. Psychiat. 128:* 241–45, 1976.

22. Bracha, S.; Hess, J. P. Death occurring during combined reserpine-electroshock treatment. *Am. J. Psychiat. 113:* 257, 1956.

23. Hill, G. E.; Wong, K. C.; Hodges, M. R. Potentiation of succinylcholine neuromuscular blockade by lithium carbonate. *Anesthesiology 44:* 439–42, 1976.

CHAPTER 7

Verbal Interventions and Behavioral Techniques

The psychotherapy of hospitalized patients has been overvalued. To our knowledge there are no scientifically rigorous, controlled studies demonstrating that psychotherapy alone is an effective treatment for any psychiatric syndrome for which people are hospitalized. Although there are some data (1–4) demonstrating the efficacy of cognitive psychotherapy for some depressions, most of the patients cited were experiencing a reactive and not an endogenous or major depression.

Nevertheless, as with physicians in any other branch of medicine, the psychiatrist's interpersonal and interviewing skills can facilitate the patient's compliance with somatic treatments. For this to occur, it is important that the patient perceive that the psychiatrist (or other specialist) cares about him and responds intelligently to his symptoms and concerns. But of all the medical specialists, the psychiatrist is particularly expected to care for his patients as people; to be skilled in comforting, educating, and advising them; to spend time with them; and to help them resolve environmental and interpersonal problems.

The Initial Diagnostic Interview

TIME ALLOTTED AND DATA NEEDED

The initial diagnostic interview sets the tone for further experiences with the patient. With the exception of emergency room interviews, most initial diagnostic interviews will take between forty-five and ninety minutes. This amount of time allows for a reasonable assessment of the patient's present illness; past personal, social, and family history; medical review of systems; and a behavioral neurologic examination. The subsequent physical examination performed by the psychiatrist or his designee will usually take fifteen to thirty minutes.

Almost as important as the data base obtained is the patient's perception that the physician has been thorough. The patient should be made to feel as comfortable as possible and should feel the examiner knows what he is doing, is interested and concerned, and is going to listen and respond to the patient's needs and reasonable requests. Subsequent contacts with hospitalized patients are usually considerably briefer but should continue to reinforce the trust established in the initial interview.

INITIAL CONTACT WITH THE PATIENT

Charts or other documents generally should not be reviewed while the patient is sitting in the office. Although starting an interview while reading a chart establishes the doctor–patient role dichotomy, it also appears cold and officious. It is better to greet the patient in a direct, friendly manner, walk with him to your office, and invite him to sit down. Many patients appreciate the physician's concern about details in their charts, but they are more appreciative of the concern shown for them face to face. Unless he is a child or teenager, the patient should be addressed by a title (e.g. "Mr. Jones," "Mrs. Smith") rather than a first name. The latter is patronizing. Children and teenagers, however, find this formality uncomfortable and generally prefer to be called by their first names.

Unless it is certain that the patient knows the purpose of the interview, a brief explanation is helpful. Usually following this (as in the initial interview in medicine or surgery), the patient should be asked a general question about why he believes he was brought to the hospital or why he came to the hospital. Occasionally, unrelated openings may be helpful. For example, one manic patient, thought to be a difficult person to examine, became a model of cooperativeness when one of us opened the interview by commenting on a green hat he was wearing—"That's a nice looking hat you have on. Where did you get it?" Other patients have responded well to such openings as "You look upset, Mr. Jones. What's happened to bother you?" and "Mr. Smith, I understand the police brought you to the hospital last night. What happened?"

THE "BODY" OF THE DIAGNOSTIC INTERVIEW

The essence of interviewing is the physician's ability to obtain a pertinent data base while simultaneously responding to what the patient is saying and doing and to the mood he is expressing. Since asking all possible questions for all psychiatric illnesses (plus covering all possible systemic illnesses as well) is impractical, the best technique is the semistructured interview, in which "screening" questions are asked and followed up only if the patient's response suggests the possibility of a particular syndrome. When a patient seems likely to have a particular condition, he is then questioned methodically for signs and symptoms of the syndrome until it is diagnosed or excluded.

For example, a fifty-three-year-old woman is admitted to a psychiatric service because of delusions. She looks worried. Given this information, the psychiatrist questions the patient thoroughly for symptoms of melancholia. In addition, screening questions for other syndromes are asked. For example, this same patient, with no apparent signs of alcoholism, could be asked, "Has anybody ever told you you were drinking too much?" and "Have you ever had medical problems from drinking, or been shaky if you couldn't have a drink?" If the answer is no to these questions, further questioning about alcoholism can be withheld or delayed unless additional evidence surfaces.

Although questions should be asked systematically, they should be asked in a friendly, relatively spontaneous and conversational fashion. Most interview questions are closed-ended. They can be answered in a word or in a sentence (e.g. "How old are you?"). However, it is useful to ask some questions that require elaboration. For example, if a patient states he has trouble sleeping, the examiner might say, "Tell me more about your sleeping problem" instead of "Are you having trouble falling asleep or are you having trouble staying asleep?"

When a patient is giving clear and pertinent answers or expressing feelings that are not impeding the progress of the interview, the interviewer should allow the patient to continue. Making an occasional empathic comment (e.g. "That must have been frightening.") is sometimes helpful. For patients with formal thinking disorders, a period of several minutes where the examiner concentrates on identifying the type or form of thought disorder (rather than the content or what the patient is talking about) is often useful. What should be avoided are district-attorney-style interrogations unresponsive to the patient's behaviors or unstructured interviews where the patient is encouraged to elaborate on "interesting" statements ad lib, to the exclusion of obtaining diagnostically important data.

The degree of interview structuring will be determined by the severity or character of the patient's condition. For example, a patient with a phobic disorder may be able to provide sufficient data without much overt interview control, whereas a patient with significant psychomotor retardation may become further inhibited by open-ended questioning and will often respond best to structured, closed-ended questions spoken in a soft voice. The examiner may also have to wait several moments for the patient to overcome his inertia and respond. We have seen several novice interviewers question depressed patients in too rapid a fashion so that the patient either appears to have nonsequitive speech (his response is to question one, whereas the interviewer has just asked question three or four) or becomes totally inhibited by the intense, overwhelming barrage of questions. In contrast, manic patients with flight-of-ideas and pressured speech may require structuring in which the examiner repeats the same question several times (just to get the patient's attention) or literally stops the patient from proceeding along a line of irrelevant associations.

The structure of the interview includes the sequence in which questions are asked. The opening questions about reasons for hospitalization or the patient's chief complaints naturally lead to further questions about the present illness, the past history related to present symptoms, and so on. Patients generally respond best when this logical sequence is followed, as it is less distracting and less anxiety-provoking. When questioning patients with a probable diagnosis of sociopathy, the logical sequence is sometimes purposely disrupted so the patient cannot anticipate questions and then prepare his answers in advance. In some cases where the elicitation of delusions is diagnostically important, some patients reluctant to reveal their delusional ideas will become somewhat anxious or irritable under deliberately disjointed questioning and begin to express their suspiciousness and eventually their delusional ideas. The corollary to this tactic is equally important. When a patient is becoming excited, the examiner should refrain from jumping from topic to topic and in a calm and reassuring manner stick to a logical sequence of questions.

The interview structure also extends to the physical actions of the examiner. Examiner restlessness and overactivity are distractions that should be avoided unless increasing the patient's anxiety or impeding his concentration is a specific interview tactic. Using a few comfortable and apparently relaxed postures is the best general approach. Occasionally leaning forward and touching a patient on the arm or shoulder is helpful in gaining the patient's attention (particularly if the patient is stuporous or has flight-of-ideas) or in comforting the patient. With some catatonics, sitting beside rather than opposite them helps disinhibit them so that they can answer questions. Regardless of the interview structure, the patient should always be treated in a respectful fashion.

Many patients ask personal questions, such as "How long have you been a psychiatrist?" or "Did you ever take drugs?" Some (usually those addressing your professional experience or qualifications) are pertinent and appropriate and should be answered briefly. When personal questions become frequent, however, they waste time and usurp some control of the interview. Personal questions asked to excess should therefore be discouraged.

Occasionally the patient's thought processes are so disturbed that the history itself is unreliable. In such circumstances the physician should take time to identify and characterize formal thinking disorders, delusional phenomena, and perceptual disturbances, and then devote considerable time to screening for cognitive dysfunctions.

CONCLUSION OF THE DIAGNOSTIC INTERVIEW

At the end of most interviews the interviewer should make a concluding statement. The usual case is one in which the physician will be providing treatment or referral. Here, unless the patient is too ill to comprehend (in which case a simple "thank you" will suffice), the physician should briefly state the working diagnosis and explain planned diagnostic testing and treatments. Explanations of treatments should usually include the rationale for the treatment and the potential side effects. Most patients appreciate thoughtful explanations, and many resent physicians who fail to provide them.

Follow-up Visits with the Patient

Following the diagnostic interview, the physician or his designee should see the hospitalized patient daily. At the morning report or a chat with one or more of the personnel attending to his patients, the physician should ascertain if there were major developments and then review recent chart entries and laboratory reports. He will be interested in changes in the patient's psychiatric status and general health, events that may affect the patient, side effects of somatic treatments, possible need for changes in the patient's privilege level, discharge planning, and anticipated patient concerns and requests. Discharge planning (e.g. where and with whom the patient will live) should start within a few days of admission.

The daily follow-up visits in the form of rounds can usually be relatively brief, lasting from several minutes in most cases to a half-hour. This is analogous to the visits of an internist or surgeon to a patient's bedside. The brevity of follow-up visits in no way implies indifference; there is no evidence that regularly scheduled half-hour to hour-long therapies improve the patient's response to treatment. Daily rounds can be conducted by walking about the unit or by seeing the patient in a consulting room on the unit.

Following an initial greeting, the main subject matter will be (1) obtaining further history, if needed, (2) current symptoms and functioning, (3) effects of treatments, (4) response to recent events on the unit or at home, (5) concerns raised by the patient, and (6) diagnostic, therapeutic, and disposition planning. This can be conducted in the form of questions by the physician (e.g. "How have you been doing?" "What's happened since I saw you yesterday?" "Are you still feeling nauseated?"), observations by the physician (e.g. "You look much more alert and vigorous today." "You seem very worried this morning."), or responses by the physician to questions or concerns of the patient. In cases where the patient is too ill to converse, he can still be greeted, briefly examined, and told about the doctor's assessment and proposed treatments.

Often there is a need for some interaction beyond a terse discussion of symptoms and treatments. The physician's supportive, empathic, or explanatory comments, as well as his willingness to listen, may be useful. Examples include challenging the patient's self-deprecatory misconceptions (one of the essentials of cognitive therapy) (5), empathizing with his suffering, sharing his pleasure at alleviation of symptoms, attempting to modify excessive guilt, letting him know that he is not alone in having particular symptoms, and explaining the meaning of certain symptoms and the reasoning behind recommended procedures and treatments. The following are some illustrations:

A twenty-four-year-old man is being treated with ECT for melancholia. He worries about "the stigma of being a mental patient" and "what my friends will say about me at work." During the ensuing discussion, the psychiatrist makes the following comments: "Nobody has to know you were depressed unless you tell them. . . . Even if they did, who'd want to be friends with someone so insensitive as to ridicule you for having been depressed? . . . In my eyes, it's an illness like any other illness, not a reflection on your character or intelligence."

A fifty-four-year-old hospitalized depressed woman reported bitterly that her twenty-one-year-old daughter (with whom she shares an apartment) invited an unemployed, "pot-smoking" boyfriend to live with them without first consulting the patient or offering to share expenses. The psychiatrist commented, "You really must feel used." The patient then cried and presented other instances wherein she felt used. Later she said, "Doctor, I'm sorry for burdening you with my troubles." The psychiatrist replied, "I *asked* you to talk about your troubles."

As the patient improves, hospital follow-up visits should help educate the patient to his illness and treatments and provide some advice about what to expect from family, friends, and employer when discharged and how to respond to these potential stressors.

Clinicians who are reasonably good interviewers in the formal doctor–patient setting often forget that *all* interactions with patients are important to the patient. When the examiner speaks to the patient, his tone of voice, manner, and choice of words are each important aspects of this informal contact on the unit or in the office waiting area. For example, a catatonic patient stood by the unit entrance each morning but was unable to say "Good morning" to any entering staff members until they had passed by him. Some staff continued to walk on without responding while others made it a point to slow down so that when the patient did say his "hello" they would be able to respond. Once recovered, the patient made a special point of thanking those staff members who were sensitive to the importance for him of the otherwise insignificant greeting. One physician never refused his patients' requests to play table tennis. His patients seemed to enjoy the interaction, and the physician said he found the games helpful in assessing his patients' motor–perceptual coordination and concentration. "He plays okay, but he can't remember the score" was a common observation.

In addition, patients often focus on the words spoken to them rather than the basic message of the statement. For example, a delusional patient, angry at being hospitalized involuntarily at his family's request, became further angered when asked why he was brought to the hospital. A rephrasing of the question to "What reasons did your family give you for their wanting you here?" ameliorated his anger, and he was then able to give a coherent history of his present illness. Nonjudgmental expressions ("How come?" rather than "Why?" or "Could there by another explanation?" rather than "I don't think so.") and more implicitly empathic phrasings ("Do people talk about you behind your back?" rather than "Do you hear voices?") facilitate patient cooperativeness.

The Patient's Family

The patient's family can play a helpful role (far less frequently, a destructive one) in his treatment. This role may include persuading the patient to accept needed treatments, visiting the patient in the hospital, and monitoring the patient's treatment following discharge.

It is therefore surprising that some physicians keep relatives at a considerable distance during the treatment process. Perhaps this stems from unproved notions about parental "causation" of major psychiatric illnesses (6–12) or the physician's anxiety that the family will interfere with or undermine his control of the patient.

In any case it is essential to establish a cordial relationship with one or more family members. The majority of patients want some explanation provided to relatives. In some cases, where a relative may act maliciously or where the admission is extremely embarrassing to the patient, keeping the family at a distance is certainly appropriate. On the other hand, in life-threatening situations requiring contact with a relative, the patient's confidentiality can be breached.

Behavioral Techniques

IGNORING UNWANTED BEHAVIORS WHILE REWARDING DESIRED SUBSTITUTE BEHAVIORS

In cases where spontaneous remission does not promptly occur or where an underlying systemic illness cannot be identified, almost all hospitalized psychiatric patients will require somatic treatments. In order that these treatments be employed in an optimal fashion, they need to be supported by the behavioral management of patients.

Behavioral management includes utilizing the following principles: (1) As attention is a powerful reinforcer of behaviors, many behaviors can be modified or partially extinguished by ignoring them. (2) Efforts should be directed to reinforcing desirable substitute behaviors to replace the unwanted ones. Reinforcers on an inpatient service include attention and conversation, trips to the canteen, unit parties, unit movies, trips off the hospital grounds, visits from friends, passes, television-watching, or a promotion within the progressive system of privileges (see Chapter 9). In some centers psychologists develop formal behavior modification systems such as token economies. These principles could be applied to the following behaviors.

Pseudosyncope or Pseudoseizures

Once systemic causes of fainting or fits are ruled out, and the patient is observed not to hurt himself when he falls, subsequent episodes are totally ignored by staff, and other patients are instructed to do the same. Normal behaviors are rewarded. This response is in contrast to the usual experience of such patients that their behavior rapidly mobilizes large numbers of concerned staff.

A thirteen-year-old boy was seen in consultation on a pediatric service because of fainting episodes in the absence of physical or laboratory signs of a systemic cause. During an initial interview he "fainted" (closed his eyes and slumped in his seat) multiple times without injuring himself. Each of these "faints" was terminated when the examiner said, "If you want to go to the playroom later, you have to wake up." On the ward he manifested stimulus-bound motor hyperactivity and borderline intelligence. An electroencephalogram showed six-per-second positive spiking. There were no other signs of psychiatric illness.

The patient was transferred to the psychiatric unit with a diagnosis of minimum brain dysfunction/hyperactivity syndrome and given methylphenidate. The staff and patients were instructed to ignore his fainting. He was praised and given privileges to go to the pediatric playroom when he did not faint or intrude in other patient activities. The fainting ceased within two days.

Low Back Pain with No Objective Findings

Many patients are admitted to orthopedic or other services with severe low back pain intensified by standing or walking. Occasionally, following an extensive evaluation, some of these patients will have absolutely no findings suggestive of disease in any structures in or near the low back, or of depression. However, the patient complains that the pain is so severe that he must remain in bed. Asked to stand or walk, he winces in pain and appears on the verge of tears. He is bedridden on the orthopedic service, receiving narcotics regularly. The differential diagnosis includes somatization disorder and malingering. He should be weaned off narcotics and presented with a regimen where all efforts to sit, stand, or walk are reinforced by enthusiastic praise and other privileges and encouraged to overcome the pain bravely.

A twenty-year-old army private was transferred from an orthopedic service to a psychiatric unit because of back pain that he claimed was so severe that he was unable to sit or walk. The orthopedic surgeons extensively evaluated the patient and found no physical or laboratory signs of systemic or orthopedic illness. Until transfer of the patient to the psychiatric unit, he was completely bedridden. Once on the psychiatric ward, he was put on a regimen of progressively increasing frequency and duration whereby he was expected to walk around the ward with a nurse. He was told that walking could not injure him; it could only strengthen his back muscles, prevent deterioration of his health, and ultimately diminish his pain. As he arose from bed and winced, groaned, or cried, he was told, "Be brave, you can do it, you can beat this thing!" His protests were ignored. At first every effort he made to walk was praised. On subsequent occasions the praise became intermittent. After several days he walked comfortably and without complaint.

ADVERSE CONSEQUENCES

Some behaviors cannot readily be ignored, and must be dealt with differently.

Breaking and Throwing Things

Breaking and throwing can sometimes be a precursor to violence directed at another person. When that is suspected, the patient should be medicated as described in Chapters 5 and 8. Whether or not it is so, if a broken article belongs to the patient, the staff or relatives should be deliberately slow in replacing it and reward attempts on the part of the patient to mend it. If food is thrown, it should not be replaced even if the patient is hungry. Periods of normal behavior should be rewarded.

Temper Tantrums or Cursing

Some patients yell, slam doors, and curse in order to receive attention or to have other needs met. If possible, staff and patients should totally ignore these behaviors, which may disappear if not reinforced. If this technique is ineffectual, to maintain order and quiet on the unit the patient may need to be discharged or placed in a seclusion room and provided with nursing care and attention only when the disruptive behaviors have been absent for a specified period of time. When the patient has quieted down for several hours, he can be released from seclusion and reinforced for normal self-controlled behavior.

SATIATION TECHNIQUES

Satiation techniques may be helpful in some situations, as in the case of hoarding. Some psychiatric inpatients hoard large quantities of primarily useless items: pieces of paper, used paper cups, washcloths, and chalk. Obviously the condition producing the hoarding requires treatment. In addition, the use of a satiation technique, whereby the staff actually adds items to the patient's hoard, may be effective. This is believed to work because these items often lose their reinforcing value when the individual has "had his fill" of them. Schaefer (13) cites the example of a towel hoarder whose rapidly successful treatment was to have the nurses regularly place towels in his room instead of removing them.

References

1. Rush, A. J.; Beck, A. T.; Kovacs, M.; et al. Comparative efficacy of cognitive therapy and pharmacotherapy in the treatment of depressed outpatients. *Cog. Ther. Res. 1:* 17–37, 1977.

2. McLean, P. D.; Hakestan, A. R. Clinical depression: Comparative efficacy of outpatient treatments. *J. Consult. Clin. Psychol. 47:* 818–36, 1979.

3. Weissman, M. M.; Prusoff, B. A.; Dimascio, A.; et al. The efficacy of drugs and psychotherapy in the treatment of acute depressive episodes. *Am. J. Psychiat. 136:* 555–58, 1979.

4. Rush, A. J.; Beck, A. T.; Kovacs, M.; et al. Comparison of the effects of cognitive therapy and pharmacotherapy on hopelessness and self-concept. *Am. J. Psychiat. 139:* 862–66, 1982.

5. Beck, A. T. *Depression: Causes and Treatment.* Philadelphia: University of Pennsylvania Press, 1967.

6. Rosen, J. N. *Direct Analysis: Selected Papers.* New York: Grune & Stratton, 1953, p. 9.

7. Searles, H. F. The effort to drive the other person crazy: An element in the etiology and psychotherapy of schizophrenia. *Br. J. Med. Psychol. 32:* 1–18, 1959.

8. Alanen, Y. O. The mothers of schizophrenic patients. *Acta Psychiat. Neurol. Scand. 124* (suppl.): 1, 1958.

9. Wynne, L. C.; Rychoff, I.; Day, J.; *et al.* Pseudomutuality in the family relations of schizophrenics. *Psychiatry 21:* 205–20, 1958.

10. Lidz, T. *The Family and Human Adaptation.* London: Hogarth Press, 1964.

11. Bateson, G.; Jackson, D. D.; Haley, J.; *et al.* Toward a theory of schizophrenia. *Behav. Sci. 1:* 251–64, 1956.

12. Arieti, S. *Interpretation of Schizophrenia.* New York: Brunner, 1955.

13. Schaefer, H. H.; Martin, P. L. *Behavioral Therapy.* New York: McGraw-Hill, 1969.

CHAPTER 8

Psychiatric Emergencies

Introduction

Psychiatric emergencies occur in a variety of clinical settings, including psychiatric and general medical and surgical inpatient units, outpatient clinics, and hospital emergency rooms. Although the diversity of psychiatric emergencies is enormous, a common feature of all is a patient who is in acute distress or whose behavior could result in immediate increased morbidity, death, injury to others, or destruction of property. Immediate remedial action is always required. A frequent early sign of an impending emergency is increasing anxiety on the part of the physician or hospital staff about a patient's condition. When the clinician recognizes these feelings, an immediate evaluation of the patient should be made.

Emergencies often present a threat to "life or limb" for patients or hospital personnel. This demands accurate and rapid assessment and the implementation of the necessary procedures and treatments to minimize the consequences from delay.

The evaluation of a patient during an emergency has the same goal as any other psychiatric examination: accurate diagnosis so that specific treatment can be instituted. In an emergency, however, elaborate laboratory testing and extensive interviewing often are not possible, and the primary treatment goal is for the clinician to reduce significantly the risks of further morbidity, injury, or death.

Often emergencies can be avoided by proper diagnosis, behavioral management, and treatment strategies. Acutely ill psychiatric patients frequently demonstrate significant cognitive impairment, and their hallucinations, delusional ideas, and language dysfunction suggest that they have deficits in information processing (1). They are often frightened by their psychopathological experiences; their anxiety, in turn, can further exacerbate cognitive deficits, resulting in a vicious circle. Because agitated, violent, and other disruptive behaviors can be precipitated or exacerbated by anxiety, procedures reducing the patient's anxiety frequently can prevent or ameliorate the emergent behavior. The following behavioral guidelines should be employed:

Interpersonal. All communication with the patient, including "Good morning" and "Nice day today," should be deliberate and specifically fitted to the individual patient. For example, many patients prefer direct statements (e.g. "You look more upset today." "You seem down in the dumps.") to the automatic phrases of social convention (e.g. "How are you?").

Communications should be simple and directed at reinforcing reality and appropriate behavior. Firmness, clarity in communications, and reality-oriented comments (e.g. "People get upset when you do that") are better than psychological "probing" (e.g. "I wonder why you're doing that?") and help reduce the patient's anxiety.

Administrative structures (to be discussed in greater detail in Chapter 9). Inpatient regulations, activities, and meetings should be organized in a clear manner. The purposes of each should be explained and reviewed with the patient. Too much activity can "overload" patients' increasing agitation and disruptive behavior. Rest periods and calm, structured activities are essential.

General Management

EVALUATION

Frequently the patient's signs and symptoms will immediately suggest a specific syndrome (e.g. mania, catatonia, acute anxiety attack) or situation (e.g. suicide attempt, delirious patient, violent patient). The two main goals of diagnosis in an emergency are to recognize the clinical presentation and then rapidly identify any life-threatening cause (e.g. pulmonary embolus, myocardial infarction) or readily treatable disorder (e.g. anticholinergic delirium, panic attack). Upwards of 40 percent of psychiatric patients have systemic illnesses undiagnosed by the referring physician yet causally related to the behaviors for which they were referred (2). Systemic examination and laboratory screening must be done whenever possible. (Chapter 10 reviews some of the specific systemic illnesses presenting as psychiatric syndromes.)

INTERVENTION

Emergency treatments include psychological and biological interventions, disposition planning, and family counseling.

The content of the psychological intervention will change depending upon the nature of the emergency, the experiental factors related to the crisis, and the life circumstances of the patient. The form of the psychological intervention should be consistent, characterized by reassurance, empathy, calmness, firmness, and reality-oriented comments. Many true emergencies (e.g. some drug intoxications) and other situations requiring immediate action (e.g. acute problems of living) can be ameliorated or resolved by simply talking to the patient in a comforting manner, allowing him to ventilate his feelings and giving him reasonable problem-solving advice (3–5).

Biological treatments for emergency situations will be described below in detail. In general principles for administering psychotropics (e.g. route of administration, dosages, drug combinations) also pertain in emergencies. Unfortunately these principles are often ignored, as when a clinician prescribes a neuroleptic when sedation is the real therapeutic goal and a sedative the agent of choice, or when an antidepressant is administered to prevent a second imminent suicide attempt, despite the fact that the therapeutic effect of these compounds requires ten to fourteen days of treatment.

Disposition planning for patients following emergency treatment is critical if the initial intervention is to be ultimately successful. Emergency treatment is generally limited to a few minutes or hours. If the effects of successful treatment are to be sustained and subsequent relapse prevented, follow-up planning should be done, taking into consideration the effectiveness of the original emergency treatment, the definitive or long-term treatment most appropriate to the individual case, and the patient's social and industrial circumstances (6, 7). Structured intervention subsequent to emergency care reduces the risk of chronicity and the rate of relapse and should be encouraged whenever possible (4, 8). Such intervention can include hospitalization; referral to a health care clinic, community agency, or special self-help organizations (e.g. Alcoholics Anonymous), or referral to individual practitioners, counselors, or clergy. With proper planning, approximately 60 percent of patients treated in an emergency room for a psychiatric disorder will comply with follow-up treatments (9).

As in all health care situations the involvement of family is helpful if treatment and disposition are to be of maximum benefit. When supportive family are available, they should be educated to the nature of the patient's condition, what treatments have been or will be given, how they can monitor subsequent treatment and symptoms, and what disposition is most appropriate for the patient.

BARBITURATES

Sedation with barbiturates is a time-honored method for controlling agitation and violent behavior. Unfortunately their use in emergencies is frequently ignored by clinicians because of the mistaken belief that these agents are somehow intrinsically more dangerous than neuroleptics. In fact barbiturates can be used in a precise manner, have a rapid onset and specific limits in duration of action, have minimal and controllable side effects, and, when administered intravenously, achieve greater sedation than neuroleptics while permitting proper diagnostic evaluation of the patient. When the emergency will probably lead to hospitalization or occurs during hospitalization, barbiturates are often the preferred initial treatment of choice for controlling behavior. Because of its rapid action and intermediate length of action, sodium amobarbital is the barbiturate of choice (10–12). When the patient is well known to the clinician, more definitive initial treatment (e.g. intramuscular neuroleptics for manic excitement) is appropriate (13).

When used in an emergency, sodium amobarbital should be administered intravenously. This can be readily accomplished even with the most violent patient, who, when restrained, usually presents with dilated superficial veins that are easily entered. A tourniquet is often not necessary. Intravenous sodium amobarbital can be delivered fairly rapidly (100 mg./15 seconds). Its sedation onset is limited only by the patient's circulation time and prior exposure to central sedatives, and dosage can be titrated to the patient's sedation threshold without undue concern about respiratory depression, which occurs at much higher doses; 500 mg. diluted in 20 cc. of sterile water or saline will suffice for most situations. The actual dose delivered will vary as the clinician stops administration only when sedation is reached. We have administered up to 1,500 mg. by this method without adverse effects. Subsequent doses (usually 250 mg.) can be administered intramuscularly every four to six hours, but more than twenty-four hours of such treatment is rarely necessary, as the risk of withdrawal seizures after cessation of treatment increases sharply after the first day (10–12).

SPECIFIC CASE MANAGEMENT

Violence Management

Although violent people often have associated psychiatric disorder, the frequency of violence among the mentally ill has been exaggerated. Most psychiatric patients are never violent. Even for the seriously ill, who frequently exhibit socially disruptive behavior, violence is uncommon. Nevertheless, when confronted with a violent or potentially violent patient, the clinician must be prepared to take appropriate steps to avoid injury to himself, other staff, and the patient.

Just as every hospital has a cardiac arrest team, every hospital with a psychiatric service should have a crisis team composed of six or seven individuals, including a physician and nursing and security personnel. The team should be prepared to respond rapidly and must be specifically trained to interact with and physically restrain the violent patient. Frequently the presence of the team—"a show of force"—is sufficient to control an impending emergency, and it is always better to overuse than underuse the crisis team.

Emergency room patients who have firearms or other lethal weapons should be isolated by immediately removing all patients and personnel and, if possible, locking the patient into the evacuated area. The police should then be called. A systematic emergency room search for weapons and dangerous objects should be part of the admission procedure.

The more common experience is that of an agitated or excited patient who is shouting, frightening other patients and staff, damaging hospital property, or attacking other patients or staff members. In this situation the crisis team should be called, and patients in the area and staff not directly involved in the emergency should be quickly removed. Unless a crisis team is present and prepared to restrain the patient, all remaining staff should stay at least 10 to 15 feet away from the patient (close enough to talk, but far enough away so as not to get hurt or provoke an attack).

The physician in charge or a designated staff member should engage the patient in conversation. The topic is not as important as maintaining a continuous interaction, which can often reduce anxiety on both sides. The staff spokesman should address the patient in as calm a manner as possible under the circumstances. He should speak slowly, clearly, and quietly and should not use psychiatric jargon. The spokesman must not patronize the patient or try to placate him by agreeing to unreasonable demands or requests, which obviously violate hospital rules. Firmness, without being agrumentative, is the best approach. On rare occasions honesty is not the best policy, and falsifications may be needed to preserve life and limb. When a patient who is to be placed in a seclusion room or is to receive an injection asks about such a decision, he should be told matter-of-factly what will happen and why. If he has an option that depends on his controlling himself, he should be told that too. Verbal threats by the spokesman are unhelpful and unprofessional, although a firm, loud, and authoritarian command can sometimes be effective.

There should be little or no unnecessary movement during the interaction with the patient. Whatever movement does take place should be done slowly and deliberately. The spokesman should tell the patient precisely what is going to be done.

Most threatening or potentially violent patients are agitated and will be moving about the room or patient area. The threat of assault can be significantly reduced if the patient can be persuaded to sit down. Occasionally the best efforts will fail and the patient will begin to approach the spokesman (or other staff) in a threatening manner. A firm command to "stop" while raising the hand like a traffic policeman becomes the last resort before retreating to safety or restraining the patient as part of the crisis team.

When the crisis team arrives, the spokesman should, if possible, continue in his role. In most cases the above approach, followed by constant reassurance and a show of force, will be sufficient to gain control of the situation. When necessary, most patients will then allow the spokesman (accompanied by the crisis team) to lead him away to his bed or to a seclusion room, where medication can be administered.

If the patient does not respond to the above approach and becomes increasingly agitated and threatening or actually attacks a team member (a rare occurrence), the team must be prepared to subdue, restrain, and seclude the patient.

The team should have a small soft (cotton) mattress (available at each nursing station) with two handles sewn to each side. This can be manned by two team members at each side and used to shield the team and force the patient into a corner. This should be done as rapidly as possible. Once pinned against a wall by the mattress, the patient can be forced to the floor with a team member restraining each limb and one member restraining the head to prevent biting. A team "leader" should be present to "direct traffic," and ideally a seventh member should be available to administer previously prepared medication. Once subdued, the patient should be restrained in padded leather restraints, medication should be administered, and then the team should place him on a stretcher and bring him to the seclusion room, where he should then be placed face down upon the mattress. Once the restraining procedure begins, it should not be interrupted or terminated until the patient is fully restrained. Abortive attempts usually lead to injury. Debates, negotiations, arguments, self-assessment, and the like have no place once the restraining process has begun.

Once in seclusion, the patient should remain in restraints until calm so that he cannot injure himself. A staff member should make a careful observation of the patient at least every fifteen minutes during the restraint period. Once sedated or calm, the patient can be removed from restraints and kept in seclusion until the physician concludes that the patient is no longer a danger to himself or to others. The physician should evaluate the patient frequently during the first few hours of seclusion and then four to six hours thereafter. Many patients will be able to leave seclusion after an hour or two. It is extremely rare for a patient to require more than twenty-four hours in seclusion.

Drug-Induced Deliria

Patients with *anticholinergic drug-induced delirium* are occasionally encountered in the emergency room and on acute medical services. Table 8–1 displays compounds (14, 15) that contain sufficient belladonna alkaloids (scopolamine, atropine) or anticholinergic properties to produce the syndrome. In addition to the medications listed in Table 8–1, there are

TABLE 8–1 Some Common Anticholinergic Substances

GROUP	GENERIC NAME	BRAND NAME
Tricyclic antidepressants	Amitriptyline	Elavil
	Imipramine	Tofranil
	Desipramine	Norpramin
	Nortriptyline	Aventyl
	Protriptyline	Vivactil
	Doxepin	Sinequan
Antispasmodics	Propantheline	Pro-Banthine
	Hyoscyamine/Atropine/Hyoscine	Donnatal
	Clidinium	Librax
	Amsotropine	Valpin
	Hexocyclium	Tral
Antihistamines	Dimenhydrinate	Dramamine
	Methapyriline	Histadyl
	Diphenhydramine	Benadryl
	Tripelennamine	Pyribenzamine
	Chlorpheniramine	Chlor-Trimeton/Ornade
	Promethazine	Phenergan
Antiparkinsonians	Benztropine	Cogentin
	Trihexyphenidyl	Artane
	Procyclidine	Kemadrin

numerous over-the-counter preparations with clinically significant anticholinergic properties (14, 15). These include *cold remedies* (Allerest, Coriciden, Romilar, Sine-Off, Contac, Sinutabs, Dristan), *analgesics* (Excedrin PM, Cope) and *hypnotics and tranquilizers* (Compoz, Devarex, Dormirex, Nytol, Sleep-Eze, Sominex).

Patients with anticholinergic deliria present with parasympathetic blockade. They have dry, hot, flushed skin, widely dilated pupils, dry mucous membranes, decreased bowel and bladder motility, mild hyperthermia, tachycardia, palpitations, and arrhythmias. These patients are severely agitated; have a clouded sensorium and diffuse cognitive impairment, rambling speech, and perceptual disturbances (illusions and hallucinations); and may be delusional. When tricyclic compounds are the offencing agents, cardiac arrhythmias are common and heart block may occur (14). A descriptive summary of these patients is mad as a hatter, red as a beet, dry as a bone, and blind as a bat.

Amphetamine psychosis may also present with severe agitation and sympathetic signs, but, unlike anticholinergic deliria, the sensorium in this state is clear.

Phenothiazines and other psychotropics with anticholinergic properties are obviously contraindicated as they exacerbate and prolong the syndrome. Emergency treatment may require restraints and sedation with intravenous anxiolytics (25 mg. chlordiazapoxide or 10 mg. diazepam intravenously). Primary treatment is physostigmine, which readily crosses the blood brain barrier and counters both peripheral and central cholinergic blockade. Related molecules such as neostigmine do not enter the central nervous system. A standard regimen is an initial 1 to 2 mg. dose administered subcutaneously repeated in thirty minutes and again at thirty- to sixty-minute intervals for a total dose of 6 to 8 mg. (16).

Drug-Induced Psychoses
(See Chapter 19 for clinical description.)

Lysergic acid diethylamide (LSD), mescaline, psilocybin, dimethyltryptamine (DMT), 2,5-dimethoxy-4-methylamphetamine (STP), phencylidine (PCP), mace and nutmeg (myristica), morning glory seeds, cannabis, amphetamine, and cocaine can each induce psychosis. Although specific psychotropic regimens have been recommended for the psychosis associated with each compound, response to a given dose of each of these agents is extremely individualized, and emergency intervention must address the requirements of each case. For example, many patients do not require pharmacologic treatment. For these individuals a quiet rest area and a reassuring person who reinforces accurate perceptions will suffice. Other patients may require additional oral anxiolytics, whereas some patients (particularly those ingesting PCP) may require hospitalization, restraints, sedation with neuroleptics and benzodiazepines, and acidification of the urine (3, 17, 18).

Definitive treatment is rarely possible in an emergency, as a comprehensive diagnostic evaluation usually is not feasible. A psychotic patient with a history of past drug use frequently tempts the practitioner to disregard the need to evaluate the patient fully and rush to administer a neuroleptic when nonspecific sedation would control the emergency and permit subsequent proper diagnosis. However, if the clinician knows the specific agent inducing the psychosis and pharmacotherapy is required, the following treatment suggestions may prove helpful:

1. Maniform drug-induced psychoses can respond to lithium carbonate or neuroleptics administered in standard doses. Phencylidine and mescaline are often associated with this type of affective syndrome (18-20).
2. Amphetamine and STP psychoses are particularly responsive to haloperidol in daily doses between 20 and 60 mg. Lithium carbonate may also be of benefit in these patients (21, 22).
3. PCP psychoses, particularly nonmaniform states, may respond to acidification of urine with 4 to 8 grams daily of ammonium chloride (to facilitate excretion of the compound), B-adrenergic blockade with propranolol 40 mg. daily (to ameliorate the severe sympathetic symptoms), and a neuroleptic in relatively low doses (e.g. haloperidol 20 mg. daily). Oral diazepam, 5 to 10 mg. TID or BID, has also been recommended. The efficacy of this polypharmacy is yet to be established (17-20, 23).

Frequently patients with drug-induced psychoses will not adequately respond to pharmacotherapy. Symptoms may persist; agitation and assaultiveness may become unmanageable; and neuroleptic-induced cognitive deficits and anticholenergic side effects (including delirium) may complicate the situation. Electroconvulsive treatment is particularly effective in drug-induced states. When a patient does not dramatically and rapidly respond to pharmacotherapy, ECT becomes the treatment of choice (20, 24).

Other Deliria

Delirium is characterized by an acutely developing, diffuse cognitive impairment and an alteration in consciousness. Common associated phenomena are distractibility, fatigue, inability to perform simple tasks, anxiety, agitation, perceptual disturbances (hallucinations and illusions), and delusional ideas. Agitation, anxiety, and resulting uncooperativeness can be severe, disrupting medical care and endangering the patient and medical staff. Head trauma, toxic and metabolic disorders, drug- and alcohol-related states, and infectious disease are the most common causes of these severe deliria requiring emergency psychiatric intervention (25–27).

When confronted with a delirious patient in the emergency room, the review of systems, systemic examination and laboratory screening are the likely means for determining etiology. With hospitalized patients, laboratory slips and medication sheets provide the decisive clues in the majority of cases (26) (see Chapter 18).

As in any psychiatric emergency the primary goal is to prevent the patient from injuring himself or others. Restraints may be required, but as delirious patients "fight" their restraints and are already in a precarious physiological state, restraining such patients is no substitute for ameliorating agitation. This can usually be accomplished by sedation with anxiolytics or barbiturates. However, the latter group is specifically contraindicated when head trauma, porphyria, or severe renal or pulmonary disease is suspected (26).

Occasionally standard behavioral and pharmacological interventions fail to relieve agitation, assaultiveness, or self-destructive behavior in a patient for whom the treatment of the underlying process (e.g. infection) has not begun to take effect. This is a life-threatening situation in which death can result from cardiovascular collapse (from initial fluid and electrolyte imbalance, compounded by struggling against restraints), the thwarting of primary treatment (e.g. pulling out IVs, ripping off surgical dressings), or self-injury (e.g. jumping out the window to escape "the voices"). ECT is the intervention of choice in this situation and has been found to be particularly useful and safe in ameliorating the symptoms of delirium. One or two treatments, using bilateral electrode placement, can resolve the agitation and permit treatment of the underlying causal process (24).

The following case vignette illustrates the effectiveness of ECT in delirium:

A fifty-six-year-old alcoholic man became agitated and confused following abdominal surgery for pancreatitis. The patient began picking at his abdominal dressing and continually pulled out his intravenous needles and foley catheter. Administration of 25 mg. intramuscular chlordiazepoxide TID and then QID had little effect. Restraints were applied, but the patient broke out of them and ripped open his abdominal wound, partially eviscerating himself. Following closure under general anesthesia, he again became agitated and confused. An encephalopathy secondary to pancreatitis was diagnosed. Injections of 25 mg. intramuscular chlorpromazine BID and then TID had little effect. He again eviscerated himself, this time partially breaking a surgical anastamosis between his pancreas and jejunum. Although the wound was again closed under general anesthesia, the patient again picked at his wound (now held together by metal retention sutures). Leaking pancreatic and abdominal juices began digesting his abdominal wall, and silver nitrate ointment was applied to the skin about the wound to prevent this. Chlordiazepoxide was added to the chlorpromazine without amelioration of his agitation and confusion.

A psychiatric consultant was requested, who recommended ECT. All psychotropic medication was discontinued, and two bilateral treatments were administered on successive days. Sufficient succinylcholine was used to prevent any motor activity during the seizures, which might have disrupted the abdominal wound.

The patient's agitation resolved, although he remained mildly confused. Further psychotropic treatment was not required. He remained in restraints for the next few days but did not struggle. A third and fourth ECT were administered at forty-eight-hour intervals, following which the patient made a slow but unremarkable surgical recovery.

ACUTE PSYCHOSES

Brief Reactive Psychosis

The brief reactive psychosis syndrome was first methodically described by Karl Jaspers (28). Although its proper place in our nosology is unclear, reactive psychosis is characterized by an acute onset episode of hallucinosis, usually with delusional ideas, following a precipitating event. Affectivity is usually intense, and thought content relates to the precipitant. The disorder rapidly resolves when the patient is removed from the stressful situation, and an underlying unspecified vulnerability is hypothesized. As agitation can be severe, emergency treatment usually involves restraints and sedation. As brief hospitalization is usually required, intravenous sodium amobarbital is the treatment of choice. Forty-eight to seventy-two hours of sedation, without the use of neuroleptics, often results in resolution of the psychosis (29). The following case vignette illustrates the syndrome:

A forty-one-year-old unmarried woman was brought to the emergency room by friends. She had been up all night, agitated and fearful. She called her friends at 3 A.M. for help and constantly asked them for reassurance that she was a good person and not a "tramp." Earlier, she had spent a rare evening out with a man, who, when escorting her into her apartment, attempted to kiss her. She rejected his advances, upon which he became angry, said she had just "teased" him, called her a whore, and left. She became progressively upset, finally calling her friends.

In the emergency room she was extremely agitated, tearful, and whining. She pleaded for reassurance, repeatedly asking: "Am I a whore?" At other times she shouted that she was a bad person and that voices were calling her bad names. She began running about the emergency room, knocking over furniture and equipment. She was restrained, sedated with intravenous sodium amobarbital, and hospitalized. She received three intramuscular doses of sodium amobarbital during the next twenty-four hours, following which she became fully alert and asymptomatic.

Excitement States (mania, catatonia)
(See Chapters 11 and 14 for additional discussion.)

Patients suffering from acute psychotic excitement can be extremely dangerous to themselves and others. Restraints or a "show of force" with a crisis team and initial sedation with sodium amobarbital are usually required. For those patients who are well known to the clinician, or whose diagnostic evaluation is complete, intramuscular neuroleptics are indicated. Specific pharmacotherapeutic details are discussed in Chapters 5 and 11. Occasionally an excited patient will not respond to even the highest doses of neuroleptic. These patients, usually manics, will race up and down hospital hallways, shouting continuously at staff, other patients, and imagined voices. Despite massive doses of neuroleptics, they continue to be hyperactive, although stiff, ataxic, and slurred in speech. Cardiovascular collapse, hyperpyrexia, and sudden death have been reported in these patients. Prior to somatic treatment this severe form of excitement resulted in the death of one out of five acutely ill hospitalized manics (30). Two bilateral ECT administered daily for two or three consecutive days can be a lifesaving procedure for such patients and should not be withheld if neuroleptics cannot control the excitement within three to five days (24).

Stupor

Stupor is a state of extreme psychomotor inhibition in which the patient hardly moves or speaks. Complete immobility and mutism can occur and are often associated with generalized analgesia. Stupor is usually a manifestation of affective disorder, particularly endogenous depression (31–33).

Stuporous patients are unable to eat or drink and, if untreated, can develop significant dehydration, hemoconcentration, hyperpyrexia, ketosis, and eventually cardiovascular collapse and death. These patients can be temporarily disinhibited by intramuscular administration of 250 mg. of sodium amobarbital. When prescribed thirty to forty-five minutes prior to meals, this medication will enable the stuporous patient to eat and drink sufficiently and cooperate during an evaluation period. However, intravenous fluid and electrolyte replacement is often required. Psychotropics rarely improve the stuporous condition, and a course of bilateral ECT serves as both the emergency and definitive treatment of choice (24).

Epilepsy

Aberrant behavior and psychopathology associated with seizure disorders most often occur during pre-, post-, and interictal periods, rather than during the seizure itself. Psychiatric emergencies associated with seizure disorders usually result when the patient becomes violent (34–36). As the patient is in an altered state of consciousness, psychological intervention is inappropriate and rapid restraint and sedation with diazepam (10 to 15 mg. intravenously) or sodium amobarbital is the best treatment (37, 38). Definitive anticonvulsant treatment can then be instituted. Repeated violent ictal-related episodes or irritable behavior and clouding of consciousness during a prodrome or preictal period are best treated by inducing a seizure. Indeed, the observation that spontaneous seizures often resulted in remission of psychosis led, in part, to the development of convulsive treatment. One or two bilateral treatments usually suffice (24).

Nonemergency Situations Requiring Rapid Action

Dystonic Reactions

Acute dystonic reactions to neuroleptic administration occur in 2 to 3 percent of patients. The risk of dystonia increases with the potency of the neuroleptic, its dose, and parenteral administration. It is more common in younger patients and men. Piperazine phenothiazines and thioxanthenes and butyrophenones are most commonly implicated.

Dystonias are distressing and painful but not dangerous. They generally occur within a few hours to a few days after neuroleptic treatment is begun and consist of acute spasmodic increased tonicity, typically of the muscles of the tongue, throat, and neck (torticollis). Dystonic movements of the body and limbs, opisthotonos, and oculogyric crises also occur.

Fifty mg. of diphenhydramine administered intravenously is the treatment of choice, with the response being almost immediate. Intramuscular benztropine (1–2 mg.) or diphenhydramine (50 mg.) is also effective. As additional dystonic reactions usually occur when the effects of the injection have worn off, oral treatment with an antiparkinsonian agent should be started at the same time and the neuroleptic dose reevaluated (39–42).

Acute Anxiety Attack (panic attack)

Not infrequently a patient suffering from an acute behavioral syndrome associated with severe anxiety is brought to the emergency room. The following case vignette illustrates such a syndrome, which is discussed in more detail in other sections of the text.

A twenty-eight-year-old man was brought to the emergency room by relatives because of chest discomfort, difficulty breathing, and uncontrollable shaking. His symptoms began at a family reunion a few hours earlier. He had had several previous episodes during the past five years and was described by a relative as "high strung" and always "nervous."

He was restless, tremulous, and fearful. He told the examiner that something terrible was happening to him, that he could not catch his breath and that he was going to die. He said he was cold. His skin was cold and clammy, and he periodically shook uncontrollably. His blood pressure was 135/85 mm. Hg. pulse was 102/min., and respirations 24/min. The remainder of the physical examination, review of systems, and laboratory screening were normal, and the patient rapidly responded to intravenous chlordiazepoxide.

Should a review of systems, a systemic examination (particularly to rule out pneumonia, hypertension, myocardial infarction, stroke, and thyroid and parathyroid disease), and laboratory screening (EKG, chest x-ray, blood glucose, urinalysis) rule out cardiovascular, metabolic, and a coarse neurologic cause of this syndrome, sedation is the primary treatment of choice. These patients often respond rapidly to intravenous or oral short-acting anxiolytics, such as chlordiazepoxide or diazepam in doses of 25 mg. and 10 mg., respectively, and can return home the same day. These compounds are not absorbed well via intramuscular administration. In most cases the patient will become drowsy and even sleep for fifteen to twenty minutes, awakening fatigued but no longer severely anxious (39, 43, 44). Occasionally a second dose will be required. Following additional reassurance and education about the syndrome, most such patients can be sent home with sufficient medication for four to six additional doses and a referral to the appropriate clinic, practitioner, or community agency.

Some patients hyperventilate when acutely anxious. The resulting respiratory alkalosis from reduction of serum carbon dioxide and increased intercellular calcium binding secondary to pH changes can result in severe perioral and hand and foot paresthesias, dizziness, muscular cramping, and syncope. This syndrome may be alleviated by having the patient rebreathe his carbon dioxide by breathing into a paper bag or a large balloon (more airtight and reliable than a paper bag) for a minute or so. Once the hyperventilation syndrome has resolved, additional anxiety symptoms can be controlled by chlordiazepoxide or diazepam in oral doses of 25 mg. or 10 mg. respectively (43, 44).

Occasionally a patient is brought to the emergency room with the label "hysterical reaction." The patient most commonly will be a woman, and the symptoms will be consistent with an acute anxiety attack in which agitation is marked and the patient is tearful and noisy. There is no evidence that severe anxiety symptoms with agitation, tearfulness, and screaming is not simply an acute anxiety attack, and treatment is identical to that described above.

Acute Alcohol Intoxication

Acute alcohol intoxication is easy to recognize. The triad of ataxia, slurred speech, and alcoholic breath are usually sufficient for a diagnosis. Nystagmus, a flushed face, red eyes, reduced concentration, poor recent memory, and rambling speech are additional clues. Confusion with hypoglycemic states, cardiovascular crises, stroke, and other intoxications can sometimes occur, and the essential review of systems, systemic examination, and laboratory screening (including blood alcohol levels) should resolve diagnostic uncertainty (45, 46).

A period of excitement can occur from depression of cortical inhibitory centers, in which the patient may become destructive to property and/or assaultive. Initial emergency treatment may require restraints and then the administration of small amounts (10–25 mg. chlordiazepoxide or 5–10 mg. diazepam) of intravenous anxiolytics (the risk of vomiting precludes the use of oral medication). This will usually ameliorate the excitement phase of the intoxication and will not significantly depress respiratory function. A "holding" area should be available in which such patients can be monitored until they are able to leave the hospital. Disposition and definitive treatment strategies will be discussed in Chapter 19 (46).

There is no adequate documentation to support the existence of the pathological intoxication syndrome in which a small amount of alcohol allegedly results in a severe excitement state, during which the patient is assaultive and acts as if "drunk." An epileptic predisposition triggered by alcohol has been hypothesized as a causal mechanism (45, 46). Careful historical study and laboratory screening for epilepsy would be critical in identifying a suspected case, and the administration of anxiolytics, as described above, is the logical initial treatment strategy.

References

1. Flor–Henry, P.; Gruzelier, J. (eds.). *Laterality and Psychopathology.* Amsterdam: Elsevier/North Holland Biomedical Press, 1983.
2. Hall, R. C. W. Medically Induced Psychiatric Disease: An Overview. In Hall, R. C. W. (ed.), *Psychiatric Presentation of Medical Illness Somatopsychic Disorders.* New York: SP Medical and Scientific Books, 1980, pp. 3–9.
3. Berger, P. A.; Tinklenberg, J. R. Treatment of Abusers of Alcohol and Other Addictive Drugs. In Barchas, J. D.; Berger, P. A.; Ciaranello, R. D.; *et al.*, (eds.), *Psychopharmacology from Theory to Practice.* New York: Oxford University Press, 1977, pp. 355–85.
4. Darbonne, A. Crisis: A review of theory, practice, and research. *Internat. J. Psychiat. 6:* 371–79, 1968.
5. Caplan, G. *Principles of Preventive Psychiatry.* New York: Basic Books, 1964.

6. Marston, M. V. Compliance with medical regimens: A review of the literature. *Nurs. Res. 19:* 312–23, 1970.

7. Wilder, J. F.; Plutchnik, R.; Conte, H. R. Compliance with psychiatric emergency room referrals. *Arch. Gen. Psychiat. 34:* 930–33, 1977.

8. Claghorn, J. L.; McBee, G. W.; Roberts, L. Trends in hospital versus community treatment of mental illness: A Texas example. *Am. J. Psychiat. 133:* 1310–12, 1976.

9. Jellinek, M. Referrals from a psychiatric emergency room: Relationship of compliance to demographic and interview variables. *Am. J. Psychiat. 135:* 209–13, 1978.

10. Shepherd, M.; Lader, M.; Rodnight, R. *Clinical Psychopharmacology.* Philadelphia: Lea & Febiger, 1968, pp. 67–75, 85–125.

11. Havey, S. C. Hypnotics and Sedatives. In Gilman, A. G.; Goodman, L. S.; Gilman, A. (eds.), *The Pharmacological Basis of Therapeutics.* 6th ed. New York: Macmillan, 1980, pp. 339–75.

12. Eichelman, B.; Estess, F. M.; Gonda, T. A. Hypnotic Agents in Psychiatric Evaluations. In Barchas, J. D.; Berger, P. A.; Ciaranello, R. D.; *et al.,* (eds.), *Psychopharmacology from Theory to Practice.* New York: Oxford University Press, 1977, pp. 270–75.

13. San Giovanni, F.; Taylor, M. A.; Abrams, R.; *et al.* Rapid control of psychiatric excitement states with intramuscular haloperidol. *Am. J. Psychiat. 130:* 1155–56, 1973.

14. Gilman, A. G.; Goodman, L. S.; Gilman, A. (eds.). *The Pharmacological Basis of Therapeutics.* 6th ed. New York: Macmillan, 1980.

15. *Physicians' Desk Reference.* 36th ed. Oradell, N.J.: Medical Economics, 1982.

16. Heiser, J. F.; Gillin, J. C. The reversal of anticholinergic drug-induced delirium and coma with physiostigmine. *Am. J. Psychiat. 127:* 1050–54, 1971.

17. Berger, P. A.; Dunn, M. J. Substance Induced and Substance Use Disorders. In Greist, J. H.; Jefferson, J. W.; Spitzer, R. L. (eds.), *Treatment of Mental Disorders.* New York: Oxford University Press, 1982, pp. 78–142.

18. Showalter, C. V.; Thornton, W. E. Clinical pharmacology of phencyclidine toxicity. *Am. J. Psychiat. 134:* 1234–38, 1977.

19. Slavney, P.; Rich, G.; Pearlson, G.; *et al.* Phencyclidine abuse and symptomatic mania. *Biol. Psychiat. 12:* 697–700, 1977.

20. Rosen, A. Case Report: Symptomatic mania and phencyclidine abuse. *Am. J. Psychiat. 136:* 118–19, 1979.

21. Cronson, A. J.; Flemenbaum, A. Antagonism of cocaine highs by lithium. *Am. J. Psychiat. 135:* 856–57, 1978.

22. Furukawa, T.; Ushizima, I.; Ono, N. Modifications by lithium of behavioral responses to methamphetamine and tetrabenazine. *Psychopharmacologica 41:* 243–48, 1975.

23. Schaffer, C. B. Treating phencyclidine intoxication. *Am. J. Psychiat. 135:* 388, 1978.

24. Taylor, M. A. Indications for Electroconvulsive Treatment. In Abrams, R.;

Essman, W. B. (eds.), *Electroconvulsive Therapy in Theory and Practice.* New York: SP Medical and Scientific Books, 1982, pp. 7–39.

25. Plum, P.; Posner, J. B. *Diagnosis of Stupor and Coma.* 2d ed. Philadelphia: F. A. Davis, 1972.

26. Varsamis, J. Clinical Management of Delirium. In Hendrie, H. C. (ed.), *Psychiatric Clinics of North America,* vol. 1/1, *Brain Disorders, Clinical Diagnosis and Management.* Philadelphia: W. B. Saunders, 1978, pp. 71–80.

27. Lipowski, Z. J. Delirium, clouding of consciousness and confusion. *J. Nerv. Ment. Dis. 145:* 227–55, 1967.

28. Jaspers, K. *General Psychopathology.* Hoenig, J.; Hamilton, M. W. (trans. from the original 1923 ed.). Chicago: University of Chicago Press, 1963.

29. McCabe, M. S. Reactive psychoses. *Acta Psychiat. Scand.* (suppl.) *259.* Copenhagen: Munksgaard, 1975.

30. Derby, I. M. Manic-depressive "exhaustion" deaths. *Psychiat. Quart. 7:* 436–49, 1933.

31. Berrios, G. E. Stupor revisited. *Comp. Psychiat. 22:* 466–78, 1981.

32. Abrams, R.; Taylor, M. A. Catatonia: A prospective clinical study. *Arch. Gen. Psychiat. 33:* 579–81, 1976.

33. Taylor, M. A.; Abrams, R. The prevalence and importance of catatonia in the manic phase of mania. *Arch. Gen. Psychiat. 34:* 1223–25, 1977.

34. Benson, D. F.; Blumer, D. Psychiatric Manifestations of Epilepsy. In Benson, D. F.; Blumer, D. (eds.), *Psychiatric Aspects of Neurologic Disease,* vol. 2. New York: Grune & Stratton, 1982, pp. 25–47.

35. Fenton, G. W. Psychiatric Disorders of Epilepsy: Classification and Phenomenology. In Reynolds, E. H.; Trimble, M. R. (eds.), *Epilepsy and Psychiatry,* Edinburgh: Churchill Livingstone, 1981, pp. 12–26.

36. Toone, B. Psychoses of Epilepsy. In Reynolds, E. H.; Trimble, M. R. (eds.), *Epilepsy and Psychiatry.* Edinburgh: Churchill Livingstone, 1981, pp. 113–37.

37. Reynolds, E. H. The Management of Seizures Associated with Psychological Disorders. In Reynolds, E. H.; Trimble, M. R. (eds.), *Epilepsy and Psychiatry.* Edinburgh: Churchill Livingstone, 1981, pp. 322–36.

38. Richens, A. Clinical Pharmacology and Medical Treatment. In Laidlow, J.; Richens, A. (eds.), *A Textbook of Epilepsy.* 2d ed. Edinburgh: Churchill Livingstone, 1982, pp. 292–348.

39. Kalinowsky, L. B.; Hippius, H.; Klein, H. E. *Biological Treatments in Psychiatry.* New York: Grune & Stratton, 1982.

40. Gulevich, G. Psychopharmacological Treatment in the Aged. In Barchas, J. D.; Berger, P. A.; Ciaranello, R. D.; *et al.* (eds.), *Psychopharmacology from Theory to Practice.* New York: Oxford University Press, 1977, p. 453.

41. Hollister, L. E. Antipsychotic Medications in the Treatment of Schizophrenia. In Barchas, J. D.; Berger, P. A.; Ciaranello, R. D.; *et al.* (eds.), *Psychopharmacology From Theory to Practice.* New York: Oxford University Press, 1977, p. 144.

42. Ayd, F. J. A survey of drug-induced extrapyramidal reactions. *JAMA 175:* 1054–60, 1961.

43. Baldessarini, R. J. Drugs and the Treatment of Psychiatric Disorders. In Gilman, A. G.; Goodman, L. S.; Gilman, A. (eds.), *The Pharmacological Basis of Therapeutics.* 6th ed. New York: Macmillan, 1980, pp. 391–447.

44. Lader, M.; Marks, I. *Clinical Anxiety.* New York: Grune & Stratton, 1971, pp. 74–77.

45. Goodwin, D. W.; Guze, S. B. *Psychiatric Diagnosis.* 2d ed. New York: Oxford University Press, 1979, pp. 118–44.

46. Goodwin, D. W. Substance-induced and Substance Use Disorders: Alcohol. In Greist, J. H.; Jefferson, J. W.; Spitzer, R. L. (eds.), *Treatment of Mental Disorders.* New York: Oxford University Press, 1982, pp. 44–61.

CHAPTER 9

The Inpatient Unit

General Considerations

The short-term psychiatric inpatient unit is analogous to other specialized hospital units (e.g. "med./surg." ICU, burn unit, trauma unit) in that, although the physician has the ultimate professional responsibility and liability for treatment, most patient care activities are carried out by other professionals (nurses, aides, technicians, social workers, psychologists). Functioning as a cohesive group, concentrating on patient care, these professionals form the core of a well-run unit. It is an unfortunate fact of the care of the mentally ill, however, that in many psychiatric units more energy is spent maintaining the spirit of cooperation of the professional staff than in treating patients. Too often many of the professional staff are more concerned with gaining control of the "best" patients for pet treatments, winning professional rivalries, amassing personal power, and ultimately controlling the unit itself, than with caring for patients (1).

These intrastaff interactions lead to an essential social structure on the unit that must be clearly understood and properly managed if patients are to receive proper care. This social structure exists in all types of hospitals—public, private, teaching, nonteaching, general, and psychiatric. Because of it, the management of the professional staff of the inpatient unit will be a continuing major task.

The professionals on the unit quickly become a social group in which professional and personal roles, status, and leadership need to be established if the unit is to function properly. Impinging upon this internal structure is the relationship of the unit to the rest of the hospital. As intragroup structures crystallize and unit functioning increases in efficiency and quality, the unit develops a sense of territory, of we-versus-them, of group loyalty, which reinforces the unit's cohesiveness and simultaneously creates problems for the unit leadership in dealing with the rest of the hospital. Physicians who ignore these factors or who assume a one-dimensional authoritarian role toward the rest of the staff will not be optimally effective in caring for their patients and may even harm them (1–3).

On well-established units varying degrees of intrastaff difficulties inevitably occur. In managing established units, it is important to identify the specific details of that unit's social structure; establish clear-cut professional roles within the unit based on the differing expertise of each discipline; identify and use specific strengths of individual staff regardless of professional identity; clearly establish a leader; and establish a daily patient care and staff program and a treatment philosophy that is clearly understood and endorsed by all staff members.

Specifically, we must recognize that psychologists, social workers, psychiatrists, and nurses traditionally fight about who works harder, who is in charge, who serves patients best, whose expertise is worth more, and who will treat which patient. Recognizing this, a primary goal of unit management must be to weld these individuals into a cohesive, mutually supportive group. A helpful first step is to encourage individual attributes of staff members that transcend professional expertise and are important in patient care. In other words, who has what interaction with a given patient may have more to do with the personality of a given staff member than with that staff member's professional training. Clearly defined professional roles also are important, and the expected contributions of the respective professionals must be explicitly stated. This is critical, because much bickering and jockeying for power arise out of the fact that professionals of one discipline deprecate what they are traditionally trained to do best and ascribe more value to what they perceive as the important treatment style (usually psychotherapy). For example, social workers too often consider social service casework a necessary but demeaning obligation and derive their real satisfaction from treating patients with psychotherapy. Similarly, nurses devalue nursing care, psychologists devalue psychological assessment and behavioral techniques, and psychiatrists devalue their medical expertise. Optimal unit functioning occurs when everyone has access to interaction with patients but each discipline is primarily responsible for its particular area of expertise, and where that expertise is valued for its utility. More psychiatric inpatients have benefited from good social service, nursing care, psychological assessment, and behavioral medicine than from psycho-therapy. This is not to say that psychotherapy is unhelpful, but special so-cial, nursing, psychological, and medical care are the main active therapeu-tic ingredients on a psychiatric inpatient unit (4).

Establishing clear-cut unit leadership is important. In some specialized units for behavior modification or alcohol rehabilitation, the psychiatrist may not have sufficient expertise to qualify for leadership. In a unit that serves patients with putative (e.g. schizophrenia, affective disorder) or recognized (e.g. psychomotor state, dementia) brain disease, however, the psychiatrist theoretically has the best combination of skill and knowledge to assume the leadership role. Obviously the best leader will be the person who combines expertise with the qualities of personality necessary for that role. We recommend, however, that the psychiatrist assume that role in a general short-term hospital unit. This leadership model also requires the establish-ment of the medical model as the specific program and treatment philosophy of the unit; that is, the unit's objective is primarily to treat patients with brain disease or dysfunction (affective disorder, schizophrenia, behavioral neurologic disease). Although there must be significant flexibility of action within this system, all staff should basically endorse it. In our view those who do not would serve themselves, the unit, and the patients best by work-ing elsewhere. The therapeutic philosophy of primarily treating patients with brain disease or dysfunction implies that such a unit is not appropriate for people who simply have problems of living (interpersonal difficulties).

The social structure of a unit also involves the goals and expectations of the staff and their professional role interactions with patients (2). Thus, a staff recruited for a unit for which the primary goal is treatment cannot be expected to launch enthusiastically and efficiently into a research project or a training program without significant preparation, discussion, and education to demonstrate that the research or training will directly or indirectly enhance patient care.

In addition, professionals have specific notions of how they and patients are to behave. Some patients, because of premorbid personality, life-style, or illness, may not adhere to the stereotyped patient roles, and the unit leadership should be prepared to recognize such situations and deal with them (see section headed "Inpatient Problems" in this chapter).

A psychiatrist who must deal with staff problems on an established inpa-tient unit, short of "firing everyone and starting over again," will find himself giving more of his time and energy to staff management than to pa-tient care. Even the private practitioner who spends relatively little time on the unit will have to deal with staff problems affecting the care of his pa-tients. Because the staff forms a more cohesive social group than do the pa-tients, intensive staff management efforts may be unavoidable.

In a newly established inpatient unit, however, much intrastaff bickering and wasted energy can be avoided if the unit's goals and treatment philosophy are clearly defined, professional roles are explicitly described, programming clearly reflects the treatment philosophy, professionally compatible staff members are recruited who endorse the unit's goals and treatment philosophy, and the staff is directed by one individual (1–3).

In the inpatient unit, which will treat primarily individuals with major mental illness, medical management (diagnosis and somatic treatment) will be the primary therapeutic approach, there being little evidence that milieu influences and psychological interventions alone are of significant therapeutic benefit to such patients (4–6). Staff working on such a unit must recognize this fact and content themselves with assuming specific professional roles that best serve such a model. Table 9–1 displays specific professional duties compatible with a medically oriented inpatient unit. In addition to the specific functions listed, all staff should engage patients in reality-oriented one-to-one and group conversations.

Program Structure

A principal goal of psychiatric hospitalization is to regulate the patient's behavior. For some patients, particularly those who are suicidal, hospitalization may literally be lifesaving and is thus in itself a treatment. An extension of this control is a program structure that provides the patient with hour-by-hour schedules, which help shape his social behaviors (4, 6, 7). This schedule contains planned activities, each with stated objectives. Frequently patients are unable to concentrate, plan, or successfully carry out daily tasks. A schedule with appropriate rest periods and free time provides the necessary daily structure until the patient is able to plan for himself. This schedule should be flexible, so that as the patient improves he can progressively assume increasing responsibilities for his own activities. This can be accomplished by a "step system" (Table 9–2), which details the specific behaviors that determine the responsibilities and privileges of a particular patient. The system (like all unit schedules and rules) should be simply stated and prominently displayed. Step changes (up or down) are usually decided each morning with input from the entire staff. Part of the step system should be a schedule of daily activities, which patients at different steps should or may attend.

Patients hospitalized in a short-term psychiatric unit differ from patients hospitalized in medical or surgical units in that they are fully ambulatory. Once they begin to improve, they will have significant needs to be physically occupied. Patients will also have to be educated about their illness and treatments and will need to deal with the social and occupational disruption their illness may have caused. Some will need behavioral programs to alter

TABLE 9–1 Specific Professional Duties on Medically Oriented Psychiatric Inpatient Service

<table>
<thead>
<tr><th align="center">NURSE</th></tr>
</thead>
</table>

1. General medical nursing care (treatments for systemic illness, preparation and escort for various laboratory procedures)
2. Administration of medication
3. General patient observation and specific observation of patients on suicidal precautions or in seclusion
4. Participation in special procedures (sodium amytal interviews, ECT, patient sedation/restraint)
5. Patient education (re: treatments)
6. Supervision of patient hygiene
7. Supervision of ward maintenance and cleaning
8. Management of ward supplies
9. Participation in on- and off-ward activities (including small groups)

<table>
<thead>
<tr><th align="center">SOCIAL WORKER</th></tr>
</thead>
</table>

1. Obtaining social, occupational, and family information
2. Identifying specific social, occupational, and family problems and recommending solutions to them
3. Educating and counseling the patient's family
4. Educating and counseling the patient about housing, work, and family problems and helping to solve these difficulties
5. Helping the patient deal with public agencies
6. Planning and carrying out patient placement
7. Participating in some of the on- and off-ward activities
8. General patient observations

<table>
<thead>
<tr><th align="center">PSYCHOLOGIST</th></tr>
</thead>
</table>

1. Cognitive and personality assessment
2. Planning and carrying out with other staff members the management of specific patient problem behaviors
3. Supervising and participating in specific ward group activities
4. Patient counseling
5. General patient observation
6. Providing in-service training to other staff

<table>
<thead>
<tr><th align="center">OCCUPATIONAL AND RECREATIONAL THERAPIST</th></tr>
</thead>
</table>

1. Planning on- and off-ward activities
2. Supervising on- and off-ward activities
3. Management of OT and RT supplies and equipment
4. General patient observation

<table>
<thead>
<tr><th align="center">PSYCHIATRIST</th></tr>
</thead>
</table>

1. General ward management
2. Patient diagnosis and treatment (medical and psychological)
3. Supervision of all patient care plans and procedures
4. Participation in specific ward activities
5. Education and counseling of patients and their families
6. Providing in-service training to other staff

TABLE 9-2 Typical Step System

STEP 1		
REQUISITES	RESPONSIBILITIES	PRIVILEGES
All new admissions Patients in seclusion, who are dangerous to themselves or others, who are assaultive, extremely disruptive or disoriented Patients who are escape risks	Must wear hospital clothes No visitors during first 24 hours No expectations	None

STEP 2		
REQUISITES	RESPONSIBILITIES	PRIVILEGES
At least 48 hours on unit No longer actively dangerous, assaultive, disruptive Not in seclusion Not extremely confused or interfering with daily activities	Making own bed Cleaning personal area Taking daily showers and appropriate self-grooming Cooperative in taking medicine and lab tests, eating meals Attending all required unit activities Must wear street clothes	May have visitors Phone time May have mail

STEP 3		
REQUISITES	RESPONSIBILITIES	PRIVILEGES
May still be hallucinating or delusional but symptoms not intrusive in daily functioning Can be on schedule Reality testing adequate	All requirements of Step 2 Must attend all activities Must help with unit activities May assume responsibility for specific unit task	All privileges of Step 2 Off-ward activities

STEP 4		
REQUISITES	RESPONSIBILITIES	PRIVILEGES
No longer obviously psychotic Must be clinically stable with only residual signs and symptoms	All requirements of Steps 2 and 3 Must assume responsibility for specific unit tasks Should be able to help with other selected patients Should be able to participate in own discharge plan	All privileges of Steps 2 and 3 May have supervised day passes for unit activities and for personal business

(Continued)

TABLE 9-2 Typical Step System (*Continued*)

	STEP 5	
REQUISITES	RESPONSIBILITIES	PRIVILEGES
Predischarge status	All requirements of Steps 2, 3, and 4	All privileges of Steps 2, 3, and 4
	Must be able to escort patients on lower steps	May have overnight and/or weekend passes

the frequency of specific behaviors, and all will need emotionally supportive interactions with various staff members. A program structure planned by unit personnel can most efficiently provide for these needs. Table 9-3 displays a typical schedule for psychiatric inpatients. Group meetings should generally be devoted to educating patients about their illness and treatments and discussing the practical interpersonal difficulties they face with family, friends, and employers. Some groups may specifically teach patients strategies for coping with some of the problems of living they may encounter. Groups should relate to the step system so that as a patient progresses, the content of the group session will also change to fit that patient's need. Thus patients in Steps 1 and 2 may be in one group, while patients in Steps 3 to 5 may be in another. Staff involved in groups should meet briefly following each session to discuss patient problems that occurred or behavioral observations that should be communicated to other staff members.

The unit meeting is for all patients and as many of the staff as can attend. The purpose of these meetings is to discuss specific unit problems and activities.

A daily hour-by-hour schedule is also needed for the unit staff. What they are supposed to do, when they are supposed to do it, and why they are doing it should be clearly and explicitly stipulated. Table 9-4 shows a typical unit schedule for staff. The morning report should include as much of the staff (all disciplines) as possible. The charge nurse for the day or the head nurse should present the nursing report from the night shift, briefly summarize any new admissions to the unit, and review any problems from the previous twenty-four hours. Potential problems for that day should be discussed, and a plan of action for each devised. Discharges for the day and last-minute discharge preparations should also be discussed.

The staff of most psychiatric units is divided into interdisciplinary teams, with each team responsible for the patients of that team's physicians. Team meetings should include all members and should function as informational, specific problem-solving, and planning sessions. In teaching hospitals, doc-

TABLE 9-3 Typical Patient Schedule[a]

Wakeup	6:30 A.M. daily
Personal hygiene	6:30– 7:00 A.M. daily
Breakfast	7:00– 7:30 A.M. daily
Cleanup of personal area and free time	7:30– 9:00 A.M. daily
Medication	9:00– 9:30 A.M. daily
Doctors' rounds	9:00–10:30 A.M., M–F
Coffee break[b]	10:30–10:45 A.M. daily
Group sessions	10:30–11:30 A.M., M, W, Th
Unit meeting	10:30–11:30 A.M., T, F
Lunch	11:30–noon daily
Free time	Noon–1:00 P.M. daily
Medication	1:00– 1:15 P.M. daily
Occupational, recreational, and activity therapies[c]	1:15– 3:00 P.M., M–S[a]
Coffee break[b]	3:00– 3:15 P.M. daily
Social skills training	3:15– 4:15 P.M., M–F
Rest period/visitors	4:15– 5:30 P.M., M–F
Dinner	5:30– 6:30 P.M. daily
Free time	6:30– 7:00 P.M. daily
Evening activity[d]	7:00– 9:00 P.M., M–Sa
Medication	9:00– 9:30 P.M. daily
Free time	9:30–10:30 P.M. daily
Bedtime	10:30 P.M. daily

[a]Sunday A.M. schedule begins one hour later. Sunday afternoon: free time or visitors. Saturday: field trips. Special diagnostic procedures and individual treatment sessions scheduled as needed.
[b]Decaffeinated coffee only, juice and snack.
[c]Includes such activities as music, exercise groups, jogging, swimming, art therapy, beauty parlor, ceramics, leather work, cooking, gardening, sewing, current events, special activities (volunteer groups putting on demonstrations, entertaining, and so on).
[d]Movies, Pokeno, a dance, a party, bingo, art therapy (twice weekly).

tors' rounds should be scheduled at the same time each weekday morning. Participants include house staff, students, and other team members (particularly a nurse and social worker). Teaching rounds should have specific training goals as the physician in charge briefly sees each new patient and reviews the progress of the other patients. In nonteaching hospitals, doctors' rounds are still important as an occasion for evaluating patients, communicating with other team members, providing mutual education, and identifying problems that require nursing and social service skills. A weekly staff meeting at which all staff members are present is also helpful in resolving unit problems, reinforcing unit philosophy, and introducing future plans. Evening and night shift staff should periodically attend these meetings, which should be scheduled close to changes of shift so that little

TABLE 9-4 Typical Staff Schedule

Nursing report	7:00– 7:15 A.M. daily
Supervision of patients' breakfast	7:15– 8:00 A.M. daily
ECT	7:30– 8:30 A.M., M, W, F
Morning report	8:30– 9:00 A.M. (some staff are supervising patient cleanup), M–F
Medication	9:00– 9:30 A.M. daily
Doctors' rounds	9:00–10:30 A.M., M–F
Group sessions/unit meeting	10:30–11:30 A.M., M–F
Group feedback	11:30–noon, M–F
Supervision of patients' lunch	11:30–noon–1:00 P.M. daily
Medication	1:00– 1:15 P.M. daily
Supervision: OT, RT, AT, social skills	1:15– 2:30 P.M., M–S
In-service training	1:15– 2:30 P.M., once weekly
Team meeting	1:15– 2:30 P.M., M, Th
Staff meeting	1:15– 2:30 P.M., W
Supervision of social skills training	3:15– 4:15 P.M., M–F
Supervision of visitors	4:15– 5:30 P.M., M–F
Supervision of patients' dinner	5:30– 6:30 P.M. daily
Medication	6:30– 7:00 P.M. daily
Evening activity supervision	7:00– 9:00 P.M., M–S
Medication	9:00– 9:30 P.M. daily
Patient bedtime	10:30 P.M. daily

time is lost. If efficiency and enthusiasm are to be maintained, educational activities should also be a regular part of the staff schedule.

The unit structure also extends to individual staff–patient interactions. What is said to a patient, how it is said, and by whom are an important part of the overall treatment plan. The specifics of this interpersonal strategy are discussed in Chapter 7.

Part of overall staff efficiency lies also in the ability to reliably observe and report psychopathology. Despite previous training, most mental health professionals need to develop additional observation and communication skills, and a system should be established for ensuring intrastaff reliability of observation. A number of clinical rating scales are available (8–10). They are short, easily learned, and extremely helpful as adjuncts to overall patient care. Table 9–5 presents one such scale (8, 9) for nurses.

Physical Structure

Unfortunately, few hospitals, let alone individual specialty units, are designed with significant input from the professionals who will use the facility. Although extant psychiatric inpatient units obviously cannot be totally rebuilt, the design of a unit and of its related clinical areas is important for its function.

TABLE 9-5   Nursing Rating Scale

Rating Instructions

1. A rating must be made for each item; therefore, the rater should make certain that the behavior defined for each item has been examined by observing and/or interviewing the patient during the time period of the rating. Read the definition of each item and the descriptions of the item numbers carefully, then write the number on the rating sheet that best indicates the intensity and pervasiveness of the patient's behavior on that item during the period of observation.
2. Evaluate each item using the description of the item and the "anchor points" at numbers 2, 4, 6, and 8 as guides. Behavior that you judge to be greater than one "anchor point" guide and less than the next should be rated at 1, 3, 5, or 7.
3. The following general concepts should be used to judge magnitude of behavior:
   a. Ratings at the 1 level are questionable and may be based on assumptions of the rater.
   b. Ratings at the 4 level are based on clearly present behavior or verbalization leaving no doubt that the behavior being rated is present. Ratings at this level should not be based on assumptions or inferences.
   c. Ratings at the 8 level are based on behavior that is extreme in both intensity and pervasiveness. Such ratings should be used when the behavior is almost impossible to interrupt even with intense intervention. This rating should not be avoided.

Scale Descriptions

I. *Depressed Mood* (Rate primarily on feelings of sadness, gloominess, pessimism; often may include feelings of helplessness, hopelessness, or low self-esteem and worthlessness; may use such expressions as being in "low spirits," "feeling blue," and "feeling empty." Use physical appearance, sad or downcast facial expression, and tearfulness to gauge degree or intensity of verbally expressed sadness.):

   0. No evidence of sadness.
   2. Mild—sadness is infrequent and/or of low intensity.
   4. Moderate—depressed mood-symptoms definite; a constant low intensity or frequent (50% of the time) periods at moderate intensity.
   6. Marked—symptoms present of at least moderate intensity more than 50% of time or occasional periods of severely depressed mood. Depressive symptoms clearly interfering with ability to function.
   8. Severe—total; a pervasive depressed mood of extreme intensity. May include feelings of being completely worthless; no hope.

II. *Suicidal Trends* (the conscious expression or clearly inferred wish of the patient to be dead and/or any self-mutilative activity):

   0. No indication of suicidal trends.
   2. Mild—vague indication of suicidal thoughts, i.e., acknowledges suicidal thoughts in past but denies any importance of these for the present, or admits thought crossed mind but dropped it. Alternatively, rater feels denial of suicidal thoughts are unconvincing.

(Continued)

TABLE 9-5 *(Continued)*

    4. Moderate—clear suicidal ideation, definitely sees suicide as a possibility. Included would be preoccupation with wish to go to sleep and not wake up or preoccupation with wish to be dead in a passive manner.

    6. Marked—constant suicidal thoughts and talking of specific plans for suicide. Wants suicide for a solution and would take action if not protected. May include less serious suicidal attempts such as wrist slashing or ingestion of small number of pills.

    8. Severe—thoughts of suicide, all-pervasive at high intensity. Serious suicide attempts.

III. *Verbal Expression of Anxiety or Fear* (Rate primarily on verbally expressed feelings of worry, nervousness, tenseness, anxiousness, fearfulness. Mild amounts include uncertainty about the future; marked amounts are feelings of something bad about to happen [impending doom]. Use physical indicators of anxiety such as pallor, hyperventilation, rapid pulse, dilated pupils, fearful facial expressions as aids in assessing degree of anxiety, but do not rate on these alone. Explore for verbal expression.):

    0. No evidence of verbal anxiety.

    2. Mild—transient verbal anxiety; intensity low and duration brief.

    4. Moderate—symptoms definitely present, moderate in intensity and present 50% of the time, or occasional episodes of marked anxiety.

    6. Marked—symptoms present more than 50% of the time of at least moderate intensity. Symptoms interfering with ability to function. Basing actions on anxious feelings.

    8. Severe—feelings pervasive; convinced something terrible is inevitable.

IV. *Expression of Anger* (Rate both the verbal and physical indicators of anger, giving each equal weight. Verbally, seen in an attitude of hostility toward others such as cutting off verbal contact, sarcasm, sharpness in tone of voice, derogation, belittlement, or threats to harm others or objects. Physically, seen in turning away from others, hostile gesturing such as clenching fists or striking out at persons or objects.):

    0. No evidence of expressed anger.

    2. Mild—intensity of expressed anger mild, duration brief.

    4. Moderate—clear expressed anger, present 50% of the time.

    6. Marked—expression of anger present more than 50% of the time. May be specifically warning others to stay out of the way. Able to check self from striking out most of the time but with great difficulty. Describes using much energy to prevent harming others or has to be removed from situations by staff to prevent striking out.

    8. Severe—extreme evidence of anger; pervasive indication of intense hostility, verbal and/or physical, which is difficult or impossible for staff to stop.

V. *Social Withdrawal* (A measure of the level of the person's social ability through participation in ward milieu, cooperation and involvement with both patients and staff. This is measured in relation to the amount of voluntary participation versus urging, and the person's general level of interaction on the unit.):

    0. No evidence of limitation in socialization.

2. Mild—some evidence of tendency to withdraw, but requires no urging to return to activities, i.e., responds readily to invitation to join others. Needs encouragement to interact verbally with others but continues conversations once begun.

4. Moderate—social withdrawal definite; tendency to wish to be alone 50% of the time. If no one urges patient to join activities, will stay alone. When with group does not continue verbal interactions begun by others.

6. Marked—clearly avoids or refuses most interactions and activities. Even with intense and continuous urging, patient does not participate as expected. Responds infrequently to verbal interactions initiated by others.

8. Severe—alone and withdrawn from all interactions and activities even with constant urging; intense isolation.

VI. *Motor Agitation* (Only rate gross movement of large parts of the body. Do not rate muscular tension or muscle flexion or teeth clenching. Rate observable evidence of increased muscular movements of any part of the body. This may be in the form of handwringing, excessive changing of position, pacing, rocking, etc. Intensity based on the ability of the patient to control the excess movement. Rate amount of movement, not speed of movement.):

0. No evidence of the above.

2. Mild—able to stop excess movement with little difficulty. Symptoms occur only occasionally under stress.

4. Moderate—obvious increased muscular movements present. May stop on questioning but always returns.

6. Marked—unable to stop all excess movement even with great effort. Symptoms interfering with ability to function.

8. Severe—pervasive, intense agitation. Totally unable to control symptoms.

VII. *Motor Retardation* (Rating based on degree of slowness of muscular movement, not amount of movement. This ranges from slowness of walk, to obvious slowing down in ability to do activities of daily living, to shuffling gait, to needing someone to help start movement, to virtual motionlessness with little response to stimulation. May include slowness of speech.):

0. No evidence of the above.

2. Mild—slowness may be just detectable. Patient may describe feeling slowed down from usual pace even though not detectable by rater.

4. Moderate—present 50% of time at moderate intensity or occasional periods of marked retardation.

6. Marked—present more than 50% of time. Clearly interfering with ability to function.

8. Severe—may have to be fed meals, etc.

VIII. *Paranoid Behavior* (Degree to which the person feels that other people are the cause of his problems and that they did this with hostile intent towards him. Do not include diffuse anger unless other persons' hostile intent is clearly inferred by patient.):

0. No evidence of the above.

2. Mild—questionable suspiciousness with no consistent or fixed statements of hostile intent of others. Intensity definitely low.

(Continued)

TABLE 9–5 (*Continued*)

      4. Moderate—tends to believe hostile intent of others with clear paranoid ideas, paranoid beliefs, or paranoid statements. Conviction "something wrong", something "uncanny" that relates to him/her. Nothing approaching a coherent plot.

      6. Marked—clear paranoid delusional system. Basing some actions on the system. Committed to the correctness of his perceptions that others have hostile intent.

      8. Severe—pervasive, fixed paranoid delusional system on which he bases most actions.

IX. *Hallucinations* (The patient experiences hearing or seeing things that the rater does not experience and rater has evidence they are not physically present.):

      0. No evidence of the above.

      2. Mild—hallucinations may be questionable and are not interrupting interactions with others. Rate 2 or 3 if patient acts as though responding to hallucinations but verbally denies that these come from outside himself.

      4. Moderate—present 50% of time; occasionally interrupting interactions with others. Patient must be able to give verbal report that sensations come from outside himself.

      6. Marked—some behavior and verbalizations guided by hallucinations. Difficult to interrupt hallucinatory process. Hallucinations frequently interrupting interactions with others.

      8. Severe—interacting with and basing virtually all behavior on hallucinations. Staff unable to interrupt the process.

X. *Thought Disorder* (Rating based on the patient's verbalization. The primary indicator should be degree of connectedness of thoughts as expressed in speech. This may include ambiguousness in speech, tangential connecting of thoughts, loosening of associations, neologisms and rhyming, and echolalia and word salad. Do not rate rapidity of speech, rate connectedness.):

      0. No evidence of the above.

      2. Mild—manifestations of ambiguity, circumstantiality and tangentialness.

      4. Moderate—loose associations or thoughts mixed up. Disconnected thoughts may be linked within sentences.

      6. Marked—very difficult to follow associations. Words patient uses together have little real meaning to the listener.

      8. Severe—echolalia, word salad, impossible to follow association, rhyming, etc.

XI. *Hyperactivity-Elation* (Rating based on three components: [1] Mood, seen in statements of wellbeing, joviality, expansiveness, grandiosity, euphoria; [2] Energy level, in pressure of activity, statements of not being fatigued even though sleeping poorly, difficulty in completing one activity before going to another; [3] thought-speech pressure—associations rapid, difficult to maintain one subject because thoughts seem to be tumbling over one another, speech may reach point of almost continuous flow, may be loud. Base ratings on any one or more of the three components. If two or more are present base rating on the highest one.):

0. No evidence of the above.
2. Mild-mood: happy, state of wellbeing. Energy: mild pressure for purposeful activities. Thought-speech: pressure to talk, may have increase in rate of speech.
4. Moderate-mood: shows moderate elation, grandiosity and/or expansiveness. Energy: moderate pressure for purposeful activities with increase in number of simultaneous projects going at once. Thought-speech: associations in rapid flow from topic to topic but able to be brought back to a subject, speech flow may be continuous.
6. Marked-mood: euphoria, marked grandiosity, expansiveness, unable to be interrupted. Energy level: impossible to sustain focused activity without external control; tries multiple different activities simultaneously. Thought-speech: continuous rapid associations virtually impossible to interrupt. Continuous speech flow.
8. Severe-mood: extreme euphoria. Energy level: constant, undirected activity. Thought-speech: continuous rapid associations with no response to staff interventions. Continuous flow of speech that is virtually impossible to understand.

XII. *Physical Complaints* (Rating based on both number of complaints about physical symptoms or sensations and on the amount of attention or preoccupation the patient gives these complaints. May include complaints of weakness, general body aches and pain, headaches, nausea, constipation, butterflies, shaking inside, etc. Do not rate on withdrawal of patient unless he specifies this due to bodily sensations or symptoms. Both number of symptoms and amount of preoccupation with the body should be considered when doing this rating.):

0. No physical complaints.
2. Mild—does not place much emphasis on specific physical complaints or general body concerns.
4. Moderate—places frequent (50% of time) emphasis on physical complaints. Moderately occupied with concerns about body.
6. Marked—constant preoccupation with physical symptoms or concern about body, somatic delusions may be present.
8. Severe—total pervasive preoccupation with physical symptoms or concern about body. Pervasive somatic delusions.

XIII. *Global Illness* (Based on intensity and pervasiveness of all symptoms and impairment of functioning. This item is the rater's assessment and is not based only on scores of preceding item.)

0. No evidence of illness.
2. Mildly ill.
4. Moderately ill.
6. Markedly ill.
8. Severely ill.

Source: N. H. French and G. R. Heninger, "A Short Clinical Rating Scale for Use by Nursing Personnel. I. Development and Design," in *Archives of General Psychiatry* 23: 233–40 (1970). (Scale covers pp. 237–40.) Copyright © 1970–73 by American Medical Association. Used by permission.

Ideally an inpatient unit should have no "blind spots." All patient areas outside of individual rooms should be visible from the nurses' station, which should be centrally located, be readily accessible to patients and staff, and contain a private staff area. A square or rectangular unit with the nursing station at one end offers maximum visibility without compromising efficiency or needs for future expansion. The unit also should be self-contained, so that when the doors are locked all patient areas are within the unit.

A seclusion area should be available in the unit. It should consist of two lockable seclusion rooms with a common anteroom and adjoining bathroom. The anteroom should be locked to the outside unit area. The seclusion room requires special construction to prevent patients from destroying wall surfaces to get at electric wires and other dangerous objects. There should be no protruding objects or moldings on the walls. The room may have a window, but it should be reinforced and double-paned with unbreakable material or covered with a metal screen. The seclusion room door should also have a reinforced glass or plastic window to permit frequent patient observation. The ceiling should be at least 12 feet high and should be constructed in such a way as to prevent a patient from jumping up and grabbing electric fixtures (one 6 foot, 3 inch manic patient of ours accomplished this in a seclusion room with a 10-foot-high ceiling). The only object in the room should be a nonflammable mattress.

An ECT suite or area should be located on or adjacent to the inpatient unit. Chapter 6 describes the ECT suite in detail. The inpatient unit should also include a treatment/examination room (with all the examination and emergency equipment available in any hospital unit), dining room (which optimally includes its own kitchen), a patient kitchen, recreational areas, sufficient office space in and near the unit, a staff conference room, and a visitors' room.

Patient bedrooms should be private or semiprivate with individual baths. All patient areas should be brightly lighted. Windows should be reinforced and made of unbreakable material. Fixtures and wall and floor coverings should be composed of material that will withstand considerable abuse, have no sharp edges or other dangerous characteristics, and yet be cheerful and not institutional in appearance. Occupational, recreation, and rehabilitation therapy services should be part of the unit or close to it. These services should be integrated into the unit's programs.

Inpatient Problems

Violence, although relatively infrequent, can be the most serious of unit problems. Discussions of violence and emergency measures in response to violence are presented in Chapters 8 and 13. More common than an actually assaultive patient, however, is a patient who is agitated and irritable and refuses to cooperate with basic unit policies, such as keeping his room and body clean and permitting a physical examination and diagnostic evaluation. In responding to such a patient, the first decision to be made is whether the patient is suffering from an illness of which his uncooperativeness, agitation, and irritability are manifestations, or whether the patient is a psychopath manipulating the hospital system. If the latter is strongly suspected, the patient should be told he must either cooperate or be discharged immediately. If he fails to cooperate he should then be discharged. If the patient is considered ill, then the lack of a physical examination and basic diagnostic tests (e.g. blood work) might be life-threatening, because a serious illness might progress undiscovered. The decision to be made at this point is whether the patient is competent to participate fully in decisions concerning his treatment. If he is competent, the reasons for the examination, diagnostic evaluation, personal hygiene, or other procedures or activities should again be explained to him; he should be told that he cannot be helped unless he cooperates and allows the staff to help him, and that he has a choice of cooperating or seeking help elsewhere. If he chooses the latter, his family or friends should be notified. If they are unable to persuade him, he should be discharged. If the patient is incompetent or dangerous to himself or others, and is not already in the hospital as an involuntary patient, his family should be informed of this assessment. If they concur, the patient should be converted to involuntary status, restrained, and sedated if necessary. He should then be examined and blood samples drawn. If x-rays and other tests are needed, they should be obtained while the patient is sedated. If the family refuses to support these procedures, which are emergency measures in that life-threatening illness may be prevented, identified, or treated, they should be asked to transfer the patient to another hospital. In our experience most families are relieved to know that firm action is being taken to find out what is wrong with the patient and will readily agree to the necessary procedures. Under no circumstances should a patient be hospitalized for longer than twenty-four hours without a physical examination and basic laboratory work.

The agitated, uncooperative patient will be on the lowest level of the step system. He may need to be sedated and possibly placed in seclusion for varying periods. Such patients, once minimal knowledge is obtained regarding their condition and there is reasonable likelihood that neuroleptic treatment is not contraindicated, should receive intramuscular neuroleptics for two to five days until no longer agitated and uncooperative. Oral neuroleptics should later be introduced, overlapping with intramuscular administration. If the patient remains agitated and uncontrollable despite several days of intramuscular medication, ECT should be administered. The procedures for these treatment strategies are discussed in Chapters 5 and 6. Uncooperativeness specifically refers to patients who are so ill that they are unmanageable. Such patients refuse to shower and clean up their personal areas. They lie on the floor, masturbate or undress in public, and generally disrupt the unit and upset the other patients. These behaviors most often reflect illness and require treatment. For the safety of the patient and those around him, such behaviors must be stopped (almost always, some degree of force is needed, from "show of force" to restraints and seclusion), and the patient must be medicated.

The overriding issue in the situations described here is to ensure that the patient does not harm himself or others. He must also be prevented from undermining his own treatments and from behaving in a manner that disrupts the unit's functioning and disturbs other patients. The obvious theme of this approach is patient control. Society continues to struggle with this issue and the degree to which individual rights can be denied to protect both the individual and society as a whole. That subject is beyond the scope of this book, but suffice it to say that once a person is identified as being ill and is hospitalized because of that illness, he has the right to treatment. If his behaviors prevent effective treatment, we believe it wrong to deny that treatment. The decision to abridge the patient's civil liberties and to treat, however, cannot be made solely by the physician. If the patient's behavior is dangerous, we are legally permitted to restrain and treat him for a limited time. Further involuntary treatment usually requires court approval. If the patient is not dangerous but is clearly psychotic or severely ill, the physician must decide whether the patient is competent to judge his own condition and the prescribed treatments. If the patient is competent, the decision to be treated is his. If the patient is incompetent, he should be treated. Court approval, however, must be obtained before definitive nonemergency involuntary treatment can be legally administered. In most instances consultation with the patient's family is helpful in obtaining the patient's consent to treatment and in reducing the risk of suit for treating the patient while court approval is being obtained. In our experience the vast majority of patients, when recovered, express their gratitude that they were stopped from doing "those crazy [embarrassing or dangerous] things" (11).

The use of intramuscular medication, restraints, and seclusion does not particularly upset or anger patients if it is clear that these methods are used as treatments and not as punishments, and that the staff involved truly cares about the patient's wellbeing. Integral to these responses to deviant behaviors are warm, caring, and concerned supportive responses to the patient's other symptoms and interpersonal needs.

Restraints

The use of seclusion and restraints is a particularly sensitive issue. Established rules for restraining and secluding patients should be clearly understood by each staff member.

Physical restraints should be used only as a therapeutic measure to protect the patient from injuring himself or others. Mechanical restraints should be used only when absolutely necessary. Restraints should never be used to punish or discipline a patient or for the convenience of the staff.

Restraints should be employed only on the written order of a physician after he has examined the patient. Orders for restraints are usually valid for up to twelve hours, at which time the patient must be formally reexamined by a physician for subsequent restraint. Nevertheless, periodic evaluation by a qualified staff member should be made every fifteen to thirty minutes. In ordering restraints, the physician should specify the duration of their application and, in an accompanying progress note, indicate the events leading to the need for restraint, the purpose of the restraint, and the length of the restraint period. In emergencies orders for restraint may be given to a nurse by telephone, or the nurse or other qualified examiner may order restraint subject to prompt confirmation (within one hour) by a physician in writing and with appropriate documentation. While in restraints the patient should be closely supervised and made as comfortable as possible. Special attention should be given to the patient's temperature and fluid intake to avoid dehydration and hyperthermia.

Rules of Seclusion

Seclusion should be used only as a therapeutic measure to prevent the patient from harming himself or others. It should not be used to punish or discipline a patient or as a convenience for the staff. When a specific seclusion room is not available, a patient bedroom may be used, provided there is one-to-one observation by nursing personnel with the room unlocked and free from furniture. All the rules applying to the ordering and monitoring of restraints also apply to the use of the seclusion room.

The Suicidal Patient

Occasionally a depressed patient will commit suicide while hospitalized. Placing a suicidal patient on "suicide precautions," although legally necessary, is often insufficient to prevent such deaths. Although we have not cared for a hospitalized patient who killed himself, we have had patients attempt suicide by hanging (using ceiling and shower fixtures), ramming the head into a wall, jumping off a clothes closet head first onto the floor, cutting the wrists with a table knife or on broken window glass, and drowning in a toilet bowl.

The suicidal patient should be placed in hospital clothes and continuously observed by a specifically assigned staff member. He may require seclusion and restraints. These patients should be on the lowest level of any step system and should never be allowed off the unit unescorted. Should a patient on suicidal precautions attempt suicide on the unit, emergency ECT should be administered as a potentially lifesaving procedure.

The Self-Mutilator

A patient will sometimes injure himself as part of a pattern of self-mutilation rather than with the desire to die. Such patients usually inflict superficial cuts and burns on their arms, legs, and chest or may insert objects into the urethra. Some of them will actually experience pleasure while harming themselves. Such a paradoxical response to pain (pain asymboly) should alert the clinician to the possibility of coarse brain disease, particularly a seizure disorder (see Chapter 18 on Behavioral Neurologic Disease). Such patients may respond to carbamazapine. Some obsessive-compulsive patients may also exhibit self-mutilating behavior. They may respond to monoamine oxidase inhibitors or imipramine. ECT may produce transient symptom relief. Self-mutilators may require restraints until a specific diagnosis can be made and treatment can be instituted (5, 12).

Although there is no known treatment for self-mutilators who do not have behavioral neurologic disease or obsessive-compulsive disorder, there is some evidence (13, 14) that they and similar patients admitted to a short-term treatment unit of a general hospital experience dramatic cessation of such behavior when transferred to a local chronic care facility. In our experience direct behavior modification techniques are rarely successful in reducing the frequency of these behaviors.

Sexual Behaviors

Most short-term inpatient units admit both men and women. Although the general experience of units that have become "coed" is the increased socialization and normalization of behavior of patients, inappropriate sexual behavior occasionally occurs. Observing overt sexual behavior in other patients is frightening to some patients, and the sexual behavior, if not immediately stopped, may lead patients to feel that the involved patients are out of control and that the staff is unable to control them. Whereas expressions of warmth and affection can be appropriate, specific sexual behavior (e.g. passionate kissing, embracing, and fondling) must be stopped immediately and treated as any other behavior that is inappropriate in a hospital or public setting. Liaisons occurring in the patient's bedrooms, although showing discretion on the part of the individuals involved, must also be prevented from recurring, because they too indicate that the participants may have lost control or that one of the participants (with diminished judgment or volition or with hypersexuality) is being taken advantage of by a patient with a less severe illness. Separation and close monitoring of the patients involved and a reevaluation of their diagnoses and treatments should be the minimal response. Continued attempts at sexual liaisons by a patient may require seclusion until specific treatment (e.g. lithium, neuroleptics) become effective. If the patient is voluntarily hospitalized and deemed not a danger to himself, discharge from the unit may be necessary. At no time, however, should overt sexual behavior be ignored. Calm but firm discussions with the participants and other patients on the unit is often helpful in reducing anxieties.

Socially Disruptive Behavior

Patients frequently behave oddly, inappropriately or annoyingly. Some examples are intruding into meetings and conversations, making importunate requests, cursing loudly, standing too close to people when talking to them. Ideally, the best response to behaviors considered inappropriate is no response, that is, to ignore the behavior, to look "through" the patient at his shoulder without making eye contact, and literally to pretend it did not happen. A negative response (e.g. saying "No. Go away" while turning away) may be reinforcing and increase such behaviors. A lack of reinforcement may reduce some patient behaviors if the staff is consistent in its approach and the behaviors to be ignored are explicitly identified. The same patient will also behave appropriately, and such behaviors should be reinforced immediately by means of some positive interaction with that patient.

Some behaviors, however, cannot be ignored, as they may adversely affect other patients. Some examples are monopolizing the phone; lying on the floor in hallways and recreational areas; hoarding common supplies, unit equipment, or other patients' property; or exhibiting pseudo-seizures. As most such behaviors are manifestations of illness, they will resolve with appropriate treatment, and simply stopping the patient from doing the behavior may suffice until the illness responds to treatment. Adjunctive behavioral techniques, if properly planned, may speed the reduction in the frequency of these behaviors and thus make the patients feel better and improve the functioning of the unit (7).

For example, the patient who monopolizes the phone may get some special privilege or treat only if the number of calls or total time on the phone is below a certain level. The patient with pseudo-seizures (medically evaluated, moved out of the way, and ignored during each pseudo-seizure) is rewarded in some fashion if the number of episodes progressively decreases with time.

Other management problem behaviors may be extinguished by forms of "massed practice" by which the patient is forced into repeating the unwanted behavior until he "cannot" do it any more. For example, a patient who hoards linen in his room would have staff members repeatedly bring linen to him until his room is filled and he can hardly live in it.

Some behaviors are not particularly disruptive but do disturb other patients. Some of these are chain smoking to the point where the patient's fingers are nicotine-stained or unsightly, and constantly drinking coffee or soda containing caffeine despite the development of caffeine reactions. Most commonly such behaviors are seen in patients who are anxious or perseverative. Although primary treatment must focus on the resolution of the patient's illness process by somatic treatment, adjunctive behavioral techniques can be of benefit. To be effective, however, behavioral techniques should include (1) specific identification of the unwanted behavior and the circumstances in which it occurs, (2) the frequency of the behavior, (3) identification of specific staff responses that are considered reinforcing for that behavior in that patient, and (4) consistent action by all staff members.

Agitation

The patient who is not assaultive but is agitated is also a management problem. Agitation is the motor expression of an intense mood. If the patient is not assaultive or irritable (see Chapters 5 and 6 for treatment strategies for these patients) the most likely cause of agitation will be depression. As the profound sadness and dysphoria of the depression improves with somatic treatment, the agitation will resolve. During the interim between admission and significant improvement from the primary treatment, sodium amytal may be of benefit. Patients with neuroleptic-induced akathisia will occasionally be mistakenly identified as agitated. The patient with akathisia, however, will describe an inner restlessness and a jumpiness in his arms and legs, which becomes overpowering unless he moves about. He may also exhibit other neuroleptic side effects. Patients with akathisia respond best to a reduction in their daily neuroleptic dose (12).

Insomnia

Most patients hospitalized on a psychiatric unit will have difficulty sleeping, particularly during the first few nights of hospitalization. "PRN" hypnotics are routinely ordered in most hospital units. However, when a patient simply cannot sleep (he is not upset or agitated) and the full hypnotic dose has been administered, the night staff should be educated to the fact that most such patients are not manipulating the system but are simply exhibiting a symptom of their illness. Rather than make an issue of their being awake—causing the patient to feel guilty and the staff angry—the night staff should allow the patient to sit up in a day area where he can read, watch TV, or talk with a staff member. The insomnia invariably improves with resolution of the illness.

Substance Abusers

Patients who are substance abusers are particularly difficult to treat in a short-term general inpatient psychiatric unit. Patients in acute alcohol withdrawal states are at increased risk for seizures and death, may require intravenous fluid and electrolyte replacement, and are generally best treated on specialized detoxification or medical units. Their treatment is discussed in Chapters 8 and 19. Patients with drug-induced psychoses are discussed in Chapter 19.

Occasionally, however, a patient addicted to opiates or barbiturates is admitted to a general psychiatric unit. These patients can cause havoc as they are frequently sociopathic. They manipulate staff and other patients, abuse other patients, demand and often receive unwarranted medication, and even may introduce street drugs to the unit's ill patients. In general all patients who are primarily substance abusers, with no psychosis or major illness such as depression, or who are simply sociopaths should be discharged as quickly as possible.

VIPs

Patients who are physicians or mental health professionals present a particular management problem. They often assume a stafflike manner and may actually be of help to other patients. Nevertheless, if they have been appropriately hospitalized (that is, if they have a major psychiatric disorder), they require the same psychological and somatic treatments as anyone else. If they are to receive the best available treatment, the staff must be educated to the tendency of these patients to act the role of treater and to the tendency of staff members to permit this, often at the expense of the patient's optimal care. A professional who is a patient can "help out" during the recovery phase of his illness, but his knowledge of his illness and treatments, his response to his illness and family, and his personal concerns should not be taken for granted. These patients deserve "full service."

Patients who are famous or exotic in some way also tempt staff members to respond to reputation or status rather than to the personal qualities of the patient and the treatment requirements of his illness.

A dramatic example occurred at a municipal teaching hospital in a ghetto. A young, attractive white actress was transferred to psychiatry from medicine following a suicide attempt. Although not endogenously depressed and fully recovered from the physiologic sequela of her overdose, she remained in the hospital for several more weeks "holding court" as literally long lines of medical students and residents from three services came to "see" her and "help her through her crisis." Her histrionic, dependent, and egocentric behaviors received unlimited reinforcement at the expense of any reasonable plan to help her deal with her problems of living. Although the staff was aware of the phenomenon, it was never discussed in a staff meeting and thus never resolved so that the patient could receive appropriate care.

Outsiders

Finally a common problem on inpatient units is that of the staff assuming an adversary relationship to "outsiders": visitors, hospital personnel from other patient care areas (e.g. medicine, emergency room), and support services (e.g. x-ray, "the lab"). The adversary attitude will develop as the unit's cohesiveness evolves. Staff behaviors suggesting such an attitude are suspiciousness and irritability toward strangers entering the unit, defensiveness and guardedness toward the families and friends of patients, expectations of "special" service from hospital support areas (e.g. expecting to obtain all requested supplies in optimal quantities, often before other patient care areas receive any supplies), and expressing unrealistically low opinions of other patient care areas (particularly other similar units or units to or from which patients may be transferred). Interestingly, these behaviors are often a sign that the unit is functioning well, but they can simultaneously lead to internecine squabbling, which reduces the unit's effectiveness as well as its needed supports from the "outsiders." Recognition and staff discussion of these behaviors, and the attitudes leading to them, usually suffice to prevent significant problems.

References

1. Stanton, A. H.; Schwartz, M. S. *The Mental Hospital.* New York: Basic Books, 1954.
2. Caudill, W. *The Psychiatric Hospital as a Small Society.* Cambridge: Harvard University Press, 1958.

3. Wing, J. K.; Brown, G. W. *Institutionalism and Schizophrenia.* London: Cambridge University Press, 1970.

4. May, P. R. A. *Treatment of Schizophrenia: A Comparative Study of Five Treatment Methods.* New York: Science House, 1968.

5. Greist, J. H.; Jefferson, J. W.; Spitzer, R. L. (eds.). *Treatment of Mental Disorders.* New York: Oxford University Press, 1982.

6. Spitzer, R. L.; Klein, D. F. (eds.). *Evaluation of Psychological Therapies, Psychotherapies, Behavior Therapies, Drug Therapies and Their Interactions.* Baltimore: Johns Hopkins Press, 1976.

7. Schaefer, H. H.; Martin, P. L. *Behavior Therapy.* New York: McGraw–Hill, 1969.

8. French, N. H.; Heninger, G. R. "A short clinical rating scale for use by nursing personnel: 1. Development and design." *Arch. Gen. Psychiat. 23:* 233–40, 1970.

9. Heninger, G. R.; French, N. H.; Slavinsky, A. T.; *et al.* "A short clinical rating scale for use by nursing personnel: 2. Reliability, validity and application." *Arch. Gen. Psychiat. 23:* 241–48, 1970.

10. Honigfeld, G.; Gillis, R. D.; Klett, C. J. "NOISE-30: A treatment sensitive ward behavior scale." *Psychol. Rep. 19:* 180–82, 1966.

11. Sierles, F. Forensic Medicine. In Sierles, F. (ed.), *Clinical Behavioral Science.* New York: SP Medical and Scientific Books, 1982, pp. 377–86.

12. Kalinowsky, L. B.; Hippius, H.; Klein, H. E. *Biological Treatments in Psychiatry.* New York: Grune & Stratton, 1982.

13. Quitkin, F. M.; Klein, D. F. Follow-up of treatment failure: Psychosis and character disorder. *Am. J. Psychiat. 124:* 499–505, 1967.

14. Grunebaum, H. U.; Klerman, G. L. Wrist slashing. *Am. J. Psychiat. 124:* 527–34, 1967.

CHAPTER 10

Consultation/Liaison Psychiatry

Introduction

Consultation psychiatrists perform individual patient evaluations to assist primary care physicians. Liaison psychiatrists, in addition to individual consultations, provide advice and teaching to the medical or surgical service as a whole. For example, a liaison psychiatrist's evaluation of a suicidal medical patient is performed within the context of a case conference, attended by internal medicine residents and students, on the subject of evaluation and management of suicidal patients on medical services.

Psychiatrists who regularly do liaison/consultation work enjoy applying their skills in general hospital settings, where there is considerable exposure to situations (e.g. postcardiotomy delirium in a patient in an intensive care unit) not ordinarily encountered in office practice. And the liaison/consultation service is a splendid setting for observing the interaction of systemic illnesses and behavior.

The concept that systemic illness and behavior are strongly related does not require a set of principles ("psychosomatic medicine") that deviate from those of medically oriented psychiatry. Behavior can affect systemic functioning (as when a diabetic teenager does not comply with dietary and insulin requirements), and systemic functioning can affect behavior (as when a patient with uremia develops a "secondary" endogenous depression), but neither fact requires the existence of intervening metapsychological phenomena such as "anger at introjects," "castration anxiety," or "unfulfilled dependency needs."

The principles and techniques of interviewing and diagnosis on the liaison/consultation service are identical to those used on the psychiatric service. What differs is the frequency of diagnoses made. For example, in a series of 170 consecutive consultations on general medical and surgical services at one of our hospitals, 8 percent of acute patients had major depression or mania as against the 30 percent of psychiatric inpatients who have major affective disorders. Table 10-1 shows the primary diagnoses made on 170 consecutive psychiatric consultations on primary care inpatient services by the consultant during a two-year period.

Because the frequencies of various diagnoses will differ, the extent to which psychopharmacologic agents or ECT are used will also vary. Although the majority of psychiatric inpatients require psychopharmacologic agents or ECT, only a small minority of medical and surgical patients will require somatic treatment. It is more likely that the psychiatrist will make recommendations such as "the patient's behavior should improve as you continue with your current vigorous medical management" or "since the patient has dysthymia, not endogenous depression, antidepressant medications are not needed."

The psychiatrist must employ an interview that elicits a thorough data base by questioning systematically and responding to patient behavior. Simultaneously he must obtain a good mental status and behavioral neurologic examination. The primary physician, regardless of training, will rarely if ever perform an adequate mental status and behavioral neurologic examination. Indeed, the importance of these examinations (and of the patient's behavior) is minimized on nonpsychiatric services. Primary physicians, as well as many psychiatrists, have a tendency to disregard the relationship of brain functioning and behavior. This is unfortunate, as psychiatric and behavioral neurologic abnormalities are common in patients on medical services (1, 2). The psychiatrist must also search for information

TABLE 10-1   Diagnostic Breakdown of 170 Consecutive Medical and Surgical Consultations

PSYCHIATRIC DIAGNOSIS	NUMBER	PERCENT
Situational reactions	55	33
Coarse brain disease	39	23
Alcohol and other substance abuse	37	22
Major psychiatric disorder	16	9
Anxiety states	6	3
Other	17	10

from such sources as the patient's doctors, nurses, relatives, friends, and laboratory tests. He must rigorously apply reliable and operationally defined diagnostic criteria, just as on the psychiatric service.

Common diagnostic problems encountered in consultation include the following: (1) the patient who simultaneously manifests systemic illness and behavioral abnormality; (2) the patient with abnormal behavior who is receiving medication known to affect the brain; (3) the patient with coarse brain disease of unknown cause; (4) the patient with symptoms of pathology where no pathology can be found; and (5) the patient whose behavior is affected by drug overdose.

Abnormal Behavior Concurrent with Systemic Illness or Medication

The patient with concomitant systemic illness and abnormal behavior is one of the commonest reasons for referral. Consultation is sought to determine if the behavior is (1) the product of the illness for which the patient was admitted; (2) due to treatment; or (3) due to coexisting psychiatric illness such as mania, major depression, or schizophrenia. In approaching these problems, the consultant should consider the following axioms: (1) If the patient has an active systemic illness known to affect the brain, the abnormal behavior is caused by that illness until proved otherwise. (2) If onset of the abnormal behavior follows onset of the systemic disease or follows treatments known to affect the brain, the behavior is more likely to be a result of that illness or treatment than of a separate psychiatric disorder. (3) The more pronounced the cognitive dysfunction, the more likely it is that the patient has coarse brain disease. (4) If the patient had prior psychiatric illness with similar manifestations or a family history of psychiatric disorder (especially affective disorder), the chances increase that the behavior is due to a coexisting psychiatric syndrome unrelated to the systemic illness. Three examples illustrate these principles:

MANIC BEHAVIOR CAUSED BY VIRAL ENCEPHALOPATHY

A twenty-four-year-old woman is admitted comatose and febrile to a medical unit. In the past three years she has been admitted twice to this unit with coma and fever followed by full recovery. Abnormal behavior was not observed during the two previous admissions. There is no history of drug or alcohol abuse and no family history of psychiatric illness. Cerebrospinal fluid reveals elevated protein and many lymphocyctes. The EEG shows diffuse slowing. The diagnosis is encephalopathy probably due to herpes simplex virus.

Emerging from coma, she remains febrile and her behavior is seriously abnormal. She sings and talks loudly to herself, yells to people passing her open door, bounces on her bed, and is emotionally labile and irritable. She exhibits significant diffuse cognitive impairment, and the psychiatric consultant diagnoses mania secondary to viral encephalopathy. He predicts her behavior will improve if her encephalopathy clears, which in fact occurs.

In this case the abnormal behavior was thought secondary to the encephalitis, because the behavior occurred simultaneously with the encephalitis and because there was no prior or family history of psychiatric illness.

A Manic Episode Following Recovery from Obstructive Pulmonary Disease in a Patient with Prior Manic Episodes

A sixty-seven-year-old man is admitted to the medical service for dyspnea associated with exacerbation of chronic obstructive pulmonary disease (COPD) of two years' duration. Past history reveals that three years before he developed recurring untreated episodes of hyperactivity, rapid and pressured speech, euphoria, and grandiose delusions. Those episodes persisted until shortly before admission and were unaffected by changes in the patient's pulmonary status or by medications for COPD. One relative had recurring psychiatric illnesses requiring hospitalization.

On the fifth day, with breathing much improved, he again manifests hyperactivity, rapid and pressured speech, euphoria, and grandiosity. Cognitive testing is normal except for mild constructional dyspraxia. EEG and CT brain scan are normal. Based on the history of psychiatric illness antedating the COPD, the family history of psychiatric illness, and the appearance of the hypomanic behavior after breathing improved, the psychiatrist diagnoses bipolar affective disorder, hypomanic episode, and recommends lithium carbonate treatment, which results in a remission of hypomanic symptoms.

In this case the manic episode was thought to be independent of the obstructive lung disease, as it began as the breathing improved, and because the patient had a history of manic episodes antedating onset of his pulmonary disease.

Delirium Following Intravenous Lidocaine Infusion

A sixty-seven-year-old great-grandmother is admitted to the medical service with a cardiac arrhythmia and a normal mental status. Fifteen minutes after an intravenous drip of lidocaine is begun, she becomes disoriented, begins hallucinating, and misidentifies objects in the room. Examination reveals significant diffuse cognitive impairment. The cardiac status improved slightly after lidocaine was initiated. The diagnosis is delirium from lidocaine toxicity; the lidocaine is discontinued. The mental status begins to improve and is normal in forty-eight hours.

In this case the abnormal behavior was thought to be secondary to the lidocaine infusion, as it occurred just after the infusion started, as lidocaine is known to cause delirium, and as there was no deterioration of her cardiac status to explain the delirium. Other drugs known to cause abnormal behavior are listed in the Appendix to this chapter.

The Patient with Diffuse Coarse Brain Disease (Organic Brain Syndrome) of Unknown Cause

Twenty percent of medical patients have diffuse cognitive dysfunction (2), and diffuse coarse brain disease is the primary diagnosis in 15 percent of psychiatric consultations on medical and surgical services. Sometimes the cause is unknown, and the referring physician is grateful for a differential diagnosis and suggestions for further evaluation. In making such recommendations, the consultant psychiatrist should consider the tests and diagnoses listed in Table 10–2.

TABLE 10–2 Evaluation of a Patient with Diffuse Cognitive Dysfunction

PROCEDURE	EXAMPLES OF DIAGNOSES IDENTIFIED BY PROCEDURE
Additional history from other sources, such as relatives, friends, old chart, additional physical examination.	All conditions
Review of medications	Drug side effects and intoxications
Complete blood count	Conditions producing insufficient, excessive, or abnormal formed elements of blood. Examples: "megaloblastic madness," basophile stippling of lead encephalopathy, thrombotic thrombocytopenic purpura, leukocytosis of meningitis, eosinophilia with parasitic infestations
Urinalysis	Glycosuria and ketonuria of diabetic acidosis, urine specific gravity of 1.010 and casts in renal failure, concentrated urine in dehydration

TABLE 10-2 (*Continued*)

PROCEDURE	EXAMPLES OF DIAGNOSES IDENTIFIED BY PROCEDURE
Chest x-ray	Hyperaeration in emphysema, neoplastic masses with potential for metastasis to brain or hormone secretion or demyelinating effects, infiltrates or consolidation with pneumonia
VDRL	General paresis, gumma in brain
Serum electrolytes (Na, Cl, K, Ca, P, Mg)	Excess or insufficiency of any of these may cause delirium. Cushing's and Addison's disease associated with abnormal Na, Cl, and K levels
Serum creatinine	Renal failure
Serum enzymes (CPK, LDH, SGOT, SGPT, alkaline phosphatase)	Hepatocellular damage, myocardial infarction
Fasting blood sugar	Diabetes mellitus
Blood gases	Hypoxia
Urine toxicology	Chemical toxins, drug side effects and intoxications, illicit drug use
EKG	Cardiac arrhythmia, myocardial infarction, electrolyte imbalance, drug toxicity, hypertension
Thyroid studies (T3, T4, effective thyroxine ratio, TSH)	Thyrotoxicosis, hypothyroidism
Serum B_{12} and folic acid	"Megaloblastic madness"
LE preparation	Systemic lupus erythematosis
EEG	Epilepsy, focal and diffuse coarse brain disease, delirium, digitalis toxicity
CT brain scan	Space-occupying lesions, hydrocephalus, atrophy in dementias
Lumbar puncture	Meningitis, encephalitis, intracranial bleeding, multiple sclerosis, neurosyphilis
Skull x-rays (unless CT scan includes an "open window" for bone study)	Skull fracture, pituitary tumor, metastasis to skull
Auditory evoked potentials	Multiple sclerosis

The Patient with Systemic Symptoms and No Diagnosable Systemic Illness

Patients are frequently referred with medically unexplained systemic symptoms, or symptoms that presented with an intensity exceeding physician expectations. In such circumstances diagnoses that should be considered include Briquet's syndrome, malingering, major depression, reactive depression, and anxiety states.

BRIQUET'S SYNDROME (SOMATIZATION DISORDER)

Occasionally the primary physician refers a patient, usually a woman, with multiple unexplained somatic complaints in many organ systems. These complaints are presented either spontaneously or in response to questions during a medical review of systems. Although most experienced physicians have seen many patients with such a clinical presentation, few are aware that they are dealing with a well-validated psychiatric syndrome. As a result, they are frustrated by the patient, whom they label a "crock," "turkey," or "hypochondriac" and welcome the diagnosis and accompanying explanation of Briquet's syndrome. When the diagnosis is made, the patient may be provided with an explanation such as the following: "You have a condition called Briquet's syndrome, which is a real illness associated with instability or immaturity in your nervous system. This makes you prone to developing many symptoms like those you have been telling me about. These symptoms are usually temporary, will usually go away by themselves, and will not kill you. Unfortunately, we cannot cure the condition, so you can reasonably expect to have more symptoms in the future, and these symptoms will usually be temporary. That does not mean you should neglect the symptoms if they are persistent or severe. But be sure if a doctor prescribes a medication, a test, or an operation for you, he gives you a good reason for it. One of the greatest risks in your condition is from getting medications or operations you don't need or that might even kill you."

An example of Briquet's syndrome, which is discussed at length in Chapter 23, is presented here.

A twenty-four-year-old woman is admitted to a medical service because of complaints of multiple foci of pain. Past history and systems review reveal forty-three medically unexplained symptoms, with symptoms in all Briquet's categories (see Chapter 23). Briquet's syndrome is diagnosed, and the patient is soon discharged to the outpatient medical clinic after being told she has Briquet's syndrome and provided with the explanation set forth above. The internist was so pleased that the diagnosis brought order out of the patient's symptomatic chaos that he wrote an article about the syndrome to inform other primary physicians.

CHRONIC PAIN

Pain that exceeds the intensity expected by the primary physician, or for which no explanation can be found, is sometimes a reason for referral. In the differential diagnosis the psychiatrist should consider primary psychiatric conditions, especially (1) malingering, (2) major depression or dysthymia, and (3) Briquet's syndrome.

When a psychiatric syndrome known to produce pain is ruled out and no other medical explanations are forthcoming, other measures are tried, regardless of proven efficacy. These include the use of fixed interval analgesic schedules, behavior modification, progressive relaxation, biofeedback, acupuncture, hypnosis, massages, warm packs, physical therapy, psychotherapy, tricyclic antidepressants (e.g. amitryptiline 150–300 mg. daily, regardless of whether the patient is depressed), or electroconvulsive therapy. Sometimes nothing alleviates pain, and here the physician must seek further consultation or explain to the patient that he must attempt to tolerate his pain.

Situations Encountered on Consultation and Liaison Services

In addition to cases where differential diagnosis may be complicated, the consultation/liaison service presents other interesting situations.

DELIRIUM AND DEMENTIA

Two syndromes associated with diffuse cognitive dysfunction are delirium and dementia. Delirium is characterized by acute or subacute onset of diffuse cognitive dysfunction, altered level of consciousness and alertness, anxiety, and agitation. Frequent accompaniments of delirium are tachycardia, irritability, muttering, suggestibility, hallucinations, illusions, delusions, asterixis (4), and generalized slowing on EEG. Delirium due to digitalis toxicity sometimes produces three-per-second EEG spikes (5). A diagnosis of delirium should be considered in patients who should be doing well but appear tired; are unable to dress, feed, and wash themselves; appear irritable and depressed despite a good "medical report"; exhibit frequent behavior changes during the day; seem intelligent but cannot follow directions; and cooperate with some procedures but not with others. Sometimes more than one cause (e.g. anemia and drug toxicity) is contributing to the delirium.

Dementia is characterized by insidious onset and chronic course of diffuse cognitive dysfunction in a patient with a clear sensorium. The EEG is sometimes abnormal but with no specific pattern. Common irreversible causes of dementia include Alzheimer's senile brain disease, CNS arteriosclerosis, and alcoholism.

Reversible dementias include nonketotic hyperposmolarity diabetic syndrome, fluid and electrolyte imbalance, normal pressure hydrocephalus, pernicious anemia and other vitamin deficiency states, malnutrition, drug reactions, thyroid disease and other endocrine disorders, environmental toxins, heart failure and arrhythmias, respiratory disease, systemic and intercranial infections, head injuries, alcoholism, space-occupying brain lesions, and brain surgery (6). In addition, there are "pseudo-dementias" (see Chapter 20) associated with major depression. Sometimes delirium and dementia coexist.

The key to management of patients with diffuse cognitive dysfunction is to identify and treat the cause. When the cause is not readily apparent, the diagnostic procedures described in Chapter 18 are in order.

Until the cause is found and corrected, or if the illness is incurable, there is a plan of management designed to prevent exacerbation, particularly at night when the environment provides insufficient orienting and supportive cues. It includes (1) using a night light; (2) redirecting lights if frightening shadows are cast on the wall; (3) having a clock and calendar in view; (4) encouraging visits by family and friends; (5) turning on television or radio; (6) making available familiar items such as photographs or newspapers; (7) prescribing, repairing, or replacing glasses or hearing aids; (8) having staff make supportive and orienting conversation; (9) keeping the patient close to or in view of the nursing station; (10) minimizing use of physical restraints—a Posey belt is preferable to full leather restraints; and (11) avoiding barbiturates and neuroleptics unless behavior is uncontrollable. In such cases haloperidol is the safest of the neuroleptics but should be avoided when delirium is caused by (1) anticholinergic toxicity (physostigmine is the proper treatment) or (2) hypnotic drug withdrawal (treatment is replacement with a hypnotic drug).

INTENSIVE CARE UNITS

Patients in intensive care units are at especially high risk for developing abnormal behavior, largely because they are among the sickest in the hospital, having conditions likely to affect brain functioning, and often receiving large amounts of potent medications. In many hospitals the setting of the intensive care unit may contribute to the problem because of the following features (7):

1. An alien environment with unfamiliar people
2. Sensory monotony, because much of the stimulation from monitors and other devices is impersonal and not thought-provoking

3. Physical discomfort due to disease
4. Crowding and lack of privacy
5. Illness and death of other patients

PATIENTS WITH VENTRICULAR IRRITABILITY

Competent consultation interviews are medically safe, with the exception of those with patients prone to ventricular arrhythmias (8). Occasionally a physician treating such a patient requests consultation because the patient's behavior jeopardizes his cardiac function. In such cases the psychiatrist should monitor the patient's pulse or EKG during the interview, especially at stressful points, and decrease the intensity of the interview or even stop it if arrhythmia develops or worsens. The following is an example where the psychiatrist must immediately "shift gears" in an interview:

A fifty-year-old man is admitted to a telemetry service with a ventricular arrhythmia due to myocardial infarction. He refuses admission to the coronary care unit (CCU); the internist asks the psychiatrist to explain the refusal. Early in the interview the patient tells the psychiatrist he was once in a semiprivate CCU where his three roommates died. The psychiatrist tells the patient, "I guess you don't want to go there because you associate it with dying."

The patient suddenly becomes pale and clutches his chest, raising his hand to convey he wishes silence. The psychiatrist, now quite anxious, says, "Okay, let's just sit a few minutes." Moments later the cardiac emergency team arrives, announcing they are responding to a ventricular tachycardia that just appeared on the monitor. But by this point the tachycardia has disappeared. The psychiatrist stops the interview several minutes later, the referral question having been vividly answered. He concludes that the patient does not want transfer to the CCU because he associates it with death and recommends continued care in the telemetry unit. He also advises that transfer should not be discussed unless the patient mentions it.

NARCOTIC ADDICTS ON MEDICAL AND SURGICAL SERVICES

Sometimes narcotic addicts are admitted to medical or surgical services for conditions (e.g. knife wound, bacterial endocarditis, lung abscess) that cannot be treated elsewhere. Although narcotic withdrawal is rarely fatal, its symptoms are uncomfortable and, if untreated, lead to noncompliance with medical and surgical care. Based on the extent of the habit, a daily dose of dolophine (Methadone), usually 10 to 20 mg. BID, can be given. This dose can be maintained throughout the patient's hospital stay or gradually tapered over one to several weeks. If the patient experiences pain (e.g. postoperative pain) unrelated to opiate withdrawal, he can be given analgesics in whatever doses would be appropriate were he not addicted. Drug addiction is discussed at length in Chapter 19.

MEDICAL/SURGICAL PATIENTS WHO REFUSE TRANSFER TO THE PSYCHIATRY SERVICE

Patients on medical/surgical services (e.g. for an "overdose") who belong on the psychiatric inpatient service will sometimes refuse transfer to the psychiatric unit while accepting medical/surgical hospitalization. The psychiatrist and primary physician have the choices of involuntary hospitalization on the psychiatric service, discharge home, or continued care on the medical/surgical service. If the patient is potentially dangerous to himself or others, involuntary psychiatric hospitalization is appropriate. If the patient is very ill but not potentially dangerous, he may be allowed to sign out against medical advice or, if he consents, permitted to remain on the medical/surgical unit for psychiatric treatment. The latter option carries some legal liability (e.g. if the patient makes a suicide attempt on the medical service) and may be contrary to hospital policy. However, if the psychiatrist and primary physician feel that better care can be provided to a relatively cooperative and noncommittable patient on a medical/surgical service than at a state psychiatric hospital or outpatient clinic, and if hospital policy permits, such treatment can be attempted on a trial basis. Such a decision requires a clear justification in the patient's chart.

SURGICAL PATIENTS

Several studies (9–12) have shown that the preoperative mental status is often predictive of postoperative morbidity and mortality from all causes. Patients with the following characteristics are prone to developing postoperative delirium (12): (1) previous or current psychiatric illness, including alcoholism, depression, coarse brain disease, or psychosis; (2) preoperative insomnia; (3) advanced age; (4) retirement adjustment problems; (5) "functional" gastroenterologic disturbance; (6) low socioeconomic status, and (7) family history of psychiatric illnesses. It is well documented that good preoperative psychological management, consisting largely of explanations of procedures and responses to questions, is associated with a better postoperative course (13, 14). Therefore, prior to elective surgery, consideration of the patient's psychiatric history and mental status by the primary physician or liaison psychiatrist, and treatment of readily treatable psychiatric conditions by a psychiatrist, are in order. Prior to any surgery the procedures and anticipated experiences of the patient should be discussed in whatever detail the patient wishes and is capable of understanding.

PLACEBOS

Outside of medical research, placebos should not be used, as about one-third of patients (15), including patients with severe illnesses such as angina pectoris (16), are placebo responders. Response to placebo does not prove the existence of a "psychiatric" or malingered cause of a symptom. One risk to using placebos is that if the patient discovers that his doctor is prescribing a placebo, he may lose trust in him.

The Mechanics of Consultations

The psychiatrist should reserve at least an hour per consultation; some of the worst consults come from five-minute "first impression" evaluations. The patient should be seen within twenty-four hours for routine consultations, and within minutes or hours for an emergency, depending on circumstances. Emergency consultations require a conversation between the primary physician and the psychiatrist, the psychiatrist specifying when he will arrive and recommending temporary measures until then. The primary physician should tell the patient a psychiatrist will arrive and should explain the reason in terms the patient can understand. The primary physician should make the psychiatrist aware of the reason for the consultation. The psychiatrist should usually extend his evaluation beyond the stated reason for the consult request.

The psychiatrist should rapidly scan the patient's chart to learn about the patient's general health, medications, lab results, past psychiatric history, and recent behaviors. He should ask the nursing staff for their observations. If he is with a resident or student, a plan of action should be made and chairs should be available for all present. The patient's privacy should be maintained whenever possible.

Once seated, the interviewer should say he is a psychiatrist and state the purpose of the interview. If the psychiatrist is with a resident or student who is trained in interviewing and diagnosis, the trainee may initiate the interview and continue for fifteen to twenty-five minutes, at which point the psychiatrist completes the interview and makes recommendations. This is usually much more efficient than having the trainee interview alone, followed by the psychiatrist's visit to the patient on another occasion. The latter strategy should be used only when the resident has previously demonstrated top-notch decision-making or when the psychiatrist runs an extremely busy service and is not immediately available.

In closing the interview, the psychiatrist should present the patient with conclusions and recommendations, adding that implementation of recommendations is the province of the patient and the primary doctor. The psychiatrist should not write orders unless requested to do so by the referring physician. Consultants traditionally make recommendations on a consultation form.

The consultation form should be filled out immediately; in rare situations where this is not possible, the psychiatrist should write in the chart, "Consultation done, note to follow today," and immediately jot down the key findings; he will forget a lot as the day wears on, especially if other interviews are done in the interim. A full consultation note, both thorough and brief, should be on the chart within several hours; postponed notes or consultations dictated into a telephone lead to unnecessary delays, which hinder the primary physician. The note should be especially detailed in the sections on differential diagnosis and recommendations, the only sections that are usually read carefully. One internist stated, "I read consults from the bottom up, and often stop at the middle." After each diagnosis is listed, it should be justified; for example, "Major depression (manifested by sustained sadness, early A.M. waking, suicidal ideas, stupor, no drugs or coarse BD)." Recommendations should also address the following points as needed:

1. Additional information needed to establish a diagnosis, (e.g. old records, history from family members, laboratory tests)
2. Degree to which current treatment may be contributing to, or ameliorating, the patient's behavioral dysfunction (e.g. advantages and disadvantages of medications being used or of interpersonal dealings with the patient)
3. Temporary and definitive medical treatments of the patient's condition, including the value of aspects of current management, addition of psychiatric (e.g. psychoactive medications or ECT) or general medical (e.g. vitamins, fluids and electrolytes) therapies
4. Noninvasive interventions (e.g. encouraging visitors, supportive conversations by nurses, visit by social worker, night light, behavior modification tactics)
5. Further involvement by the psychiatrist, if needed (e.g. follow-up visits on the ward or outpatient clinic, transfer to the psychiatry service)
6. Recommendation about further psychiatric care or discharge (e.g. "no need to postpone surgery for psychiatric reasons," "do not let patient leave the hospital," "no reason to keep patient in hospital for psychiatric reasons"). The recommendations should be explicit enough that a follow-up call from the primary physician will rarely be necessary. For example, "I have instructed patient that between 9 A.M. and 4 P.M. on the day after discharge, he should call our outpatient

clinic at 777–7777 to request an appointment with Dr. Jones for follow-up. I gave him this number and I will tell Dr. Jones about him."

The differential diagnosis and recommendations must be written by (or under intense supervision of) an experienced psychiatrist. If the consult was an emergency, the primary physician should be telephoned immediately; if not, conversation between consultant and primary physician about the case should occur only if it is likely to enhance or reinforce what the consultant has written.

Liaison Services

The psychiatrist may provide consultations only or may also do liaison work, during which he evaluates new patients, makes rounds with the primary physicians, gives lectures or case conferences on the primary service, or does research with the primary physicians. At one of our hospitals the liaison team (an attending psychiatrist working quarter-time, and one resident psychiatrist and one medical student half-time) provide (1) morning rounds once weekly on a ten-bed medical service with a medicine team consisting of an attending internist and several students and residents; (2) initial evaluation of all newly admitted medical patients; (3) a biweekly case conference in which a medical patient is interviewed in the presence of all residents and students from psychiatry and medicine; (4) one to ten formal consults per week; and (5) an ongoing research project on cognitive functions and diagnoses of medical patients. One study (17) has demonstrated better postoperative outcomes for orthopedic patients routinely seen by a liaison psychiatrist than for a matched control group of orthopedic patients not routinely seen by a psychiatrist.

One element of an effective liaison service is the primary service's desire to work with the psychiatrists. Ideally the primary service asks the psychiatrist to begin the liaison, rather than the reverse. It is also helpful if the joint morning rounds are conducted as teaching (not business) rounds with mutual desire to share principles pertinent to the patient and illness being discussed. Ideally, the level of teaching is high enough for the psychiatrists to enjoy the rounds only if the primary care subject were discussed, and the primary doctors to enjoy rounds only if psychiatric aspects of the primary specialty were covered.

"Reverse liaison" (where the psychiatry service is the primary service and the liaison physicians are from another specialty) is not yet popular but has important potential. In one study of state psychiatric hospital patients (18), 46 percent had a nonpsychiatric illness causing or intensifying the behavioral disorder, and an additional 34 percent had coexisting medical illness that could not explain the psychiatric problem.

APPENDIX: Some Drugs That Cause Psychiatric Symptoms

DRUG	REACTION	COMMENTS*
Amantadine (*Symmetrel*)	Visual hallucinations, nightmares	Occasional; more frequent in elderly
Aminocaproic acid (*Amicar*)	Acute delirium, with auditory, visual, and kinesthetic hallucinations	Immediately following bolus injection
Amitriptyline (*Elavil*; others)	Anticholinergic psychosis	*see* Atropine
Amphetamines	*see* Dextroamphetamine	
Amphotericin B (*Fungizone*)	Delirium	IV and intrathecal use
Anticonvulsants	Tactile, visual and auditory hallucinations, delirium, agitation, depression, paranoia, confusion, aggression	Usually with high doses or high plasma concentrations
Antihistamines	Anxiety, hallucinations, delirium	Especially with overdosage
Asparaginase (*Elspar*)	Confusion, depression, paranoia, bizarre behavior	Occur frequently in some studies
Atropine and anticholinergics	Confusion, memory loss, disorientation, depersonalization, delirium, auditory and visual hallucinations, fear, paranoia. Sudden incoherent speech, delirium with high fever, flushed, dry skin, visual and tactile hallucinations	More frequent in elderly and children and with high doses From eye drops, with high or repeated doses, and particularly when mistaken for nose drops, leading to overdosage
Baclofen (Lioresal)	Visual and auditory hallucinations, paranoia, insomnia, nightmares, mania, depression, anxiety, confusion	Sometimes with treatment, but usually after sudden withdrawal

204

Drug		Frequency
Barbiturates	see Phenobarbital	
Belladonna alkaloids	see Atropine	
Benztropine (*Cogentin*)	see Atropine	
Bromocriptine (*Parlodel*)	Mania, delusions, visual hallucinations, paranoia, aggressive behavior	Occasional, not dose-related symptoms may persist 6 weeks after stopping the drug
Chlordiazepoxide (*Librium*)	Probably same as diazepam	
Chloroquine (*Aralen*)	Confusion, agitation, violence, personality change, delusions, hallucinations	Several cases, one within 2 hours of single 1-gram dose
Cimetidine (*Tagamet*)	Visual and auditory hallucinations, paranoia, bizarre speech, confusion, delirium, disorientation, depression	Many reports; usually with high dosage, more frequent in elderly and with renal dysfunction
Clonazepam (*Clonopin*)	Probably same as diazepam	
Clorazepate (*Azene; Tranxene*)	Probably same as diazepam	
Contraceptives, oral	Depression	15% in one study
Corticosteroids (*prednisone, cortisone, ACTH*, others)	Mania, depression, confusion, paranoia, visual and auditory hallucinations, catatonia	More common with high dosage or rapid increase but can also occur with low dose for short periods
Cyclopentolate (*Cyclogyl*)	see Atropine	Eye drops
Cycloserine (*Seromycin*)	Anxiety, depression, confusion, disorientation, hallucinations, paranoia	Common

---

*Frequency is unknown with many drugs; adverse effects are usually underreported.

(*Continued*)

DRUG	REACTION	COMMENTS
Dapsone (*Avlosulfon*)	Insomnia, irritability, uncoordinated speech, agitation, acute psychosis	Occasional, even with low doses
Desipramine (*Pertofrane*)	Anticholinergic psychosis	*see* Atropine
Dextroamphetamine	Bizarre behavior, hallucinations, paranoia	Usually with overdose or abuse, but can occur with lower doses
	Depression	On withdrawal
Diazepam (*Valium*)	Rage, excitement, hallucinations, depression, suicidal thoughts	Can occur with usual doses; depression and hallucinations can occur on withdrawal
Diethylopropion (*Tenuate*)	*see* Dextroamphetamine	
Digitalis glycosides	Nightmares, euphoria, confusion, delusions, amnesia, belligerence, visual hallucinations, paranoia	Usually with excessive dosage or high plasma concentrations; more frequent in elderly
Disopyramide (*Norpace*)	Agitation, depression, paranoia, auditory and visual hallucinations, panic	3 patients, within 24–48 hours after starting treatment
Disulfiram (*Antabuse*)	Delirium, depression, paranoia, auditory hallucinations	Not related to alcohol reaction
Doxepin (*Adapin; Sinequan*)	Anticholinergic psychosis	*see* Atropine
Ephedrine	Hallucinations, paranoia	Excessive dosage
Ethchlorvynol (*Placidyl*)	Agitation, confusion, disorientation, hallucinations, paranoia	Continued use or on withdrawal
Ethosuximide (*Zarontin*)	*see* Anticonvulsants	

Fenfluramine (*Pondimin*)	*see* Dextroamphetamine	
Halothane (*Fluothane*)	Depression	Postoperative period
Imipramine (*Tofranil*; others)	Anticholinergic psychosis	*see* Atropine
Indomethacin (*Indocin*)	Depression, confusion, hallucinations, anxiety, hostility, paranoia, depersonalization	Especially in elderly
Isoniazid (*INH*; others)	Depression, agitation, auditory and visual hallucinations, paranoia	Several reports
Ketamine (*Ketalar*; *Ketaject*)	Nightmares, hallucinations, crying, delirium, changes in body image	Frequent with usual doses
Levodopa (*Dopar*; others)	Delirium, depression, agitation, hypomania, nightmares, night terrors, visual and auditory hallucinations, paranoia	More frequent in elderly; risk increases with prolonged use
Lidocaine (*Xylocaine*)	Disorientation	
Methamphetamine	*see* Dextroamphetamine	
Methyldopa (*Aldomet*)	Depression, hallucinations, paranoia, amnesia	Several reports
Methylphenidate (*Ritalin*)	Hallucinations	In children
Methysergide (*Sansert*)	Depersonalization, hallucinations	Occasional
Metrizamide (*Amipaque*)	Confusion, disorientation, hallucinations, depression	Can occur frequently
Nalidixic acid (*NegGram*)	Confusion, depression, excitement, visual hallucinations	Rare

(Continued)

APPENDIX (*Continued*)

DRUG	REACTION	COMMENTS*
Niridazole (*Ambilhar*)	Confusion, hallucinations, mania, suicide	More likely with higher doses
Nortriptyline (*Aventyl*)	Anticholinergic psychosis	*see* Atropine
Pentazocine (*Talwin*)	Nightmares, hallucinations, disorientation, panic, paranoia, depersonalization, depression	During treatment
Phenelzine (*Nardil*)	Paranoia, delusions, fear, rage, aggressive behavior	Symptoms may resolve quickly after drug is stopped
Phenmetrazine (*Preludin*)	*see* Dextroamphetamine	
Phenobarbital	Excitement, hyperactivity, visual hallucinations, depression, delirium tremens-like syndrome	On withdrawal, or with usual doses in some children and the elderly, or with overdosage in epilepsy
Phentermine (*Fastin*; others)	*see* Dextroamphetamine	
Phenylephrine (*Neo-Synephrine*)	Depression, visual and tactile hallucinations, paranoia	Overuse of nasal spray
Phenytoin (*Dilantin*, others)	*see* Anticonvulsants	
Primidone (*Mysoline*)	*see* Anticonvulsants	
Procainamide (*Pronestyl*)	Paranoia, hallucinations	Uncommon
Procaine Penicillin G	Terror, hallucinations, disorientation, agitation, bizarre behavior	Probably due to procaine; occurs occasionally, 33 patients in 1 report

Drug	Effects	Comments
Propoxyphene (*Darvon*)	Auditory hallucinations, confusion	Usually with high doses
Propranolol (*Inderal*)	Depression, confusion, nightmares, visual and auditory hallucinations, paranoia	Several reports, with usual doses and after dosage increase
Protriptyline (*Vivactil*)	Anticholinergic psychosis	*see* Atropine
Quinacrine (*Atabrine*)	Bizarre dreams, anxiety, hallucinations, delirium	Can occur with usual doses but more common with high doses
Rauwolfia aklaloids (*reserpine: Serpasil*, others; *rauwolfia: Raudixin*, others)	Depression	Occurs commonly with doses higher than 0.5 mg. daily; may continue for months after drug is stopped
Scopolamine (*Hyoscine*)	*see* Atropine	*see* Atropine
Sulindac (*Clinoril*)	Paranoia, rage, personality change	Reported in 5 patients
Thiabendazole (*Mintezol*)	Hallucinations	Occasional
Tricyclic antidepressants	Anticholinergic psychosis	*see* Atropine
Trihexyphenidyl (*Artane*)	*see* Atropine	*see* Atropine
Trimipramine (*Surmontil*)	Anticholinergic psychosis	*see* Atropine
Vinblastine (*Velban*)	Depression	Occasionally
Vincristine (*Oncovin*)	Hallucinations	Less than 5% of patients, high doses

Source: *The Medical Letter on Drugs and Therapeutics* 23 (1981): 9–12. Used by permission.

References

1. Knights, E. B.; Folstein, M. F. Unsuspected emotional and cognitive disturbance in medical patients. *Ann. Int. Med. 87:* 723–24, 1977.
2. Sierles, F. S.; Taylor, M. A.; Herschberg, S.; *et al.* Cognitive deficits in medical inpatients. Manuscript in preparation, 1984.
3. (Unsigned). Some drugs that cause psychiatric symptoms. *The Medical Letter* New Rochelle, N.Y. *23:* 9–12, 1981.
4. Wells, C. E.; Duncan, G. W. *Neurology for Psychiatrists.* Philadelphia: F. A. Davis, 1980, p. 51.
5. Douglas, E. F.; White, P. T.; Newlson, J. W. Three per second spike wave in digitalis toxicity. *Arch. Neurol. 25:* 373–75, 1971.
6. Wells, C. E. The Organic Brain Syndromes. In Strain, J. J. (ed.), *Psychiatric Clinics of North America: The Medically Ill Patient.* Philadelphia: Saunders, 1981.
7. Kimball, C. P. Psychosomatic Theories and Their Contributions to Chronic Illness. In Usdin, G. (ed.), *Psychiatric Medicine.* New York: Brunner/Mazel, 1977.
8. Lown, B.; Desilva, R. A.; Reich, P.; *et al.* Psychophysiologic factors in sudden cardiac death. *Am. J. Psychiat. 137:* 1325–35, 1980.
9. Kimball, C. P. Psychological responses to the experience of open heart surgery. *Am. J. Psychiat. 125:* 348–52, 1969.
10. Abram, H. S.; Gill, B. Predictions of post-operative psychiatric complications. *New Eng. J. Med. 265:* 1123, 1961.
11. Kennedy, T.; Bakst, H. The influence of emotion in the outcome of cardiac surgery: A predictive study. *Bull. N.Y. Acad. Med. 42:* 311, 1966.
12. Morse, R.; Litin, E. Post-operative delirium: A study of etiologic factors. *Am. J. Psychiat. 126:* 388, 1969.
13. Lazarus, H.; Hagens, T. Prevention of psychosis following open heart surgery. *Am. J. Psychiat. 124:* 1190, 1968.
14. Egbert, L.; Battet, G.; Welch, C.; Bartlett, H. Reduction of post-operative pain by encouragement and instruction of patients. *New Eng. J. Med. 270:* 825, 1964.
15. Beecher, H. K. *Measurement of Subjective Responses.* New York: Oxford University Press, 1959.
16. Evans, W.; Hayle, C. The comparative value of drugs used in the continuous treatment of angina pectoris. *J. Med. 2:* 311–38, 1933.
17. Levitan, S. J.; Kornfeld, D. S. Clinical and cost benefits of liaison psychiatry. *Am. J. Psychiat. 138:* 790–93, 1981.
18. Hall, R. C. W.; Gardner, E. R.; Stickney, S. K.; *et al.* Physical illness manifesting as psychiatric disease: 2. Analysis of a state hospital inpatient population. *Arch. Gen. Psychiat. 37:* 989–95, 1980.

PART III

CLINICAL GROUPS

CHAPTER 11

Affective Disorders

The affective disorders are highly prevalent in the general population, with estimates ranging as high as 25 percent in one door-to-door sampling of the population of New Haven (1). Most patients identified as ill in such studies are suffering from milder forms of depressive illness and are rarely treated in the hospital. Recent studies using modern operational diagnostic criteria report private hospital admission prevalence rates of about 25 percent (2) with a large excess of depressives over manics. But in many public hospital units for the treatment of acutely ill psychiatric patients, the majority of affective admissions will suffer from mania (3). In one study of 465 consecutive patients admitted to an acute treatment university service of a public hospital (4), 26 percent received a research diagnosis of mania and 9 percent one of depression.

Although the syndromes of depression and mania were well known to nineteenth-century psychiatrists, it was Emil Kraepelin who synthesized the available information and defined the clinical entity of manic-depressive illness, linking the two syndromes in a single diagnosis. At the same time he was able to separate manic-depressive illness from the other major functional psychosis, dementia praecox, by demonstrating important differences in symptoms, course, and outcome for the two entities. Of these, course and outcome were most compelling, with manic-depressives exhibiting a phasic pattern of recurrent attacks of illness, restoration of premorbid levels of

213

functioning between attacks, and a nondeteriorating course, contrasting sharply with the relentless progression of dementia praecox, which terminated in a permanent defect state.

Kraepelin also observed that affective disorders tend to run in families, and numerous investigations over the years have confirmed the genetic transmission of manic-depressive illness (5). The risk for developing affective disorder in any first-degree relative of an affectively ill proband is variously estimated at 8 to 42 percent (mean = 18.4 percent), approximately seven times that for the general population. The mode of transmission is probably multifactoral, requiring the summation of several independent factors to exceed the threshold for manifestation of the illness. Nongenetic factors doubtless also play a role, and one of the most influential is the sex of the patient. Women are at considerably greater risk for affective disorder (unipolar or bipolar) than men, and this observation cannot generally be explained by sex-linked transmission (6). Probably certain biological (hormonal?) patterns peculiar to the female sex predispose to the development of affective illness, but these factors are at present obscure.

Much research into the biology of the affective disorders has yielded few hard facts. Certainly the simplistic view of depression as a deficiency (and mania an excess) of catechol- or indole-amines remains unsubstantiated almost twenty years after it was first proposed (7), and more complex variations on this basic theme have also so far failed to provide a viable hypothesis for the etiology of the affective disorders. The fact that both mania and depression are responsive to the same agents (e.g. lithium, ECT) militates against any simple deficiency/excess model, and the failures of the cerebral amine precursors (L-dopa, tryptophan, 5-hydroxytryptophan) to relieve depression and of the amine antagonists (methysergide, alphamethyldopa) to relieve mania have rendered the amine hypotheses mainly of historical interest. Neuroendocrine investigations have been somewhat more rewarding, demonstrating excessive cortisol production in melancholia with resistance to suppression by exogenous steroids (8)—although contradictory data exist (9)—and a blunted response of the pituitary in releasing thyroid-stimulating hormone after provocation with thyrotropin-releasing hormone (10) or growth hormone after hypoglycemia (11).

Depressive Syndromes

There are several dichotomous classifications of the depressive syndromes, doubtless reflecting a genuine bimodal distribution of depressive symptoms in any large unselected sample of depressed patients. The *primary/secondary* dichotomy was introduced by the Washington University group in order to isolate a homogeneous sample of depressives for research purposes (12).

The group defined primary depression as occurring in a patient who either had never been ill before or had received only a prior diagnosis of affective disorder. Secondary depression occurred in a patient who had received a prior diagnosis of a nonaffective illness (e.g. alcoholism, personality disorder). By limiting their research samples to primary depressives, the investigators were able to reduce the variance introduced by an underlying nonaffective illness and to increase the probability of demonstrating familial differences among depressives, patients with other diagnoses, and normal control samples. This proved very useful for selecting research samples, but the group of primary depressives is nonetheless clinically heterogeneous. A substantial number of recently bereaved persons, for example, satisfy criteria for primary depression, but neither they nor their physician believe they are either ill or in need of treatment (13). Moreover, about half of all primary depressives suffer from reactive depression (14), a fact that makes the treatment and prognosis of primary depression extremely variable.

The *unipolar/bipolar* dichotomy was introduced by Leonhard (15), who reported different familial transmission in depressed patients with and without a prior diagnosis of mania, a finding confirmed by Perris (16). Perris's data showed a preferential loading of bipolar illness in first-degree relatives of bipolar probands, and the analogous finding for relatives of unipolar probands. Although this classification is widely used and firmly ensconced in modern diagnostic systems, there is increasing evidence that it may not be valid. Several recent genetic studies have failed to find any significant difference in the morbid risk for unipolar and bipolar affective disorder in the first-degree relatives of unipolar and bipolar probands (5), suggesting that Kraepelin's original description of a single disorder may well have been correct.

Another dichotomy is *bipolar I/II* (17), introduced to differentiate depressed patients with a clear history of treated mania (bipolar I) from those with a history of manic symptoms mild enough to go untreated (bipolar II). No significant biological, familial, or treatment-response differences between bipolar I and II patients have ever been conclusively demonstrated, and certainly no clinical purpose is served in observing this separation.

A trichotomous classification has been introduced by Winokur and associates (18), based entirely on familial data. In their system *pure (or familial) depressive disease* arises in a patient who has a family history of depression; *depressive spectrum disease* in a patient with a family history of alcoholism or antisocial personality; and *sporadic depressive disease* in a patient with a family history negative for any psychiatric illness. This classification has proved heuristically valuable in that it has succeeded in accurately identifying those depressed patients who fail to suppress their endogenous cortisol production in response to an oral dose of dexamethasone. In this study most of the nonsuppressors were in the familial group, with a smaller number in the sporadic group and none in the spectrum group. If those results are confirmed, the classification will have great research power. It is unclear at this writing whether it will also have important treatment implications.

The *endogenous/reactive* dichotomy is the oldest. It originally implied that there were two types of depressive patterns, one characterized by reactivity of mood and one that arose from within, as an unexplained and an ununderstandable phenomenon. The validity of the endogenous/reactive dichotomy derives from several sources. A number of investigators have applied factor, regression, or discriminant function analyses to checklists of depressed patients, and related the symptom clusters obtained to the response to ECT or tricyclic antidepressants (19). In most instances the clinical features correlating best with a favorable response to treatment were those of endogenous depression, whereas failure to respond correlated with features of reactive depression. Two laboratory measures, described in more detail below, have also been used to separate the two types. In the sedation threshold test (20) endogenous depressives are relatively sensitive to the central effects of intravenously administered barbiturates, while the reverse is true for reactive depressives. In the dexamethasone suppression test, almost all depressives with a positive test have the endogenous syndrome, and almost none of the reactive depressives show a positive test (8).

Overlapping to a large extent with the endogenous/reactive dichotomy is the division of depressed patients into *neurotic or psychotic* groups. As generally used, neurotic depression approximates reactive depression, but psychotic depressives are a narrower group than endogenous depressives, defined by the presence of hallucinations or delusions, yielding a pure group of psychotic endogenous depressives and a mixed group of nonpsychotic endogenous depressives plus reactive depressives, with the latter group exhibiting a heterogeneous outcome in response to somatic treatments.

For the clinician the most useful classification is that which serves as a guide to treatment and prognosis, and for this purpose the endogenous/reactive dichotomy works best. It is important to note that the terms endogenous and reactive have no etiologic implications. In fact, both types of depression are equally likely to have been preceded by an identifiable environmental stress or precipitating event (21). The two terms merely identify symptom clusters, or syndromes, and might just as well be called Type I and Type II depression. The term melancholia, as described in *DSM-III*, is probably preferable to the phrase "endogenous depression," as it avoids any suggestion of etiology. Dysthymic disorder is the closest *DSM-III* approximation to reactive depression but lacks the specificity of symptoms described in the classical literature and is clearly not coterminous with the latter class.

Tables 11–1 and 11–2 show the clinical features differentially associated with endogenous and reactive depression. Many of the endogenous symptoms are "vegetative" in nature and presumably relate to dysfunction in the

TABLE 11-1   Characteristic Features of Endogenous Depression (Melancholia)

Depressed Mood
Distinct quality, different from "normal" feelings of depression
Not reactive or responsive to environment
Relentless; patient does not experience any "good" days
Diurnal variation, worse in A.M.
Anhedonia, total loss of enjoyment in usual activities, friends, even family

Thought Content
Guilt, self-reproach, self-blame
Worthlessness, low self-esteem
Hopelessness
Suicide, fatal attempts typical
Loss of insight into abnormal nature of experiences

Physiological
Insomnia, with early morning waking (difficulty staying asleep)
Anorexia, must be strongly encouraged to eat
Weight loss, usually >5 lb. in two to three weeks
Loss of libido
Decreased intestinal secretions/motility, constipation
Inability to cry, no tears
Oligomenorrhea, amenorrhea

Motor
Retardation, may progress to stupor
Agitation
Omega sign (fixed, furrowed brow)
Veraguth's folds (fixed, distant, or hollow stare)
May have catatonic features

Cognition
Impaired attention concentration, can't read or watch TV
Impaired memory, forgetfulness
Slowed thinking, delayed verbal responses

Psychosis
Delusions or hallucinations of guilt, sin, poverty, ill health, death

Premorbid Personality
Stable, may be obsessional

Laboratory Tests
Positive dexamethasone test
Blunted TRH response to TSH
Blunted growth hormone response to amphetamine
Low sedation threshold

Response to Treatment
ECT: Excellent
Tricyclic antidepressants: good–excellent
Lithium: good–excellent
MAOIs: poor
Insight-oriented psychotherapy: poor

TABLE 11-2 Characteristic Features of Reactive Depression (Dysthymia)

Depressed Mood
Quality similar to "normal mood swings"
Reactive to environment
Fluctuating; patient has some "good" days
Tendency to anhedonia responds to suggestion/persuasion
Anxiety, lability, irritability, and dysphoria may also be present
Weeps easily; lachrymose

Thought Content
Tendency to blame others or outside circumstances for troubles
Self-pity
Helplessness
Suicide, nonfatal attempts typical
Full insight into abnormal nature of experiences

Physiological
Insomnia with difficulty falling asleep, followed by tendency to oversleep
Anorexia, but eats "because I know I have to" (may overeat)
Weight loss, <5 lb. in two to three weeks (may gain weight)

Premorbid Personality
"Neurotic" traits in childhood, adulthood
Unstable, histrionic, impulsive, hypochondriacal

Laboratory Tests
Negative DST
High sedation threshold

Response to Treatment
ECT: poor
Tricyclics: poor–fair
Lithium: unknown
MAOIs: good–excellent
Cognitive psychotherapy: good–excellent

autonomic and neuroendocrine systems controlled by the hypothalamus (22). Thus alterations in circadian (diurnal) rhythms occur, affecting the sleep–wake cycle; the menstrual cycle and libido are affected; appetite, G–I secretions, and motility are impaired; and there are measurable alterations in heart rate, sweating, and body temperature. These symptoms are lacking in reactive depression, which in turn is characterized predominantly by characterological abnormalities, inadequacies, and a variety of anxiety-related symptoms (19).

Specific criteria which we have found useful in the diagnosis of melancholia (5) require the presence of a sad or dysphoric mood, plus any three of the following: early waking, worse in the A.M.; >5-lb. weight loss in three weeks; retardation or agitation; suicidal thoughts or behavior; and feelings of guilt, hopelessness, or worthlessness.

DIAGNOSTIC PROCEDURES

There are several investigative procedures that have been used in the differential diagnosis of affective disorder.

Sedation Threshold Test

Developed in an attempt to predict response to ECT, the sedation threshold test was found also to differentiate endogenous from reactive depression (20). The test is performed by preparing a 10 percent solution of sodium thiopental and slowly injecting it intravenously at a rate of 5 mg./kg./minute until the sedation threshold is reached. This threshold has been defined differently by different investigators, using clinical, electroencephalographic, and electrodermal end points. The clinical end point is reached when the patient develops a fine horizontal nystagmus or slurred speech; the electroencephalographic end point is defined by a sharp fall-off in the rate of increase in barbiturate-induced high-voltage beta activity; and the electrodermal end point occurs when the galvanic skin response is abolished (23). A total administered dose of 3.5 mg./kg. or less is associated with a diagnosis of endogenous depression and a favorable response to ECT, and 4.0 mg./kg. or more with reactive depression and an unfavorable ECT response. This method is better than 90 percent accurate in separating these groups, yet it is rarely used. The problem is that the clinical end point is not reliable, and the electrophysiological end points require expensive equipment and someone to operate it while the physician performs the test. At present the test is mainly of theoretical interest.

Dexamethasone Suppression Test (DST)

There is ample evidence that endogenous depressives exhibit elevated serum cortisol levels and a shift in peak cortisol secretion levels to earlier in the day, much like patients with diencephalic Cushing's syndrome (8). The fact that the excessive cortisol secretion fails to suppress in response to exogenously administered steroids forms the basis for what has recently been optimistically described as "a specific laboratory test for the diagnosis of melancholia": the DST (8). Borrowed from the internists, the DST is performed by administering 1 mg. dexamethasone at 11:30 P.M. and obtaining plasma cortisol levels at 4:00 P.M. and 11:00 P.M. the next day. A cortisol level at either time greater than 5 mcg./dl. is defined as abnormal and is 96 percent specific and 67 percent sensitive in diagnosing endogenous depression in psychiatric inpatients. False positive test results occur under various circumstances, including pregnancy, Cushing's disease, malnutrition, administration of barbiturates and other enzyme-inducers, and major systemic illness. Abnormal DSTs are reported to return toward normal with successful treatments (24). One recent study, however, failed to confirm the diagnostic accuracy of the DST (9).

Thyroid-Stimulating Hormone (TSH) Response to Thyrotropin-Releasing Hormone (TRH)

Although less widely studied than the DST, the response of TSH to TRH has been observed by several workers to be blunted in about one-third of endogenous depressives (10).

The procedure is done as follows: after an overnight fast, a baseline sample of blood is obtained and 500 mg. of TRH administered intravenously in a bolus. Repeated blood samples are then obtained at fifteen, thirty, sixty, and ninety minutes. A peak value of less than 6 mcU./ml. is considered blunted.

There is some evidence that combining the results of the DST and TSH response tests provides greater discriminating ability than using either one alone (10).

HOSPITAL MANAGEMENT

Endogenous depressives, in contrast to reactive depressives, usually require hospitalization, most often because of the presence of serious suicidal ruminations or attempts in the former group or other severe symptoms such as profound anorexia and weight loss, retardation or stupor, or psychosis. Such seriously depressed patients should be treated in a locked unit under close observation. Even in the absence of specific suicidal ideation or behavior, melancholics present a markedly increased suicidal risk (25), particularly if they are older, have lost a spouse, or are in poor physical health. No attempt should be made to engage them in group or occupational therapy, as their inability to participate in such activities only makes them feel worse. All forms of exploratory and interpretive psychotherapy are also interdicted. These patients feel guilty and worthless enough as it is without being informed that their problems really result from "anger turned inward against the self." On the contrary, patients should be informed that their illness has a biological basis that is not under their voluntary control, and that there is every expectation that they will make a speedy and full recovery. The message may have to be repeated frequently during the hospital stay, as the patient's self-doubts and guilty ruminations quickly erase the modest effects of such comforting medical reassurance. Once recovered, however, many patients will describe the gratitude they felt but were unable to express for such support.

The role of the nursing and other professional staff with regard to severely depressed patients is to provide the much-needed support and reassurance, to encourage the patients' acceptance of and compliance with the primary treatment offered, to observe and record the patients' behavior, and to prevent them from committing suicide. Acutely suicidal patients may require continual one-to-one observation, and staff must be aware that it is possible for a determined patient to kill himself by running at full speed and ramming his head against the wall.

Patients should be weighed daily and their sleep carefully charted, both to document alterations in these critical areas and to provide a baseline for assessing improvement. Severely depressed patients should not be permitted prolonged visits with family until significant improvement has occurred. Many endogenous depressives are unable to feel any emotion even for their loved ones, and seeing them only increases their guilt and self-reproach. Nighttime sedation should be administered liberally in the presence of severe insomnia, and the barbiturates (e.g. 360 mg. sodium amobarbital, q H.S.) are more effective hypnotics than the newer anxiolytic sedatives such as flurazepam.

ECT, tricyclic and tetracyclic antidepressants (TCA), and lithium are the mainstays of treatment in endogenous depression. Each method is described in detail elsewhere in this volume (see Chapters 5 and 6). In general, we believe that if a patient is severely depressed enough to require inpatient care, he should be offered ECT as the initial treatment. This is all the more true for those who have already failed a course of TCA prior to admission. Those who refuse ECT may be treated with TCA or lithium but should be informed that the treatment will take longer and may not provide as thorough a result.

The following cases illustrate some of these points.

A twenty-five-year-old single black medical student was admitted, stating: "I'm depressed. I don't know whether I can function in medical school." For two months prior to admission he had not gone to school and had remained at home all day. There were insomnia and feelings of hopelessness and worthlessness, but no anorexia or weight loss. One week prior to admission he took an overdose of medication, having left a suicide note, but he was treated in a local emergency room and released.

His first illness episode, of which the present one was really an extension, had begun five months earlier with feelings of apprehension, fear over meeting new people, and an impulsive, wrist-slashing suicide gesture. Hospitalization for a month resulted in little change, and he remained at home after discharge until the present illness began.

On admission to hospital he demonstrated marked psychomotor retardation, a sorrowful facial expression, and feelings of guilt, worthlessness, and hopelessness.

Imipramine, 200 mg. p.o., H.S., was started on the third hospital day, with improvement noted after twelve days of treatment. He became cheerful at times and lost the feelings of guilt, hopelessness, and worthlessness. He went on home leave without any problems and was discharged, markedly improved after one month in hospital, on imipramine, 200 mg. p.o., H.S.

He attended an outpatient clinic, where imipramine was discontinued after one month because he had maintained his improvement. Two weeks later he became increasingly taciturn and expressed delusional ideas of guilt: "I am just evil and spent too much time chasing girls." "I turned loose all the gold in the world." "Troops are coming to get me." He rarely left his room and neglected his personal hygiene. Imipramine was restarted at the same dose, but without effect. Two weeks later he was readmitted and advised to have ECT, but he and his family refused. Imipramine was continued, but on the seventh hospital day he was found in his bedroom attempting to hang himself with his belt. There was profound psychomotor retardation and the patient spoke only three sentences in fifteen minutes: "What is happening to everybody?" "What did they do to Arthur Ashe?" "I can't watch the news, it's so depressing." His mother's consent was obtained and emergency ECT given that afternoon. A week later he smiled appropriately, had a normal rate of speech, and felt he could do well in medical school. After the fifth ECT he appeared happy and expressed an active interest in things. He was discharged, fully recovered, after six ECT. (N.B.: One year later he was admitted in a state of acute mania, which responded to lithium therapy.)

This case is of interest in that it demonstrates a reasonably good response to tricyclic antidepressants in a nonpsychotic endogenous depression, but failure of the identical regimen (and a dramatic response to ECT) in the same patient when he developed psychotic symptoms.

Although the specific indications for lithium versus tricyclic antidepressants have yet to be defined, the following case illustrates the striking effects that can be achieved with lithium alone in endogenous depression:

A twenty-two-year-old married white woman was admitted after slashing her throat because "it was all there was left to do." She had become depressed about a month prior to admission and received amitriptyline, 150 mg./day, from a local physician. Despite this her symptoms progressively worsened, and she told her husband that "God keeps telling me I'm guilty of causing all the suffering and death of the little children."

There was no prior history of psychiatric illness, although the husband described her as having rapid mood swings.

On admission to hospital she was agitated, perplexed, and showed impaired concentration and markedly slowed thinking. She felt "guilty for all the world's troubles and sin" and wanted "to be punished." There were complete auditory hallucinations, thought insertion, and thought broadcasting: "I'm embarrassed at the thoughts you are hearing."

Lithium therapy was started on the fourth hospital day at 1,200 mg./day, and by the end of one week she had improved markedly. By the end of the second week she had recovered completely, at a serum lithium level of 0.83 mEq/L, and was discharged home on maintenance lithium therapy.

A course of six to nine bilateral ECT is generally sufficient to induce a full remission in most endogenous depressives. Where the clinical presentation is unequivocal and uncontaminated by complicating or atypical features such as obessionality, hypochondriasis, or mood-incongruent psychotic symptoms, 95 to 100 percent of patients should be fully restored to their normal state of health, as illustrated by the following patient:

A thirty-five-year-old single, white physical therapist was admitted, complaining "The world is coming to an end." "I am no good." "I did a lot of bad things." "The whole world gangs up on me." For the week prior to admission he had been agitated, constantly pacing about the house, and experienced anorexia as well as initial and terminal insomnia. He heard voices calling him "no good," felt depressed and guilty, and told his father "Eternity is here." The night before admission he awakened a neighbor to tell him, "The world is coming to an end."

He first became ill ten years prior to admission, when he was mute and depressed, and recovered with ECT. He remained well until a year prior to admission when he again became depressed and told people, "The end of the world is coming." Treatment with a combination of neuroleptics and tricyclic antidepressants was only partially effective, and he remained intermittently symptomatic until the present admission.

In hospital he appeared sad and retarded. There were complete auditory hallucinations and delusions of guilt: "I hear voices of men and women who say I am no good—a murderer, a pervert, a child molester." He claimed he had sold himself to the devil: "I smell brimstone and hell." "I saw a dead man walking on the road, am bad and no good, am in a different dimension."

Bilateral ECT was started five days after admission, and by the third treatment there was complete resolution of delusions, hallucinations, depressed mood, and psychomotor retardation. A total of six ECT were given, after which he became very active in recreational and occupational therapy and exhibited a transient euphoria. He was discharged three and a half weeks after admission, fully recovered, to return to his home and work.

The presence of so-called schizophrenic symptoms in no way alters the favorable response to ECT in endogenous depression (26), as demonstrated by this case:

A forty-seven-year-old white maintenance man was brought to the hospital because of "unusual behavior." Several days prior to admission he claimed the TV was talking directly to him and asked his mother to "shoot me with a gun." Later he claimed his mother was dead, heard "noises in my head," and refused to speak. He felt his thoughts were broadcast aloud for others to hear and that they came "from Satan." On the day of admission he claimed he could "control the destiny of the Earth and change people."

He first became ill at age twenty-three, at which time he received ECT and insulin coma therapy for depression and for saying he was "going to straighten Russia out." A second brief hospitalization occurred at age forty-one, after the death of his father, followed by two more hospitalizations for depression at ages forty-four and forty-five.

On admission he was initially mute, perplexed, and agitated and had a vacant stare. Gait was slow and hesitant, and at one point he fell to his knees in a prayerful posture. When he spoke, he exhibited blocking, derailment, and nonsequiturs, as well as grandiose delusions. During the first week of hospitalization he exhibited intermittent muteness and posturing, with interspersed echolalia and verbigeration. On the tenth day he had to be removed from the top of a locker in his room where he had climbed in an apparent suicide attempt. The following day he was given two bilateral ECT spaced several minutes apart; the day after the procedure he was improved, and over the next two or three days showed rapid resolution of his symptoms without further ECT. He began to eat well; became alert, oriented, and cheerful; and expressed a sense of hopefulness about the future. He dressed in street clothes and was given full privileges, which he handled successfully. He was discharged, fully recovered, three weeks later, having received no further treatment.

Following a successful course of ECT all patients should be given a three- to six-month course of maintenance drug therapy in order to prevent relapse. Either TCA or lithium may be used, as both have been shown to reduce the relapse rate significantly (27). TCA dosages for post-ECT maintenance are the same as those used in treating acutely ill depressives (e.g. imipramine or amitriptyline, 200–250 mg./day), and if plasma levels are monitored, these should be kept in the standard therapeutic range (see p. 134). The dose of lithium should also be adjusted to maintain a serum level close to 1.0 mEq/L. These drugs are equally effective in preventing relapse in unipolar and bipolar depressives.

Perhaps 10 percent of patients will relapse despite maintenance drug therapy. Such patients are candidates for maintenance ECT (see p. 134).

Reactive Depression

It is quite clear from the literature as well as general clinical experience that reactive depressives do not respond well to ECT or TCA and may even feel worse after receiving such treatments (28, 29). They tolerate poorly the side effects of both methods, developing a host of complaints that serve as foci for hypochondriacal ruminations. Reactive depression is part of a group of disorders in which lifelong personality attitudes (e.g. histrionic, impulsive) interact with a variety of neurotic traits and psychophysiological symptom patterns. Other related disorders include anxiety neurosis and agoraphobia, both of which may also present with depressive symptoms. Monoamine oxidase inhibitors (MAOIs) are effective pharmacological agents in the management of reactive depression and are also of use in the anxiety and phobic disorders mentioned (30). Phenelzine is the most widely used MAOI and the compound for which the best efficacy data exist. Phenelzine should be initiated at 45 mg./day orally, in two divided doses, and increased by 15 mg. a day to a total daily dose of 75–90 mg./day (about 1.2 mg./kg. body weight). MAOIs may take longer than TCAs to exhibit their effects, and treatment should be continued for at least three weeks before declaring it a failure. The response rate is about 60–70 percent. There is increasing evidence that, in contrast to melancholia, reactive (nonendogenous) depressives are responsive to psychotherapy (31). The specific method that has been successful in controlled trials is cognitive therapy, a procedure in which the patient is made aware of the inappropriate way in which he views himself in relation to others and is encouraged to alter this self-defeating self-image. There is some evidence that combined pharmacotherapy–psychotherapy is more effective than either method alone (31, 32), hence such combined therapy should probably be considered the treatment of choice in reactive depression.

Bereavement (Mourning)

Recently bereaved persons may experience many symptoms of depression, including some endogenous symptoms as well. However, such persons do not feel "ill" and generally do not seek psychiatric care (33). The symptoms of bereavement are best resolved within "the bosom of the family" if such family exists, and not by removal of the bereaved person to the unfamiliar environment of the hospital. If the bereaved person has no family or friends to fall back on, a brief period of hospitalization with sedation and sympathetic discussions may help tide him over a difficult period.

Depressive Pseudodementia

It is now well established that primary endogenous depression in older patients may initially present as a dementing disorder, with diffuse decrements in cognitive functioning, most marked in the areas of attention, concentration, and registration (34). Such patients are often incorrectly diagnosed as having senile dementia by physicians who have failed to note, or have discounted, the presence of insomnia, weight loss, retardation, and other features of endogenous depression. Sadness or despondency may be absent, and the patient may simply appear perplexed or bewildered. Scores on the Mini-Mental State Examination (p. 42) average around 20 points (range 15–25) and may be in the demented range. These individuals, often living alone, in their confusion neglect to feed and clothe themselves properly, presenting a misleading picture of profound organic deterioration.

ECT is the treatment of choice in depressive pseudodementia and may produce very striking improvement after only a few treatments. Along with the clinical improvement comes improvement in the cognitive dysfunction, and any fears that ECT might worsen the memory disturbance are unwarranted. So long as depressive symptoms are present, the marked confusion and memory loss that may be noted are a strong indication, rather than a contraindication, for ECT.

Mania

Mania is entirely subsumed under the rubric of bipolar affective disorder, for which the presence of one manic episode is both necessary and sufficient. The risk for mania in the general population is about 0.1 percent (5), and manics constitute up to 25 percent of acute public psychiatric hospital admissions (35). It is not surprising that one recent population prevalence study found no manics in a door-to-door survey of New Haven (1). Most are far too ill to remain at home.

There is no equivalent for mania of the endogenous/reactive dichotomy, although cases of secondary mania are well known (36) and may occur in relation to such exogenous causes as viral infections, toxic states, head trauma, and cerebral hemorrhage. Kraepelin classified mania into various stages ranging from hypomania to delirious mania (37). This classification has neither practical nor theoretical significance, as it merely represents a continuum along a severity axis.

The diagnosis of mania by American psychiatrists fell into eclipse in the middle years of this century, *pari passu* with a universal tendency reflexively to diagnose all mentally ill individuals as suffering from schizophrenia. All patients received neuroleptic drugs or ECT, and manics were simply the "schizophrenics" who recovered. But the rapidly spreading use of lithium carbonate in Europe and Great Britain during the 1960s changed matters considerably, as not only did this salt exert more or less specific antimanic properties, but it did so without causing the permanent neurological sequelae widely acknowledged to occur with the neuroleptics, such as the syndrome of tardive dyskinesia. The publication in 1969 of the monograph *Manic Depressive Illness* (12) sparked the American rediscovery of mania as a clinical entity, and when lithium was introduced specifically for mania in this country in 1972, there was no dearth of patients to receive it. In the same year the Washington University operational criteria were introduced (38), precluding a diagnosis of schizophrenia in the presence of prominent affective symptoms, and within a few years the process was complete and the diagnosis of mania was fully restored to its rightful place in the nomenclature.

DIAGNOSIS OF MANIA

The classic triad of euphoria, overactivity, and pressured speech provides the core of the manic state, to which may be added the frequently occurring grandiosity and flight-of-ideas. Mood is not inevitably elevated, however, and irritability and lability are extremely common. Table 11–3 lists a number of the characteristic features of mania, and it is striking how many of the signs and symptoms reflect frontal lobe dysfunction. Impaired attention and concentration, distractibility, the stimulus-bound attitude, perseveration, loss of social inhibitions, and *Witzelsucht* are all seen in syndromes of the frontal lobe, particularly after damage to the orbitomedial areas (39). In mania, however, these phenomena are functional and state-related, as they remit with successful treatment.

Illness onset is usually acute, with the first episode generally appearing in the late teens or early twenties. In one of our studies the modal age at onset for fifty consecutive patients was only eighteen years. The disorder is more common in women, by a factor of 3:2 or more, and exhibits strong familial aggregation (40). A depressive episode is not commonly the harbinger of bipolar disease, as only 5 percent of patients go on to develop a manic episode later in their course (41). About 40 percent of manic patients never have a depressive episode, but these "unipolar manics" do not differ from those with both manic and depressive episodes in any important way (42).

TREATMENT OF THE MANIC STATE

Acute mania always requires urgent treatment and not infrequently presents a medical emergency. Excitement, overactivity, and elation may rapidly be replaced by irritability, argumentativeness, and aggressive/assaultive behavior, which presents a real and present danger to other patients and the staff. Intrusive, importunate, and demanding patients may become extremely vexed at only slight provocation; where persecutory delusional ideas are present, the risk of violent attack is sharply increased. Such patients may be observed pacing the hallways and muttering angrily to themselves, or even cursing at other patients and staff. Under no circumstances should potentially assaultive, uncooperative patients be inter-

TABLE 11-3   Phenomenology of Mania

Affect

Intense
Broad
Labile
Related

Mood

Euphoric, elated, expansive
Irritable, hostile, labile
Transient depression

Thought and Speech

Rapid, pressured, flight-of-ideas
Clang associations, rhyming, punning, joking, *Witzelsucht*, grandiosity

Dominant Themes (Content)

Religion
Sex
Business/financial
Persecution
New theories/inventions

Cognitive

Distractability
Stimulus-bound
Short attention span
Impaired concentration

Behavior

Hyperactive, hypergraphic, restless, agitated
Intrusive, importunate, demanding
Loud, vulgar, obscene, verbally abusive
Aggressive/assaultive, threatening/menacing
Sexually provocative/seductive
Nudity, sexual exposure
Incontinence of urine/feces
Fecal smearing
Self-decoration, head decoration ("Mohawk" haircut, turban, earrings, wigs)
Laughing, singing, dancing, gesticulating, saluting, military and sporting gestures,
    poses, postures

Social Behavior

Extravagance
Bad checks
Big bills
Sudden trips
Gifts
Gambling

Vegetative Signs

Insomnia (feels less need for sleep)
Increased libido
Increased appetite

viewed alone in a closed office, nor should any staff member, no matter how experienced or self-confident, be permitted to attempt to "talk the patient down" as the initial or sole treatment method. Neuroleptic therapy and seclusion are the safest and most rapidly effective measures and should be instituted without delay once the diagnosis is confirmed. It is a serious error to administer oral medication under such circumstances, regardless of the dose. We have witnessed numerous instances when manic patients have injured others despite high-dose oral neuroleptics, but never after receiving an initial intramuscular dose of 20–30 mg. haloperidol.

At least five staff members are needed to medicate an uncooperative, potentially assaultive patient: one to hold each limb, and one to give the injection. Ideally, a sixth should be present to restrain the head and prevent biting. If inadequate numbers of staff are present, additional help should be recruited from other units or from the hospital security personnel before approaching the patient. In most instances a patient confronted with five or six determined staff members accepts medication without a struggle. Even so, he should be placed in a locked seclusion or quiet room for an hour's observation after receiving medication to permit the full effect of the drug to develop. Such a procedure is mandatory in patients who must be physically restrained in order to medicate them.

Our drug of choice under these circumstances is haloperidol, 20–30 mg., given deep in the gluteal muscle (43). The large volume of solution (4–6 ml.) may require that two injections be given, one in each buttock, and the nursing staff should prepare the necessary syringes and paraphernalia well in advance. Some authors have recommended lower dosages (e.g. 5–10 mg. haloperidol) administered at hourly intervals until the desired effect is achieved. We have never seen the point of such a regimen. If the immediate aim of treatment is to reduce rapidly the psychotic excitement state and the risk of injury to patients and staff, then the correct dose is the one most likely to be effective yet not incur significant risk to the patient. A 20–30 mg. injection of haloperidol is much more rapidly effective than two or three 10 mg. injections at hourly intervals, and we have never observed any serious side effects from the higher doses either in a formal study (43) or in the subsequent clinical management of hundreds of patients.

Our standard order is for 20 mg. haloperidol IM, "Stat and B.I.D." This is continued for at least forty-eight hours even if there is a dramatic response to the first injection, as too hasty a switch from parenteral to oral administration frequently results in a rapid return of symptoms. The vast majority of acutely ill manics respond well to such a regimen, although an occasional patient may require 20 mg. IM, TID, or 30 mg. IM, BID. It is poor practice simply to give a "stat" dose of a neuroleptic and prescribe subsequent injections on a "p.r.n." basis. Such a method only ensures that patients will be permitted to develop all their acute symptoms again between doses.

Once the decision to treat has been made, it should be carried out systematically to provide continuous relief of symptoms.

When the change to oral medication occurs, there should be a brief period of overlap with parenteral therapy in order to smooth out the transition. For most patients a single nighttime oral dose of a neuroleptic can be instituted at a dosage 50 percent greater than the parenteral one. This dose (e.g. 60 mg. haloperidol orally in patient receiving 40 mg. parenterally) should be given for two nights before discontinuing the parenteral dosage. The increase in dosage is to counter the reduced efficacy of the oral versus the parenteral route of administration.

By the end of the first week of neuroleptic treatment most manic patients are fully stabilized, and lithium therapy can be instituted. Combined therapy with lithium and the neuroleptic dosage is routine while the neuroleptic is being tapered off prior to discontinuation. Fears of such combined therapy are generally unwarranted. The 1974 report (44) of permanent neurotoxic damage secondary to the lithium/haloperidol combination has never been confirmed, although several reports of increased toxic side effects have appeared (45). It is possible that lithium potentiates the extrapyramidal side effects of the neuroleptics, and for this reason it is prudent to lower the dosages or discontinue one or the other medication should an excessive or severe extrapyramidal syndrome develop during their combined administration.

The following case illustrates the approach described above:

A twenty-seven-year-old married white man was admitted stating: "I have these special powers, and I feel like I'm going to misuse them and hurt someone." For several weeks prior to admission he noted a decreased need for sleep, often staying up all night, and recently had stopped eating entirely, losing 20 pounds. On the day of admission he appeared in a physician's office without appointment and demanded an immediate consultation. He was loud and verbally abusive to the receptionist, and the police were called to bring him to the hospital.

There was no prior psychiatric history and no evidence of alcohol or drug abuse.

On admission he was irritable and agitated, with loud, rapid, and pressured speech and a euphoric mood with extreme lability. He exhibited flight-of-ideas and claimed to have vast wealth and "a string of offices across the country." Affect was expansive, and he claimed increased awareness of his own abilities. He said: "There's a millionaire and some other people I'm going to destroy, including my wife." He claimed there was nothing on Earth he could not do and no one whom he could not control with his "special powers." Hallucinations and first-rank symptoms were absent, and cognitive functions were intact.

Due to increasing irritability, agitation, and hostility, he was started the next day on haloperidol, 20 mg. IM, B.I.D., which was changed to the oral form after three days, at which time marked improvement had occurred. At the same time, lithium carbonate was started at a dose of 1,500 mg./day. Five days later his lithium level was 1.4 mEq/L. He was pleasant and cooperative, and displayed no grandiosity. Haloperidol was discontinued and lithium reduced to 1,200 mg./day. He remained well and was discharged two weeks after admission, fully recovered, on maintenance lithium therapy.

About 10 percent of acute manic patients do not respond to even the most intensively administered pharmacotherapy and may progress to a toxic, dehydrated, and febrile state if measures are not taken to interrupt the process. If five days of parenteral, high-dose neuroleptic therapy have not terminated the acute phase of the illness, medications should be discontinued and ECT given without further delay. Two ECTs may have to be given daily for the first two or three days in order to bring the illness to a halt. When this has been accomplished, usually by the second or third session of two bilateral ECTs, the remainder of the course is given at the usual frequency. Manics require more ECTs than depressives, the usual course being eight to twelve treatments. Even if the patient recovers earlier, say by the fifth or sixth treatment, it is wise to continue to at least eight treatments in order to avoid rapid relapse.

A forty-one-year-old married white woman was admitted because of "talking senselessly." She had been functioning well until two weeks prior to admission, when she developed early morning waking, irritability, and lability. She soon became agitated and hyperactive, wept suddenly for no reason, and wandered about the house at night appearing confused.

She had first become ill at age nineteen, at which time she received ECT for a severe depression. A second episode at age twenty-nine also responded well to ECT. At age thirty-four she had the first of four manic episodes, characterized by hyperactivity, flight-of-ideas, clang associations, pressured speech, and "confusion," all responding to neuroleptic drugs.

On admission she was agitated, hyperactive, and frequently attempted to embrace the interviewer. Affect was broad, labile, and intense, and mood alternated between euphoria and brief episodes of lachrymose morosity. Speech was rapid, pressured, and characterized by flight-of-ideas, tangentiality, and nonsequiturs. She insisted she was to be "killed at dawn tomorrow."

After three days of observation she was started on haloperidol, 20 mg. IM, BID, with no appreciable reduction in symptoms over forty-eight hours. On the third day of treatment she developed catalepsy, echopraxia, and automatic obedience. Haloperidol was increased to 20 mg. IM, TID, and continued for two more days, at which time it was discontinued for lack of improvement. ECT was begun, and although there was rapid and marked improvement for several hours after each treatment, sustained improvement did not occur until the seventh treatment. A total of ten ECT were given, with full recovery, followed by lithium carbonate maintenance therapy, 1,200 mg./day, and she was discharged on this regimen, in full remission, three weeks after starting ECT.

This case is also of interest because it illustrates the not infrequent occurrence of catatonic features following the administration of parenteral neuroleptics.

There is a strong trend in this country to encourage voluntary admission to mental hospitals, reflected in the official policies of many institutions that admit both voluntary and involuntary patients. The question of admission status frequently arises where manic patients are concerned, as they often lack insight into their abnormal behavior and unrealistic plans, yet may readily sign for voluntary admission in an impulsive, magnanimous gesture. Where there is such impaired judgment, or where the patient is delusional, hallucinated, or potentially assaultive, involuntary commitment should be obtained *even if the patient is willing to sign for voluntary admission.* Such involuntary admission must be, of course, compatible with widely varying state laws but, if permitted under the local mental health code and hospital policy, it is far wiser than the voluntary status, which is invariably withdrawn by the patient immediately when he realizes his physician actually intends for him to reside on a closed unit and even take medication. The advantage of involuntary commitment for such psychotic patients is that in most states they may be medicated involuntarily, permitting a rapid and uneventful resolution of their psychosis and a speedy return to society. Voluntary patients may not be so treated (unless there is demonstrable danger to life or limb), and their illness may rapidly get out of hand during the obligatory period of converting them to involuntary status and arguing the issue with the local mental health lawyer. Civil rights are rarely at issue here; psychotic patients are often simply unable to assess adequately the nature of their illness and its treatment, are often combative or assaultive, and must frequently be treated against their will for their own benefit.

Mania/Hypomania

Where there is no urgency by reason of extreme excitement, overactivity, or assaultive behavior, and the patient is willing to accept oral medication, therapy should be initiated with lithium carbonate. As there is a five- to seven-day lag before the onset of significant antimanic activity with this medication, the staff (and the other patients) must be able to tolerate the frequently annoying and occasionally disruptive behaviors typical of manic patients. In a healthy individual without history of renal, thyroid, or cardiac disease, lithium therapy can be started as soon as the blood is drawn for the initial laboratory tests without waiting for the results to come back. A dose of 1,200–1,800 mg./day will usually produce a blood level within the therapeutic range (1–1.5 mEq/L.) by the end of seven to ten days, and serum lithium levels should be obtained twice weekly until a stable therapeutic level is achieved. If a therapeutic level is not achieved within a reasonable time at a dose of 1,800 mg./day, three possibilities should be considered: (1) The patient is not swallowing all of his medication; (2) polyuria with excessive lithium loss is occurring; and (3) the dose is too low. Manic patients with grandiose or persecutory delusions frequently prefer not to take medications and find tablets or capsules of lithium easy to sequester in the cheek or under the tongue for subsequent disposal. Such patients are readily identified as the ones who rush to the water fountain or bathroom as soon as they have "swallowed" their pills, and they should be given the liquid (citrate) form of lithium.

The anti-ADH effect of lithium described elsewhere in this volume leads some patients to excrete a large volume of dilute urine, carrying with it a considerable load of lithium and making it difficult or impossible to achieve a therapeutic level. Chlorothiazide 500–1,000 mg./day may be prescribed to block the anti-ADH effect, reducing urinary output and increasing serum lithium levels (46). Needless to say, patients should be closely observed for signs of lithium toxicity during this maneuver and serum lithium levels should be more frequently monitored.

When these two potential causes of lithium therapy failure are ruled out, a small group of patients remains who simply require more than 1,800 mg./day of lithium to achieve a therapeutic level. Such patients typically exhibit no side effects at 1,800 mg./day, and a stepwise increase in dosage is indicated until therapeutic levels are obtained. The highest dose we have ever administered in such circumstances was 2,700 mg./day. The patient responded well to this regimen without significant side effects.

The following case illustrates successful use of lithium alone in acute mania:

A forty-six-year-old white housewife was brought to the hospital complaining that "my phone has been tapped and drug rings are trying to control the market and are putting drugs into children's cookies." She had been discharged from the hospital one month prior to admission after successful treatment of a manic episode with lithium carbonate but had discontinued this medication on her own soon after returning home. One week prior to admission she again became intrusive and verbally abrasive at home, disrupting the neighborhood by incessant talking and yelling about a "drug ring."

The patient first became ill at age twenty-eight, when she developed a depression immediately following the birth of her first child. Each subsequent childbirth was followed by a more severe depression, and five years after the birth of her youngest child she developed her first of several manic attacks.

On admission to the hospital the patient was neat, clean, and alert but uncooperative. She was agitated and hyperactive, and exhibited rapid and pressured speech. Affect was broad, and mood was euphoric and labile, quickly becoming sad or irritable. She talked and joked incessantly and exhibited pronounced flight-of-ideas, tangentiality, and circumstantiality. There were no hallucinations or first-rank symptoms.

Lithium carbonate was started on the seventh hospital day at a daily dose of 1,500 mg., achieving a serum level of 1.69 mEq/L. after five days. At this time she was much improved, and the dose was reduced to 900 mg./day because of nausea and vomiting. She was discharged home on the seventeenth hospital day, at which time she was described as calm, alert, cooperative, and without agitation or hyperactivity. Affect was broad and stable, with appropriate mood, and speech was moderate in rate and productivity. There was no circumstantiality, tangentiality, or flight-of-ideas, and no delusions were present.

After ten or twelve days at therapeutic lithium levels most patients who ultimately respond favorably to this medication will already have experienced a significant reduction in symptoms. If a patient has exhibited no improvement after two weeks at a lithium level in the neighborhood of 1.5 mEq/L., there is no point in persisting with this therapy alone. Addition of a neuroleptic drug at this point may yield the desired improvement, although it is unclear whether this results from the combined therapy or merely the neuroleptic. The point of continuing lithium at this stage of the treatment process is that although those patients who require additional treatments stay longer in hospital, they are no less improved than the "lithium only" group at discharge and can be released almost as frequently on lithium alone (47).

The following patient, however, required combined therapy in order to be discharged:

A twenty-one-year-old white man was voluntarily admitted because of "restlessness and short attention span." Two weeks prior to admission he began to pace about the house and developed insomnia, mood swings, and emotional lability. He was noted to be laughing or crying for no apparent reason, talked and mumbled to himself, and said things that were difficult to follow.

He first became ill three years prior to admission with "agitation and hyperactivity," which did not respond to neuroleptics but remitted after ECT. Two subsequent episodes in the next year and a half also responded to ECT.

On admission to hospital the patient was hyperactive, pacing, and distractible. Affect was broad and labile, rapidly switching from making jokes to weeping. He exhibited punning and clang associations and believed he could think "five times faster than normal" and read minds. On the ward he was intrusive and demanding and paced continually. Three days after admission, haloperidol was initiated at 20 mg. IM, BID, with only modest effect. Lithium carbonate was then started at 1,800 mg./day, and the haloperidol was discontinued when therapeutic lithium levels were achieved (range of 1.16–1.36 mEq/L.). No further improvement was seen over the next two weeks at this dosage. He remained intrusive, labile, and demanding. Haloperidol, 60 mg./day oral was restarted in combination with lithium, and he was shortly noted to be less intrusive, slowed down, and sleeping more. He went on several weekend passes without any problems and was discharged after six weeks in hospital, on lithium 1,500 mg./day and haloperidol 20 mg./day, to return to his work as a TV repairman.

LITHIUM FAILURE

The causes of lithium failure are not well understood, and several in-vestigators have failed to define any specific, reproducible variables that predict a poor response to this drug. One group reported that "rapid cyclers" who had four or more episodes per year were likely to be lithium failures (48), and another group found such failures to be most prevalent among pa-tients with "paranoid–destructive" symptoms (49). We examined these and other variables in a sample of manics who responded to lithium alone, in comparison with a group who required coadministration of neuroleptics or who had to be switched to ECT to achieve remission. Unable to confirm rapid cycling or paranoid–destructive behavior as poor prognostic features, we concluded that social factors, especially premature termination of treat-ment by the patient or his family, were primarily responsible for lithium failure (47).

An alternative method employs the anti-manic properties of car-bamazepine, a drug of choice in treating temporal lobe epilepsy (50). Car-bamazepine is started at an initial dosage of 200 mg. PO, BID, increasing by 200 mg./day, as tolerated, to a total daily dosage of 1,200 mg. (range = 600–1,600 mg./day). The aim is to maintain serum carbamazepine levels between 8.0 and 12.0 mcg./ml., a range similar to that recommended in the treatment of epilepsy. Patients who respond to carbamazepine usually show significant improvement by the end of the first week of treatment at therapeutic levels and a two-week trial is adequate to assess its effects in a given patient. Although there is some evidence for a prophylactic antimanic effect of carbamazepine (51), there are as yet inadequate data to support its routine use for this purpose.

Lithium maintenance should be continued regardless of any relapses dur-ing the first year, as the relapse rate decreases in subsequent years in patients who persist with treatment (48). Manic and depressive episodes alike are reduced in frequency and severity with lithium maintenance as a function of the direct action of the medication and because frequent clinic visits permit early detection and treatment of recurrent symptoms before they have developed momentum. Manics who fail lithium prophylaxis, alone or com-bined with neuroleptics, should be placed on maintenance ECT. Manics are the only patients for whom a prophylactic effect of ECT has been demonstrated (52), albeit in an uncontrolled trial. Treatments are given at biweekly to monthly intervals for a period of time directly related to the fre-quency and severity of past attacks. As for maintenance ECT in depressive illness, the procedure should be limited to about six months, after which time a treatment-free observation period should be instituted or maintenance lithium therapy tried again. ECT and lithium should not be combined:

Lithium increases the neuromuscular block with succinylcholine, and instances of prolonged apnea have resulted (53).

Mixed Affective States

Bipolar patients not infrequently present with a clinical mixture of manic and depressive symptoms or develop such a presentation at some time during their hospital course (37). This syndrome is not simply the frequently reported occurrence of brief depressive symptoms or emotional lability in manic patients; it is a true combination of states that may have stability over time and is more difficult to treat than either state alone. Such mixed states also occur during the "switch" process (54) from depression into mania and in bipolar patients with prominent diurnal variation, who may be depressed in the morning and pass through a mixed state, even becoming hypomanic, by evening. A trial of lithium therapy is worthwhile in patients with such mixed states, as the following case illustrates, but if major improvement is not obtained by the end of two weeks, a course of ECT should be given in preference to adding a neuroleptic drug:

A fifty-year-old white single woman was admitted because "voices told me to come to the hospital." She had been well until one day prior to admission, when she told her brother she was hearing voices and repeatedly said to herself: "Help me to your God."

She was first hospitalized at age thirty-four at which time she received insulin coma therapy and ECT for "paranoid schizophrenia," remaining for three years in a state hospital. Two other admissions to state hospitals followed over the next seven years, characterized by symptoms of depression accompanied by auditory hallucinations. During the second episode she was treated with trifluoperazine plus imipramine and remained hospitalized for two years.

On admission to hospital the patient was agitated and slightly hyperactive, and kept her eyes closed while rubbing prayer beads continually. Rate and pressure of speech were increased, and she complained of persistent auditory hallucinations and thought broadcasting. There was perseveration of speech with loosening of associations and word approximations. Over the next few days her mood fluctuated rapidly between euphoria and depression, with lability, sudden weeping, and a generally expansive, intense affect.

Lithium carbonate, 1,200 mg./day, was started on the tenth hospital day, and gradual, progressive improvement was observed beginning after four days. Two weeks after starting lithium she went on pass without any problems, and she was discharged fully recovered after a total of five weeks in hospital.

Cyclothymia

The term cyclothymia or cyclothymic personality traditionally described a person who was characteristically endomorphic (pyknic), extroverted, outgoing, cheerful, and optimistic, but also impulsive and subject to sudden unexplained fits of moodiness during which he would be depressed, irritable, or short-tempered (55). Many authors described an increased frequency of premorbid cyclothymia in manic-depressive patients, and a few even considered cyclothymia to be a *forme fruste* of the latter disorder.

In recent years the term has been used increasingly to describe a mild form of manic-depressive illness, rather than an abnormal personality, and the *DSM-III* criteria for cyclothymia portray what is essentially a partial form of the major disorder, one that often does not require specific treatment. Cyclothymia so diagnosed is reported responsive to lithium carbonate (56) which damps the mood swings and provides stability in an otherwise often chaotic life. Lithium is reported similarly effective in "emotionally unstable character disorder" (57), a disused but evocative term, which describes patients who in fact may have cyclothymic characteristics. In any case, whether cyclothymia is a personality type or a disease, it rarely leads to hospitalization. Where the behavioral characteristics cause suffering in the individual or those around him, lithium is certainly worth a try.

References

1. Weissman, M.; Meyers, J.; Harding, P. Psychiatric disorders in a U.S. urban community: 1975–1976. *Am. J. Psychiat. 135:* 459–67, 1978.

2. Ries, R.; Bokan, J.; Schuckit, M. Modern diagnosis of schizophrenia in hospitalized psychiatric patients. *Am. J. Psychiat. 137:* 1419–21, 1980.

3. Hohman, L. B. A review of one-hundred and forty-four cases of affective disorders: After seven years. *Am. J. Psychiat. 94:* 303–8, 1937.

4. Abrams, R.; Taylor, M. A. Differential EEG patterns in affective disorder and schizophrenia. *Arch. Gen. Psychiat. 36:* 1355–58, 1979.

5. Taylor, M. A.; Abrams, R. Reassessing the bipolar–unipolar dichotomy. *J. Aff. Dis. 2:* 195–217, 1980.

6. Taylor, M. A.; Abrams, R. Gender differences in bipolar affective disorder. *J. Aff. Dis. 3:* 261–77, 1981.

7. Schildkraut, J. J. The catecholamine hypothesis of affective disorders: A review of supporting evidence. *Am. J. Psychiat. 122:* 509–22, 1965.

8. Carroll, B. J.; Feinberg, M.; Greden, J. F.; *et al.* A specific laboratory test for the diagnosis of melancholia: Standardization, validation and clinical utility. *Arch. Gen. Psychiat. 38:* 15–22, 1981.

9. Amsterdam, J. D.; Winokur, A.; Caroff, S.; *et al.* The dexamethasone suppression test in outpatients with primary affective disorder and healthy control subjects. *Am. J. Psychiat. 139:* 287–91, 1982.

10. Targum, S. D.; Sullivan, A. C.; Byrnes, S. M. Neuroendocrine interrelationships in major depressive disorder. *Am. J. Psychiat. 139:* 282–86, 1982.

11. Gruen, P. H.; Sachar, E. J.; Altman, N.; *et al.* Growth hormone responses to hypoglycemia in post-menopausal depressed women. *Arch. Gen. Psychiat. 32:* 31–33, 1975.

12. Winokur, G.; Clayton, P. J.; Reich, T. R. *Manic Depressive Illness.* St. Louis: C. V. Mosby, 1969, p. 5.

13. Clayton, P. J.; Desmarais, L.; Winokur, G. A study of normal bereavement. *Am. J. Psychiat. 125:* 168–78, 1968.

14. Nelson, J. C.; Charney, D. S.; Vingiano, A. W. False-positive diagnosis with primary-affective-disorder criteria. *Lancet 2:* 1252–53, 1978.

15. Leonhard, K. *Aufteilung der Endogenen Psychosen.* 2d ed. Berlin: Akademie Verlag, 1959.

16. Perris, C. A study of bipolar (manic-depressive) and unipolar recurrent depressive psychoses. *Acta. Psychiat. Scand.* (suppl. 194) *42:* 1–188, 1966.

17. Dunner, D. L.; Gershon, E. S.; Goodwin, F. K. Heritable factors in the severity of affective illness. *Biol. Psychiat. 11:* 31–42, 1976.

18. Schlesser, M. A.; Winokur, G.; Sherman, B. M. Hypothalamic–pituitary-adrenal axis activity in depressive illness: Its relationship to classification. *Arch. Gen. Psychiat. 37:* 737–43, 1980.

19. Abrams, R. Clinical prediction of ECT response in depressed patients. *Psychopharm. Bull. 2:* 48–50, 1982.

20. Shagass, C. S.; Naiman, J.; Mihalik, J. M. An objective test which differentiates between neurotic and psychotic depression. *Arch. Neurol. Psychiat. 75:* 461–71, 1956.

21. Forrest, A. D.; Fraser, R. H.; Priest, R. G. Environmental factors in depressive illness. *Br. J. Psychiat. 111:* 243–53, 1965.

22. Pollitt, J. *Depression and Its Treatment.* London: Wm. Heinemann, 1965, pp. 12–13.

23. Perez-Reyes, M.; Cochrane, C. Differences in sodium thiopental susceptibility of depressed patients as evidenced by the galvanic skin reflex inhibition threshold. *J. Psychiat. Res. 5:* 335–47, 1967.

24. Albala, A. A.; Greden, J. F. Serial dexamethasone suppression tests in affective disorders. *Am. J. Psychiat. 137:* 383, 1980.

25. Guze, S. B.; Robins, E. Suicide and primary affective disorders. *Br. J. Psychiat. 117:* 437–38, 1970.

26. Abrams, R.; Taylor, M. A. The importance of mood-incongruent psychotic symptoms in melancholia. *J. Aff. Dis. 5:* 179–81, 1983.

27. Perry, P.; Tsuang, M. T. Treatment of unipolar depression following electroconvulsive therapy. *J. Affect. Dis. 1:* 123–29, 1979.

28. Carney, M. W. P.; Roth, M.; Garside, R. F. The diagnosis of depressive syndromes and the prediction of ECT response. *Br. J. Psychiat. 111:* 659–74, 1965.

29. Kiloh, L. G.; Garside, R. F. The independence of neurotic depression and endogenous depression. *Br. J. Psychiat. 109:* 451–63, 1963.

30. Robinson, D. S.; Nies, A.; Ravaris, C. L.; *et al.* The monoamine oxidase in-

hibitor, phenelzine, in the treatment of depressive anxiety states: A controlled clinical trial. *Arch. Gen. Psychiat. 29:* 407-13, 1973.

31. Di Mascio, A.; Weissman, M. M.; Prusoff, B. A.; *et al.* Differential symptom reduction by drugs and psychotherapy in acute depression. *Arch. Gen. Psychiat. 36:* 1450-56, 1979.

32. Blackburn, I. M.; Bishop, S. Changes in cognition with pharmacotherapy and cognitive therapy. *Br. J. Psychiat. 143:* 609-17, 1983.

33. Clayton, P. Bereavement. In Paykel, E. (ed.), *Handbook of Affective Disorders.* Edinborough: Churchill Livingstone, 1982, p. 411.

34. Folstein, M. F.; Folstein, S. E.; McHugh, P. R. "Mini-mental state": A practical method for grading the cognitive state of patients for the clinician. *J. Psychiat. Res. 12:* 189-98, 1975.

35. Hohman, L. B. A review of one-hundred and forty-four cases of affective disorders: After seven years. *Am. J. Psychiat. 94:* 303-8, 1937.

36. Jampala, V. C.; Abrams, R. Mania secondary to left and right hemisphere damage. *Am. J. Psychiat. 140:* 1197-99, 1983.

37. Kraepelin, E. *Manic Depressive Insanity and Paranoia.* Barclay, R. M. (trans.). Edinburgh: E. & S. Livingston, 1921, pp. 54-74.

38. Feighner, J. P.; Robins, E.; Guze, S. B.; *et al.* Diagnostic criteria for use in psychiatric research. *Arch. Gen. Psychiat. 26:* 57-63, 1972.

39. Benson, D. F.; Blumer, D. *Psychiatric Aspects of Neurologic Disease.* New York: Grune & Stratton, 1975, pp. 157-59.

40. Taylor, M. A.; Abrams, R.; Hayman, M. A. The classification of affective disorders: A reassessment of the bipolar–unipolar dichotomy—A clinical, laboratory, and family study. *J. Affect. Dis. 2:* 95-109, 1980.

41. Winokur, G.; Morrison, J. The Iowa 500: Follow-up of 225 depressives. *Br. J. Psychiat. 123:* 543-48, 1973.

42. Abrams, R.; Taylor, M. A. Unipolar mania revisited. *J. Affect. Dis. 1:* 59-68, 1979.

43. SanGiovanni, F.; Taylor, M. A.; Abrams, R.; *et al.* Rapid control of psychotic excitement states with intramuscular haloperidol. *Arch. Gen. Psychiat. 130:* 1155-56, 1973.

44. Cohen, W. J.; Cohen, N. H. Lithium carbonate, haloperidol, and irreversible brain damage. *JAMA 230:* 1283-87, 1974.

45. Jefferson, J. W.; Greist, J. H. *Primer of Lithium Therapy.* Baltimore: Williams & Wilkins, 1977, pp. 112-13.

46. MacNeil, S.; Jennings, G.; Eastwood, P. R.; *et al.* Lithium and the antidiuretic hormone. *Br. J. Clin. Pharmacol. 3:* 305-13, 1976.

47. Krishna, R. N.; Taylor, M. A.; Abrams, R. Manic states: Responders and nonresponders to lithium. *Biol. Psychiat. 13:* 601-6, 1978.

48. Dunner, D. L; Fieve, R. R. Clinical factors in lithium carbonate prophylaxis failure. *Arch. Gen. Psychiat. 30:* 229-33, 1974.

49. Murphy, D. L.; Beigel, A. Depression, elation and lithium carbonate responses in manic patient subgroups. *Arch. Gen. Psychiat. 31:* 643–48, 1974.

50. Ballenger, J. C.; Post, R. M. Carbamazepine in manic-depressive illness: A new treatment. *Am. J. Psychiat. 137:* 782–90, 1980.

51. Post, R. M.; Uhde, T. W.; Ballenger, J. C.; *et al.* Prophylactic efficacy of carbamazepine in manic-depressive illness. *Am. J. Psychiat. 140:* 1602–4, 1983.

52. Geoghegan, J. J.; Stevenson, G. H. Prophylactic electroshock. *Am. J. Psychiat. 105:* 494–96, 1949.

53. Hill, G. E.; Wong, K. C.; Hodges, M. R. Potentiation of succinylcholine neuromuscular blockade by lithium carbonate. *Anesthesiology 44:* 439–42, 1976.

54. Bunney, W. E., Jr.; Goodwin, F. K.; Murphy, D. I. The "switch process" in manic depressive illness: 1. A systematic study of sequential behavioral changes. *Arch. Gen. Psychiat. 27:* 295–302, 1972.

55. Akiskal, H. S.; Dekerminjian, A. H.; Rosenthal, R. H.; *et al.* Cyclothymic disorder: Validating criteria for inclusion in the bipolar affective group. *Am. J. Psychiat. 134:* 1227–33, 1977.

56. Schou, M. Lithium in psychiatric therapy and prophylaxis. *J. Psychiat. Res. 6:* 67–95, 1968.

57. Rifkin, A.; Levitan, S. J.; Galewski, J.; *et al.* Emotionally unstable character disorder: A follow-up study. 1. Description of patients and outcome. *Biol. Psychiat. 4:* 68–88, 1972.

CHAPTER 12

The Suicidal Patient

The Frequency and Preventability of Suicide

Suicide is the tenth leading cause of death in the United States, resulting in almost 30,000 deaths annually (1). Because 95 percent of patients who commit suicide have diagnosable psychiatric illnesses and often visit doctors shortly before they kill themselves (2, 3), it follows that suicide is often preventable.

In one study (3) two-thirds of the patients who committed suicide had visited their family doctor in the month before their death, and 40 percent had done so in the prior week. In another study (2) 54 percent had received care for psychiatric illness in the year before committing suicide, and 31 percent had received such care in the final month.

Problems in Suicide Prevention

Despite these opportunities for suicide prevention, suicide continues to be common. In the United States the rate is 12.1 per 100,000 population per year (4). In Austria, West Germany, Hungary, Japan, Denmark, Finland, Sweden, and Switzerland it is even higher, exceeding 25 per 100,000 per year (5). In some cases the reason is inadequate diagnosis or treatment (2, 3). For example, many patients who commit suicide have been treated successfully for prior major depressive episodes with ECT (2, 3), but they or their doctors choose not to repeat this therapy during the depression that leads to the suicide. Some patients receive inadequate doses of tricyclic antidepressants (3), and others are given barbiturates or neuroleptics unnecessarily (3) because of sleep problems in the former, and overdiagnosis of schizophrenia in the latter. Another consideration is the lethality of tricyclic antidepressants, barbiturates, neuroleptics, and lithium when taken in large overdoses. In more than half of cases of suicide by overdose, the substance taken had been supplied during a recent visit to a physician (6). And some patients simply do not come to medical attention. There may be no caring friends or relatives available. If available, they may not realize the lethal potential of the situation, may not be able to persuade the patient to accept treatment, or may not be aware of their right to seek involuntary hospitalization for the patient.

Sources of Information About Suicide

Few physicians have extensive experience treating patients who kill themselves while under their care. This requires that physicians learn much about suicide from retrospective studies of sizeable numbers of completed suicides. Three such studies, those of Robins (2), Barraclough *et al.* (3), and Dorpat and Ripley (7), are available. The Robins study is particularly noteworthy, as it details the case histories of 134 suicides. There is also one prospective study, that of Borg and Stahl (8).

The Clinical Approach to the Patient

Despite the anxiety inherent in dealing with these potentially fatal situations, treating suicidal patients can be particularly gratifying, as so many suicidal patients are curable, often dramatically so.

Suicide is not itself an illness; it is a behavior that most often results from severe psychiatric illness. But the assessment of suicide risk is similar to the process of diagnosis of illness, beginning with a thorough history and mental status examination. The clinician should be alert to the possibility of suicide in any patient who has serious psychiatric illness or who conveys intense sadness, intense guilt, hopelessness, or significant agitation. The following are specific factors associated with high and low suicide risks, respectively:

HIGH RISK

    I. Suicidal ideation and intent
   II. Diagnoses, including the following:
      A. Endogenous depression

     B. Alcoholism
     C. Serious systemic illness (particularly those which are chronic or painful), including:
       1. Renal failure
       2. Emphysema
  III. Middle age or elderly
  IV. Male sex
   V. Mental status phenomena
     A. Hopelessness
     B. Sustained sadness
     C. Severe agitation or motor retardation
     D. Psychosis
  VI. Single, widowed, divorced, or separated
 VII. White or American Indian
VIII. Protestant
  IX. Prior suicide attempt
   X. Family history of suicide
  XI. Unemployed or in financial difficulty

Low Risk

   I. No suicidal ideation
  II. Mood improves as interview progresses and is reactive to environmental stimuli
 III. Good general health
 IV. Child
  V. Pregnant

Probably the most important factors are the presence of suicidal intent coupled with a diagnosis associated with high suicide risk, especially major depression.

Two patients, for whom psychiatric consultations were called to assess suicide risk, illustrate the assessment process:

An eighteen-year-old single Catholic student at a broadcasting college, two months pregnant, is admitted to an internal medicine service because of ingestion of "five to ten" anxiolytic sedatives. She was well until several days prior to the overdose, when she learned that her mother, with whom she lives and upon whom she depends for moral support, was contemplating a move to Missouri, where the patient's stepfather was trying to find work. The patient does not want her family to move, because she feels she needs her mother's moral support and because Missouri has no college for future broadcasters. On admission, she stated to her mother, "If you move, I'll kill myself."

The mental status reveals a mildly obese, attractive, cooperative, articulate, normoactive young woman. At the beginning of the interview she is in tears; at the end, she is euthymic and even joking. The rest of the mental status examination is normal.

The patient was diagnosed as having no major psychiatric illness, and was discharged home two days after admission upon learning that the family would not move to Missouri and therefore retracting her threat to commit suicide.

A seventy-year-old single, retired white Protestant man is admitted to an internal medicine service for dehydration and a 20-pound weight loss due to decreased drinking and eating in the past two months. On the medical ward he states that he will kill himself if someone gives him an opportunity to do so. In recent months he has had trouble falling asleep and trouble returning to sleep after awakening early in the morning. He has had two prior hospitalizations for major depression since age sixty, during both of which he responded well to ECT.

The mental status reveals a gruff, dehydrated, gaunt white man who is hypoactive and minimally spontaneous. His mood is dysphoric and angry and remains so throughout the interview. His thought content is extremely pessimistic. His concentration is impaired, but there are no other cognitive abnormalities. The rest of the physical examination and the laboratory tests reveal no systemic medical illness or coarse brain disease. This man was diagnosed as having major depression and thought to be suicidal. He was transferred to the psychiatric service where he recovered after six ECT treatments.

The characteristics of the first patient that led to the conclusion of relatively small suicide risk were (1) young, (2) female, (3) Catholic, (4) pregnant, (5) *not psychiatrically ill*, (6) *retracted suicide threat*. The characteristics of the second patient that led to the conclusion of relatively high suicide risk were (1) elderly, (2) white, (3) male, (4) Protestant, (5) single, (6) *endogenously depressed*, (7) *continued suicidal ideation*.

As is the case in psychiatric diagnosis, of course, the variables must be considered summatively: No single factor should be taken alone. Thus, it is certainly possible for a teen-age girl to commit suicide. The odds of this would clearly increase if she were endogenously depressed.

A third example, quoted verbatim from Robins (2), is a case of a man who did commit suicide.

This 63-year-old black railroad carpenter had suffered from arthritis for some years. About two years prior to his death his arthritis worsened somewhat although he was still able to work. One year before his death, his symptoms changed. He developed headaches, pains throughout his body and extremities, epigastric discomfort, dizzy spells, visual blurring, chronic fatigue, feelings of weakness, anorexia, insomnia (requiring sedation), constipation, and complete absence of sex drive. Associated with these symptoms were marked despondency, self-blame for his illness, a belief that he would never get well, self-disgust, nervousness, diminished motor activity, undertalkativeness with occasional periods during which he would not talk at all, concern that he was losing his memory, and many ideas of suicide and death. These latter ideas included preoccupation with suicidal and accidental deaths as reported in the newspapers, and statements that he wanted to die and was going to commit suicide. He told his wife of his great concern that she might die first, leaving no one to take care of him, and that he might have a stroke. He constantly reminded his wife that she was not to spend too much money for his burial.

He saw physicians for these complaints on two occasions, six months and three months before his death. Aside from moderate hypertension and osteo-arthritis, there was no positive evidence of other medical disease. Just before see-ing the first physician he had remained in bed for three weeks. At that time his job aggravated him greatly, but he changed to a more congenial job without any lessening of his symptoms. Other than the possible aggravation of his work, the informants knew of no other life stresses.

His wife said that he had been an excessive drinker for many years. This ex-cessive drinking was demonstrated by the information that his wife objected to his drinking, that he believed he drank too much, that he got into trouble at work because of drinking, and that he had been arrested at least twice for drinking and peace disturbance. It was of interest that during his last illness his drinking diminished.

On the morning of his suicide he told his wife not to buy a new summer hat or new clothes for him because he would not need them. A few minutes later he hung up his hat and coat, took off his glasses, went down to the basement and hanged himself. His meticulous preparations had led his wife to believe that he was only going to tidy up the yard or basement [2].*

Correlates of Suicide

Having mentioned factors associated with suicide, we shall now discuss them in detail:

Suicidal Ideation and Suicidal Intent

The majority of patients, 69 percent in the Robins study (2) and 55 percent in the Barraclough sample (3), communicate suicidal intent to one or more peo-ple. In reading the Robins case histories, the reader is struck by the (retrospective) obviousness of the messages conveyed by the suicides, such as: "On the night before his suicide, he brought home some poison which he said he intended to use to kill himself." "He mentioned suicide several times, asking his wife where she had hidden the shotgun, and saying he wished a car would run over him" (2).

Because of the tendency of suicidal patients to convey their suicidal thoughts (9), it is almost always imperative that the physician ask the patient if he is contemplating suicide, using questions such as the following: Would

*From *The Final Months: A Study of the Lives of 134 Persons Who Committed Suicide*, by Eli Robins. Copyright © 1981 by Oxford University Press, Inc. Reprinted by permission.

you like to go away and never come back? Would you like to go to sleep and never wake up? Would you like to end it all? Would you be better off dead? Do you want to die? Are you thinking of suicide? When you feel this way, do you consider killing yourself?

For patients who answer yes to such questions, it is useful to follow up with questions about suicidal intent, such as these: Have you actually planned how you would do it? How would you go about killing yourself? Do you feel you need to be in a locked room, or under close supervision, to prevent you from doing it?

For the suicidal patient these questions are often reassuring, as they reveal the doctor's awareness of the patient's desperation and the doctor's concern for preservation of the patient's life. Although data are mostly anecdotal (10, 11), there is no evidence that these questions stimulate suicidal patients to commit suicide. On occasion, however, a malingerer might threaten suicide or make a superficial suicide gesture in order to gain admission. In these latter cases the examination usually reveals that the patient is neither acutely ill nor suffering intensely.

One means of conveying suicidal ideation, suicidal threats, and suicidal intent is the suicide note, found in 39 percent (3) of completed suicides. Although the suicide note can be extremely helpful in identifying a risk and assessing its lethality, it rarely has preventative value, as it is usually found postmortem or with a dying patient (3). Not all such notes are evidence of serious suicidal intent. In the following case a desire to be rescued is revealed:

A thirty-three-year-old married insulin-dependent diabetic mother of two children became annoyed at her husband following a disagreement with him about childrearing. Instead of taking her usual 20 units of NPH insulin in the morning, she took 30 units. Late in the afternoon, about an hour before her husband was to return from work, with her two children present in the house, she ate a large afternoon snack and left her husband a note stating how much insulin she had taken that morning and how many calories she had ingested that day. She then took a nap in anticipation of her husband's return.

PSYCHIATRIC ILLNESS

In the Robins (2), Barraclough (3), and Dorpat (7) studies, the diagnoses were as follows:

Barraclough et al. (100 Suicides)

Depressive illness	70%
Alcoholism	15%
Schizophrenia	3%
Phobic anxiety state	3%

Barbiturate dependence	1%
Acute schizo-affective disorder	1%
Not mentally ill	7%

Dorpat and Ripley (108 Suicides)

Depressive illness	28%
Alcoholism	26%
Schizophrenia	11%
Personality and sociopathic disorders	9%
Organic brain syndrome	4%
Miscellaneous	3%
Unspecified illness	15%
No psychological information	5%

Robins (134 Suicides)

Affective disorder	47%
Alcoholism	25%
Organic brain syndrome	4%
Schizophrenia	2%
Drug dependence	1%
Undiagnosed psychiatric illness	15%
Terminal medical illness	4%
Well	2%

The diagnoses most highly associated with suicide are depression and alcoholism. Even in Dorpat's study (7), where a diagnosis of "depressive illness" was made in only 28 percent of cases, the authors noted that *all* the patients had some depressive symptoms. Robins's study, the only one of the three to use modern research criteria, demonstrated that most depressed patients had primary affective disorder, depressed type. Most of them would correspond to a diagnosis of major depression.

Of all the myriad syndromes of psychiatry, major depression is most highly associated with death by suicide; indeed, about 15 percent of patients with major depression eventually commit suicide (12). The degree to which reactive depression (dysthymic disorder) is associated with suicide is not known; a small percentage of cases diagnosed by Robins as having primary affective disorder, depressed, may have had reactive depression.

Alcoholism is also highly correlated with suicide. Interestingly, many of the alcoholics in Robins's case histories (2) had some signs and symptoms of major depression. Unfortunately, Robins did not present data sufficient to document the extent to which the alcoholic suicides had depressive illnesses. The evidence is certainly not striking that alcoholism *per se* (alcoholism unaccompanied by mood change or psychosis) is an immediate and direct cause of suicide. One would not hospitalize a patient as a suicide risk simply because he was alcoholic.

Using RDC criteria for schizophrenia, Wilkinson (13) reported a ten- to fifteen-year suicide rate of 8 percent in thirty-nine patients with schizophrenia. Robins's study (2) also reveals a suicide rate for schizophrenics higher than that in the general population. Borg and Stahl (8) report a significantly increased risk of suicide in drug abusers.

Anxiety neurosis, obsessional neurosis, and uncomplicated Briquet's syndrome occur less frequently among suicides than they do in the general population (2). There is only one reported case of suicide in a patient with Briquet's syndrome (14).

SIGNIFICANT SYSTEMIC ILLNESS

Compared to the general population, larger numbers of patients who commit suicide have significant systemic illness (2, 7). The frequency of suicide in one sample of hemodialysis patients was 400 times greater than the national average (15). The frequency of suicide in patients with Huntington's chorea is also very high (16). The risk of suicide in male cancer patients is somewhat higher than the national average for men (17). Hackett (18) reports an increased frequency of suicide in tic douloureux and cluster headache patients, but he does not cite the source of this information. Interestingly, most of these conditions are associated with brain dysfunction. However, two conditions not usually associated with brain dysfunction, rheumatoid arthritis (21 percent of Dorpat's cases) and peptic ulcer (15 percent of Dorpat's cases) are more common in patients who commit suicide than for the general population (7). However, the figures for the latter two conditions are not corrected for age.

PHENOMENA OBSERVED IN THE MENTAL STATUS EXAMINATION

Mental status (e.g. sustained sadness) and other physical (e.g. hemodialysis shunt) findings will point to diagnoses associated with high suicide risk. Some findings are of concern regardless of diagnosis: hopelessness, profound guilt, severe agitation, and psychosis. There is some evidence that the finding of hopelessness can be independent of depressive illness as a predictor of suicide risk (19, 20). This might explain some of the suicides in alcoholics who do not have major depression. Severe agitation could be an immediate predictor of suicide risk.

AGE

The risk of suicide increases with age, and the majority of suicides occur among the middle-aged and the aged (2, 3, 5, 21). Pfeiffer and Busse write:

"When an old person attempts suicide, he almost always fully expects to die" (21). The risk of suicide is extremely small in early childhood. Although suicide is far less common in adolescents than in the middle-aged and elderly, it is the third leading cause of death in adolescents (22). That is partly because adolescents rarely die from age-related illnesses such as myocardial infarction and cerebrovascular disease.

Sex

The frequency of death by suicide is greater for men than for women, regardless of diagnosis (2). This is striking, because major affective disorders are more common in women than in men and suicide *attempts* are more common for women than for men (2, 5). The male:female ratio for suicide is 3.5:1 (2). For patients with affective disorders, it is 2.5:1 (2). The reasons for these sex differences are not known (21).

Racial/Ethnic Differences

The frequency of suicide is greater for American Indians than for American whites (23). The white:black suicide ratio in the United States is approximately 2:1 (2, 24). Since suicide is as common for blacks in adolescence and early adulthood as at middle age and the geriatric ages (24), the differences in white:black suicide rates consist of differences among the middle-aged and elderly (24). The reasons for these racial/ethnic differences are not known; there is no evidence that these ethnic differences in suicide are income-related.

Religion

The frequency of suicide for Protestants is higher than that for Catholics (5). The suicide rates in predominantly Catholic countries are lower in general than those for predominantly Protestant countries, but this is not uniformly so. For example, Austria, a predominantly Catholic country, has a high suicide rate (5). One hypothesis for the relatively low rate of suicide among Catholics is the strong association with "mortal sin" among Catholics, but this has not yet been proved to be a causal relationship.

Psychiatric Hospitalization and Discharge

Suicide can occur on psychiatric units or when the patient is on pass. In Robins's study (2), about 27 percent of the sample of the suicides who had been hospitalized killed themselves in the hospital.

Seventy-five percent of suicides of patients discharged from psychiatric inpatient units occur within the first six months following discharge (25). That is probably because the first six months are the time of greatest risk for recurrence of major depression, a likely time for discontinuation of antidepressant medications, and obviously a time of risk if the patient continues to be ill. Thus the time of hospitalization and the months following discharge should be periods of special vigilance.

PRIOR SUICIDE ATTEMPTS

In every study of suicide, suicide attempts are associated with increased risk for future suicide. Eighteen percent of the Robins subjects (2), 30 percent of the Barraclough suicides (3), and 33 percent of the Dorpat suicides (7) had made prior attempts. Hendin (5) quotes a figure of 60 percent but does not state his source. Among suicides women (32 percent) are more likely to have made prior attempts than men (19 percent) and more likely (13 percent for women, 3 percent for men) to have made multiple suicide attempts (2).

LETHALITY OF SUICIDE ATTEMPTS

By definition, people who kill themselves do so by using biologically lethal means. In one study 6.4 percent of patients making serious suicide attempts will commit suicide some time within the following five years, as against 3.2 percent of patients making suicide attempts judged to be nonserious (10). For people who have made nonfatal suicide attempts, the correlation between physiological lethality and suicidal intent *at the time of the attempt* is surprisingly low ($r = + .19$). That is because many patients do not know the biological lethality of certain modes of suicide (26). When the patient has an accurate conception of the actual biological lethality of an intended suicidal act, the correlation between suicidal intent and medical lethality is strong ($r = + .73$) (26). Thus knowledge of actual plans for suicide may help the clinician, albeit to a small degree, to predict immediate suicide risk.

OTHER CORRELATES OF SUICIDE

Other correlates of suicide are also of interest. Suicide rates increase during times of economic hardship, the highest rates in United States history being during the Great Depression (4). The highest suicide rates for occupations occur among police (11), dentists (11), musicians (11), lawyers, (11) and female physicians (27).

Initial Triage and Management

When the suicidal patient is first seen, the primary goals are to protect him from harming himself while working vigorously at establishing a diagnosis and initiating appropriate treatment.

THE SERIOUSLY SUICIDAL PATIENT

For the seriously suicidal patient psychiatric hospitalization should always be recommended. If such a patient refuses hospitalization, the physician is justified in hospitalizing the patient involuntarily; in fact, he is expected to do so. On the hospital unit the physician must continue to provide protection for the patient. Such protection might include any of the following: continuous one-to-one staff observation; restraints; seclusion room; sleep-induction with sodium amobarbital, and emergency ECT.

On the hospital psychiatric unit the psychiatrist's concern about the safety of a suicidal patient is conveyed (1) by discussion of the suicide risk and precautions with the nursing staff, whose vigilance will then be heightened, and (2) by writing orders for suicide precautions. The order "suicide precautions" is insufficient by itself. The doctor should specify the precautions to be employed. For the seriously suicidal patient, one of the following precautions should be considered: (1) A staff member should be with the patient continuously, even when the patient is in the bathroom, or (2) the patient should be placed in a seclusion room and observed every fifteen minutes at least. For such patients emergency ECT should be considered. In most hospitals the suicide precautions are formalized in a written protocol.

Hospital studies reveal that the majority of patients committing suicide in the general hospital were admitted for nonpsychiatric illnesses (28–31), probably because medical and surgical personnel are not as likely to search for suicidal ideation, and because medical and surgical units are not well suited (e.g. no locked units, no seclusion rooms, insufficient personnel for continuous observation) for managing suicidal patients. Thus psychiatric consultants should attempt to transfer suicidal patients to psychiatric units if it is medically safe to do so. For reasons of medical or administrative necessity (e.g. many psychiatric services won't accept patients with intravenous lines), some patients must be treated on the medical/surgical services. In such cases the nursing staff should be informed of the risk and instructed to observe the patient at specified intervals. If the suicide risk is serious, the patient may have to be restrained or will need a relative to remain with him and be responsible for him while he is not restrained. Some hospitals have a close relative sign a document informing him of the suicide risk and of the limitations of protecting a medical/surgical patient. He or she is also asked to sign a consent to stay in the patient's room when the patient is not restrained.

THE PATIENT WHO IS CLEARLY NOT SUICIDAL

At the other end of the suicide risk spectrum is the young patient who has attempted suicide (sometimes referred to as a "pseudosuicide" or "parasuicide") (26) to gain attention, win concessions from others, or hurt someone's feelings. Usually such a patient does not have an acute or serious psychiatric illness. Sometimes he has no illness at all. Frequently, following emergency room treatment, he states that he is no longer suicidal. This "change of heart" usually occurs because of some combination of the following: the aversive effect of the gastric lavage or induced emesis; the attention and sensitivity of the emergency room staff; and the accomplishment of the purposes for which the "pseudosuicide" is intended or the realization that the goals of the "pseudosuicide" will not be forthcoming. These patients should usually be discharged home directly from the emergency room, intensive care unit, or medical ward. As these patients often continue to experience the stress leading to their "pseudosuicide," follow-up evaluation and psychological/social intervention are usually necessary and may prevent chronicity of such behavior. Emergency rooms receive more "pseudo-suicidal" patients than seriously suicidal patients.

THE PATIENT WHOSE SUICIDE RISK IS UNCERTAIN

The Patient Seen Shortly After an Overdose

When patients take overdoses, false positive drug-caused signs of endogenous depression may occur. For example, the overdose may transiently produce a sustained dysphoric mood or psychomotor retardation. These patients should be hospitalized on the medical service until the effects of the overdose have dissipated. After about twenty-four hours, the psychiatrist should not be surprised to find a significant improvement in mood and activity level.

The Endogenously Depressed Patient with No Suicidal Intent

Hospitalization should still be strongly recommended for endogenously depressed patients without stated suicide intent. But the patient could be discharged if the following circumstances occur concurrently:

1. The patient and his family refuse further hospitalization.
2. The family promises to be vigilant in observing the patient at home.
3. The patient shows motivation for outpatient treatment.
4. The patient is willing to sign an "against medical advice" form after he and his family are informed of the risk of prolonged illness and suicide.

Here is an example:

A twenty-five-year-old single employed man is seen in consultation on an outpatient basis. He has major depression with occasional suicidal ideation but states, "I wouldn't kill myself." He and three close family members vehemently oppose hospitalization on the grounds that the stigma of psychiatric hospitalization would be intolerable. Having been fully informed of the risks, they all agree that the patient will be brought thrice weekly for electroconvulsive therapy and that the family will stay with him continuously. This is feasible, for both his father and his sister volunteer to take one month's leave from work. The family keeps its promise, and the patient's depressive episode remits following twelve outpatient electroconvulsive treatments given over a four-week period.

The "Parasuicidal" or Reactively Depressed Patient Who Maintains That He Is Still Suicidal

One fairly common and somewhat difficult problem occurs in the case of the "pseudosuicidal" or reactively depressed patient who maintains that he is still suicidal. Rarely, if ever, should a "parasuicidal" patient be admitted to the hospital. Only a minority of reactively depressed patients should be admitted. Reflexively admitting such patients because of suicide threats may positively reinforce the use of such threats to obtain desired goals in the future. In triaging such patients, it should be noted that more than 99 percent of all patients discharged after suicide attempts are alive at the end of one year (32).

In these circumstances the physician should consider the following:

1. Reassess the patient in terms of the correlates of suicide discussed earlier in this chapter.
2. Discuss whether the patient feels his life would be worth living once the current personal crisis is resolved.
3. Discuss the patient's short-term and long-term plans if the current crisis were resolved.
4. Discuss what would be the patient's short-term and long-term plans if he were to be discharged from the hospital immediately.
5. Ask the patient whether he feels he could be assisted by outpatient treatment or hospitalization.

6. Ask the patient whether, if discharged, would he return to the hospital if he felt he was on the verge of killing himself.
7. Consider possible reasons for the patient to be malingering (e.g. trying to be discharged from the military, being undomiciled).
8. Assess the sincerity with which the patient claims to be suffering and needing to seek relief by suicide. Is the suicide threat presented in a seemingly rehearsed or dramatized way?
9. Obtain information and opinions from a family member or friend who is accompanying the patient (or is immediately available by phone).

In these cases, factors that would speak against hospitalization are:

1. Low suicide risk according to criteria described earlier in the chapter, especially the absence of serious psychiatric or medical illness
2. Suspected malingering
3. Insincerity of the expression of suffering or suicidal intent
4. Expression of hope for improvement by resolution of the current crisis or by treatment
5. Motivation to stay alive despite suicidal ideation
6. Diagnosis of sociopathy
7. Family member's or friend's doubts about seriousness of suicide risk

The following is an example of a patient who was thought not to be suicidal despite his statements that he was suicidal:

A nineteen-year-old single white Army artillery trainee was seen with the chief complaint, "If you don't let me out of the Army, I'll kill myself." He also stated that when discharged from the Army, a caring fiancée, loving parents, and a job awaited him in his home town. The mental status revealed a young man with a euthymic mood and no signs of endogenous depression or other significant psychiatric disorder. He was immediately returned for duty in his military unit.

When a patient thought to be malingering or insincere about suicidal intent states, "If you discharge me, I'll kill myself," he can be told, "I hope that you don't kill yourself when you go home. It's up to you, not to me."

In cases where a reactively depressed patient is felt to be suffering considerably and in need of hospitalization, he should be triaged the same way as the "endogenously depressed patient with no suicidal intent" discussed previously. Of course, the definitive treatments for reactive and endogenously depressed patients will be different.

Definitive Treatment

In the context of adequate protection for the suicidal patient, proper diagnosis and treatment are essential. Indeed, the patient's short- and long-term survival, in terms of suicide *as well as other causes of death* (33), hinges upon whether adequate treatment is provided. For endogenously depressed patients, the category at highest risk for suicide, the mortality rates for causes of death (e.g. cancer, infection, cardiovascular disease) other than suicide exceed that for the general population (33, 35).

The patient with major depression is best treated with ECT. Survival rates for adequate tricyclic antidepressant treatment are better than for no treatment or for inadequate antidepressant treatment (33). Lithium carbonate is another possibility. Prescription of tricyclic antidepressants or lithium carbonate for depressed and suicidal patients should occur only in the hospital or under the circumstances described in Chapter 11, and the patient should have access to no more than one week's supply of medication, carefully monitored by a family member.

For the patient with an endogenous depression secondary to coarse brain disease, the underlying disease, if it can be remedied, should be the main focus of treatment, as in the following example:

A fifty-four-year-old single white Catholic man was admitted to an internal medicine service with uremia secondary to obstructive uropathy caused by benign prostatic hypertrophy. As the uremia developed prior to admission, so too did a severe endogenous depression associated with appetite and weight loss, early morning wakening, and feelings of hopelessness and worthlessness. The patient stated that he was suffering so severely that he wanted his doctors to kill him or to discharge him home to die. He had no past history or family history of psychiatric illness. The physical examination revealed pallor and an enlarged suprapubic mass (his bladder), palpable to the umbilicus. His mood was of sustained sadness with crying, and he manifested hopelessness and worthlessness. He was felt to be imminently suicidal and detained in the hospital against his wishes. Twenty-four hours later two close friends convinced him to undergo Foley catheterization and prostatectomy. Within twenty-four hours after a Foley catheter was inserted, his mood improved and his suicidal ideation ceased.

The patient with reactive depression should be treated with MAO inhibitors and/or cognitive psychotherapy. Prescription of MAOIs for reactively depressed patients should occur only in the hospital or in the presence of circumstances 1 to 4 listed on page 253. Reactively depressed outpatients should have access to no more than one week's supply of medication, carefully monitored by a family member. Patients with alcoholism or schizophrenia should be treated as discussed in Chapters 19 and 15 respectively.

In referring the patient to another physician for outpatient care, the referring physician should simplify the referral process as much as possible for the patient before the first visit. If the referring physician is concerned about the patient's suicide risk, he should call the outpatient physician or the patient to be sure the patient has kept the first appointment. Failure to keep a first appointment should be a cause for concern, and a follow-up call to the patient or a relative is in order.

Maintenance Treatment

Once the acute episode leading to the suicidal risk is remitted, steps should be taken to maintain the patient's recovery. For the patient in remission following treatment of major depression, maintenance tricyclic antidepressants, lithium carbonate, or ECT should be prescribed as described in Chapters 4–6 and 11. For the patient successfully treated for an endogenous depression secondary to coarse brain disease, ongoing treatment should be continued if the underlying coarse disease has not been resolved. Patients with schizophrenia should usually be maintained on neuroleptic drugs for about one year following initial prescription of neuroleptics. Whenever possible continuity of care with regular visits to a physician should be maintained for at least one year.

At any point in the management of the suicidal patient there are several other considerations. First, as in any other difficult situation the psychiatrist should feel free to request a colleague's consultation. Second, as in all other medical situations the psychiatrist should write careful notes, ensuring that his actions have been clearly explained in writing. For example, if a patient for whom suicide risk has been an issue is sent home or given a pass, the doctor should note that the patient is "not imminently suicidal," "not actively suicidal," or "not suicidal," if such is in fact the case. Third, the doctor need not absolutely honor the patient's confidences if disclosure of the patient's suicidal risk might save his life. For example, if a potentially suicidal patient elopes from the hospital, the doctor should notify a relative, a close friend, or the police.

References

1. Teuting, P.; Koslow, S. H.; Herschfeld, R. M. A. *Special Report on Depression Research.* DHHS pub. no. (ADM) 81–600024, 1982.
2. Robins, E. *The Final Months.* New York: Oxford University Press, 1981.
3. Barraclough, B.; Bunch, J.; Nelson, B.; *et al.* A hundred cases of suicide: Clinical aspects. *Br. J. Psychiat.* 125: 355–73, 1974.
4. Gregory, I.; Smeltzer, D. J. *Psychiatry: Essentials of Clinical Practice.* Boston: Little, Brown, 1977, p. 197.
5. Hendin, H. Suicide. In Freedman, A.; Kaplan, H. (eds.), *Comprehensive Textbook of Psychiatry.* Baltimore: Williams & Wilkins, 1967, p. 1173.

6. Murphy, G. E. The physician's responsibility for suicide: 1. An error of commission. *Ann. Int. Med.* 82: 301–4, 1975.

7. Dorpat, T. L.; Ripley, H. S. A study of suicide in the Seattle area. *Comp. Psychiat.* 1(6): 349–59, 1960.

8. Borg, S. E.; Stahl, M. Prediction of suicide: A prospective study of suicides and controls among psychiatric patients. *Acta Psychiat. Scand.* 65: 221–32, 1982.

9. DeLong, W.; Robins, E. The communication of suicidal intent prior to psychiatric hospitalization: A study of 87 patients. *Am. J. Psychiat.* 1127: 695–705 (1961).

10. Littman, R. E.; Farberow, N. L. Emergency Evaluation of Self-destructive Potential. In Farberow, N. L.; Shneidman, E. S. (eds.), *Cry for Help.* New York: McGraw–Hill, 1961.

11. Shader, R. J. Assessment of Suicide Risk. In Shader, R. J. (ed.), *Manual of Psychiatric Therapeutics.* Boston: Little, Brown, 1975, p. 306.

12. Guze, S. B.; Robins, E. Suicide and primary affective disorders. *Br. J. Psychiat.* 117: 437–38 (1970).

13. Wilkinson, D. G. The suicide rate in schizophrenia. *Br. J. Psychiat.* 140: 138–41, 1982.

14. Morrison, J. R. Suicide in a case of Briquet's syndrome. *J. Clin. Psychiatry* 42: 3, 1981.

15. Abram, H. S.; Moore, G.; Westervelt, F. Suicidal behavior in chronic dialysis patients. *Am. J. Psychiat.* 127: 1199–1204, 1971.

16. Beckford, J. A. R.; Elleson, R. M. The high incidence of Huntington's chorea in the Duchy of Cornwall. *J. Ment. Sci.* 99: 623, 1953.

17. Fox, B. H.; Stanek, E. J., III; Boyd, S. C.; *et al.* Suicide rates among cancer patients in Connecticut. *J. Chronic Dis.* 35: 89, 1982.

18. Hackett, T. P. The Pain Patient: Evaluation and Management. In Hackett, T. P.; Cassem, N. H. (eds.), *Handbook of General Hospital Psychiatry.* St. Louis: C. V. Mosby, 1978, pp. 41–63.

19. Pokorny, A. D.; Kaplan, H. B.; Tsai, S. Y. Hopelessness and attempted suicide: A reconsideration. *Am. J. Psychiat.* 132: 954–56, 1975.

20. Beck, A. T.; Kovacs, M.; Weissman, A. Hopelessness and suicidal behavior: An overview. *JAMA* 234: 1146–49, 1975.

21. Pfeiffer, E.; Busse, E. W. Affective Disorders. In Busse, E.; Pfeiffer, E. W. (eds.), *Mental Illness in Later Life.* New York: American Psychiatric Association, 1973, p. 125.

22. Hollinger, P. Violent deaths as a leading cause of mortality: An epidemiologic study of suicide, homicide, and accidents. *Am. J. Psychiat.* 137(4): 472–76, 1980.

23. Glickman, L. The Phenomenon of Suicide. In Simons, R.; Pardes, H. (eds.), *Understanding Human Behavior in Health and Illness.* Baltimore: Williams & Wilkins, 1977, p. 612.

24. Hendin, H. *Black Suicide.* New York: Harper & Row, 1969.

25. Pokorny, A. D.; Kaplan, H. B. Suicide following psychiatric hospitalization. *J. Nerv. Ment. Dis.* 162: 119–25, 1976.

26. Beck, A. T.; Beck, R.; Kovacs, M. Classification of suicidal behaviors: I. Quantifying intent and medical lethality. *Am. J. Psychiat.* *132:* 285–87, 1975.

27. Pitts, F. N., Jr.; Schuller, A. B.; Rich, C. L.; *et al.* Suicide among U.S. women physicians, 1967–1972. *Am. J. Psychiat.* *136:* 694–96, 1979.

28. Reich, P.; Kelly, M. J. Suicide attempts by hospitalized medical and surgical patients. *New Eng. J. Med.* *294:* 298–301, 1976.

29. Farberow, N. L.; Schneidman, E. S.; Leonard, C. K. Suicide among general medical and surgical hospital patients with malignant neoplasms. *Med. Bull. V. Adm.* *9:* 1–11, 1963.

30. Pollack, S. Suicide in a General Hospital. In Shneidman, E. S.; Farberow, N. L. (eds.), *Clues to Suicide.* New York: McGraw–Hill, 1957, pp. 152–63.

31. Farberow, N. L.; McKelligott, J. W.; Cohen, S.; *et al.* Suicide among patients with cardiorespiratory illness. *JAMA 195:* 422–28, 1966.

32. Ettlinger, R. W. Suicide in a group of patients who had previously attempted suicide. *Acta Psychiat. Scand. 40:* 363–78, 1964.

33. Avery, D.; Winokur, G. Mortality in depressed patients treated with electroconvulsive therapy and antidepressants. *Arch. Gen. Psychiat. 33:* 1029–37, 1976.

34. Bratfos, O.; Haug, J. L. The course of manic-depressive psychosis: A follow-up investigation of 215 patients. *Acta Psychiat. Scand. 44:* 89–112, 1968.

35. Kerr, T. A.; Schapira, K.; Roth, M. The relationship between premature death and affective disorders. *Br. J. Psychiat. 115:* 1277–82, 1969.

CHAPTER 13

The Violent Patient

We define a violent person as one having an increased likelihood of injuring somebody in circumstances not permitted by law (e.g. war, self-defense). Ninety percent of people arrested for felonies (many of which are violent crimes) have a psychiatric syndrome, particularly sociopathy (1). A review of the list of these syndromes leads to the unfortunate conclusion that most felons (e.g. sociopaths without underlying affective disorder or drug-induced psychosis) cannot be effectively treated for their behavioral problems by physicians. Society must deal with them.

Despite the lack of a standard, effective treatment for violent people, violent patients are often evaluated or treated by mental health professionals. In a survey of 115 psychiatrists on a university faculty, 42 percent reported having been assaulted by a patient (2). In another survey of mental health professionals, 24 percent of 101 therapists had been attacked by at least one patient during the year prior to the survey (3). Eighty-two percent of psychiatrists and psychologists in a California survey (4) reported having seen at least one patient per year whom they considered to be potentially dangerous, with the mean number of dangerous patients seen per year being fourteen. In a survey of Boston psychiatrists (5) 35 percent saw violent patients on the average at least once a month; 8 percent of these evaluated more than 50 percent the total number of violent patients. Interestingly, the youngest and least experienced among them had the greatest exposure to violent patients.

There has been a steady increase in the rate of violent crimes during the past decade (6). The estimated frequency of crime in general and violent crime in particular is presented in Table 13-1. Homicide is the eleventh leading cause of death in the United States and is the second leading cause of the death of adolescents (7).

The Literature on Long-term Violence Prediction

The literature on the long-term prediction of violence contains statements that the mental health field has shown "an abysmal failure to predict violence accurately" (8). Such conclusions are based upon studies (9–13) of inmates in institutions for the criminally insane, who upon discharge were evaluated largely through arrest records in nonpenal settings or in the community. "Only" 14–35 percent of those individuals were eventually arrested for violent acts. These data are summarized by Monahan (14) and shown in Table 13-2.

From these studies it has been claimed that "the state of the art is that for every 100 people we classify as dangerous, no more than one-third subsequently engage in violent behavior" (15). Thus a prediction that a given individual in an institution for the criminally insane will be violent is more likely to be wrong than right. The extent to which data from institutions for the criminally insane can be extrapolated to the general hospital is unknown. However, a psychiatrist testifying at a commitment hearing should not state with *certainty* that a person will injure someone else. Rather, he should state that compared to the general population, the patient is statistically more likely (or not more likely) to be violent, and give reasons. Predictors of violence will be discussed later in the chapter. One reason it is difficult to predict whether a given person will be violent is that in studies of violent individuals the independent contribution toward violence of individual factors (e.g. gender, ethnic group, age, and diagnosis) is rarely determined statistically by employing matched control groups.

Although there are no controlled studies on the prediction of violence in critical situations (14), physicians are obligated to provide treatment to violent patients during emergencies, even if it means involuntary hospitalization, as in this case:

A seventeen-year-old single black woman was brought to an emergency room by six relatives after she attempted to stab her brother. She was sleepless for three days and had no history of drug abuse. The mental status revealed irritable mood, hyperactivity, and pressured speech. Testing of cognitive functioning and a brief physical ex-

TABLE 13-1 National Crime, Rate, and Percent Change

Crime Index Offenses	ESTIMATED CRIME 1980		PERCENT CHANGE OVER 1979		PERCENT CHANGE OVER 1976		PERCENT CHANGE OVER 1971	
	Number	Rate per 100,000 Inhabitants	Number	Rate	Number	Rate	Number	Rate
Murder	23,040	10.2	+ 7.4	+ 5.2	+22.7	+15.9	+29.6	+18.6
Forcible rape	82,090	36.4	+ 8.0	+ 5.5	+44.7	+37.9	+94.2	+77.6
Robbery	548,810	243.5	+17.5	+14.8	+30.6	+24.4	+41.6	+29.5
Aggravated assault	654,960	290.6	+ 6.6	+ 4.1	+33.4	+27.1	+77.6	+62.5
Burglary	3,759,200	1,668.2	+13.9	+11.3	+21.7	+15.9	+56.7	+43.4
Larceny-theft	7,112,700	3,156.3	+ 8.1	+ 5.6	+13.4	+ 8.0	+60.8	+47.1
Motor vehicle theft	1,114,700	494.6	+ 1.6	− .8	+16.4	+10.9	+17.6	+ 7.6
Violent	1,308,900	580.8	+11.1	+ 8.5	+32.7	+26.4	+60.3	+46.7
Property	11,986,500	5,319.1	+ 9.2	+ 6.7	+16.2	+10.7	+54.2	+41.1
Total	13,295,400	5,899.9	+ 9.4	+ 6.9	+17.6	+12.0	+54.8	+41.7

Source: *Uniform Crime Reports for the United States, 1980.* Washington, D.C.: U.S. Department of Justice, Federal Bureau of Investigation.

TABLE 13-2 Validity Studies of the Clinical Prediction of Violent Behavior

STUDY	PERCENT TRUE POSITIVE	PERCENT FALSE POSITIVE	PERCENT TRUE NEGATIVE	PERCENT FALSE NEGATIVE	NUMBER PREDICTED VIOLENT	NUMBER PREDICTED NONVIOLENT	FOLLOWUP YEARS
Kozol et al. (1972) (9)	34.7	65.3	92.0	8.0	49	386	5
Steadman and Cocozza (1974) (10)	20.0	80.0	—	—	967	—	4
Cocozza and Steadman (1976) (11)	14.0	86.0	84.0	16.0	154	103	3
Steadman (1977) (12)	41.3	58.7	68.8	31.2	46	106	3
Thornberry and Jacoby (1979) (13)	14.0	86.0	—	—	438	—	4

NOTE: A "true positive" is a person who was thought to be dangerous and then does commit a violent act; a "false positive" is one thought to be dangerous who does not eventually commit a violent act; a "true negative" is one who is thought nondangerous and later is nonviolent; a "false negative" is a person thought not to be dangerous who some time later does act violently.

SOURCE: John Monahan, Table 3, p. 79 in *Predicting Violent Behavior*. Copyright © 1981 by Sage Publications, Inc. Reprinted by permission.

amination revealed no abnormalities. The working diagnosis was bipolar disorder. The family agreed that the patient should be in the hospital, but she refused. She was then hospitalized involuntarily as being potentially violent.

The Assessment of the Patient

The assessment of risk of violence begins with a thorough, sensitively taken history, which should include questioning about past violent acts (e.g. "What's the most violent thing you've ever done?") as well as inquiries about the following:

Current violent thoughts
Current violent intentions
Past felonies
Likelihood of drug or alcohol
  intoxication
Jealous or persecutory feelings
  or delusions
Ownership and availability of
  weapons
Divorces and separations
Employment status
Parental or other family violence

Command hallucinations
Thoughts of suicide
Symptoms of alcoholism
Symptoms of drug dependence
Symptoms of sociopathy
History of enuresis, firesetting,
  or cruelty to animals
Symptoms of epilepsy and other
  coarse brain disease
Symptoms of mania or
  depression
Hospitalizations for
  psychiatric illness

When available, additional history should be obtained from hospital records, family and friends, physicians, and other informants. A thorough physical (including a thorough mental status) examination should be performed. Particular attention should be paid to signs of drug or alcohol intoxication, tattoos, needle-tracks, motorcycle-gang style of dress, agitation, pacing, muscle-clenching, menacing gait, threatening gestures, anger or irritability, and rapidity or pressure of speech; revengeful, jealous, or threatening thought content; delusions of persecution; alterations of consciousness; automatic behavior; or postictal delirious behavior. When laboratory investigations are to be done for a potentially violent patient, an electroencephalographic study (with nasopharyngeal leads if possible) should be performed to rule out the presence of a seizure disorder.

Behaviors specifically associated with imminent risk for violence include the following, which commonly precede the violence:

1. Recent assaultiveness
2. Homicidal or assaultive threats or intent
3. Pacing, muscle-clenching, or menacing gestures
4. Agitation, rage, shouting, or irritability

The occurrence of one or more of these demands a rapid therapeutic response, as described in the sections on violence and agitation in chapters 5, 8 and 11.

Factors predictive of the long-term risk of violence (also influencing the acute situation) include:

1. Past criminality (particularly violent crime) or violent behavior
2. Diagnosis of one of the following:
   A. Antisocial personality (sociopathy)
   B. Somatization disorder (Briquet's syndrome)
   C. Mania
   D. Epilepsy
   E. Alcoholism
   F. Drug dependence
3. Abnormal EEG

Factors decreasing the risk of violence include:

1. No past crime or violent behavior
2. No psychiatric illness

Three case reports illustrate factors that predict violence.

Case 1

The patient was a thirty-three-year-old white, married (once divorced) former fireman hospitalized, on an inpatient unit devoted to stress disorders, because of recurring intense daydreams and nightmares of a fire seven years prior to admission in which he was unable to rescue an elderly man from a burning building. Since the fire, he lost interest in some of the activities he had enjoyed before it, had trouble falling asleep, and felt guilty that he had survived the fire. Also since the fire, he had been fired several times and had quit jobs without another job prospect. He had six fights during his adult life. Once he tried to shoot a stranger who insulted him. He beat his wife several times.

After enlisting at age seventeen to fight in Vietnam, he occasionally became angry and cut off fingers of dead Vietcong soldiers. Also in Vietnam he began drinking heavily, and he continued to do so until his admission. He occasionally drank before breakfast, had blackouts, and had several episodes of tremulousness when he couldn't drink. Once he was arrested for destroying property while drinking. He missed work because of drinking and was hospitalized several times because of drinking.

One of his childhood hobbies was hunting. He was arrested for assault when he was sixteen. An older brother had had several hospitalizations for drug abuse.

His mental status was essentially normal throughout his hospital stay, and three electroencephalograms were normal. He was diagnosed as having alcoholism, sociopathy, and post traumatic stress disorder. He refused disulfiram. Because of the unit's belief that he had a stress disorder, he was hospitalized for five months for treatment of his recurrent daydreams. During the hospital stay he had taken six passes, five of which had been without incident. On his fourth pass he drank and expressed suicidal thoughts, and on his seventh pass, while drinking and without prior warning, he got into an argument with his brother and shot him to death.

Important factors in this case included prior violence and diagnoses of alcoholism and sociopathy. His long-term risk for violence was greater than for the general population, but he was not thought to be immediately homicidal. This case illustrates how difficult it can be to predict violent behavior at a given time. It also illustrates the futility of protracted hospitalizations of patients of normal mental status with no curable illness.

Case 2

The patient was a thirty-four-year-old single white man who was hospitalized two weeks after release from prison at the urging of his parole officer, who was afraid the patient might harm the patient's mother. The patient said that God had told him there was a Nazi plot to take over the media and that a lot of blood would be shed as a result.
As a child he ran away from home and was suspended from school. He had chronic problems keeping a job. He was arrested several times for shoplifting and served two jail terms for attempted homicide by stabbing. He used a variety of drugs, including phenyclidine, amphetamine, cocaine, and LSD.
The admission mental status examination revealed delusions and incomplete auditory hallucinations. The diagnosis was sociopathy and drug-induced psychosis. He requested several times to sign out against medical advice but rescinded this decision all but the last time. Because he was felt to be potentially dangerous, he was held on the unit awaiting a commitment hearing. After learning of the impending commitment, he began refusing to take medication. His refusal was permitted on the grounds that despite the patient's history he retained the right to refuse medication. He then shaved his head into a "Mohawk" haircut and started pacing the halls. The following morning, he stabbed his doctor in the chin with a plastic knife secreted from the ward kitchen.

Important factors in this case included two prior violent felonies, diagnosis of sociopathy, and an intensifying unmedicated drug-induced psychosis associated with head-shaving, loss of compliance, and pacing. The risk of short-term violence was progressively increasing in this case; the safety of the ward doctor was also a civil right, which should have been honored well before the stabbing by medicating the patient involuntarily with haloperidol.

Case 3

The patient was a twenty-three-year-old single, unemployed Hispanic man admitted to a psychiatric inpatient service following an episode during which he attempted, without provocation, to choke his mother. He had no recollection of this attempted matricide, which so frightened his family that they said they would not let him return home after discharge from the hospital.

He was receiving diphenylhydantoin and phenobarbital for grand mal seizures that began several years previously with the onset of tuberous sclerosis. In recent months the seizures had been less frequent. An uncle had died from tuberous sclerosis.

The physical examination revealed adenoma sebaceum of the face and shagreen patches on the skin of the back and neck. The mental status revealed sullenness, an understandable pessimism about his condition, borderline intelligence, and no other abnormalities.

On the fifth hospital day, the patient was observed by several patients to be staring for several minutes with his eyes deviated, following which, for no apparent reason, he hit a fellow patient and had to be restrained. An EEG revealed bilateral temporal lobe spiking, and a diagnosis of partial complex seizures due to temporal lobe epilepsy was made. Treatment with carbamazepine was then initiated.

Important factors in this case were a history of prior violence, diagnosis of psychomotor epilepsy, and an abnormal electroencephalogram. The lifetime risk of violence in such individuals is greater than that of the general population. By a year after discharge, the patient had committed no more violent acts.

Predictors of Violence

Past History of Criminal or Violent Behavior

All studies of the prediction of violent behavior show the predictive value of past violence (1, 14, 16–19). In one study of murdered children, in 90 percent of cases the victims, their siblings, or both had been physically abused or neglected before the killings (16). Among maladjusted Vietnam combat veterans under psychiatric evaluation, those most likely to act violently had committed violent acts (e.g. torturing prisoners, attacking officers with grenades, mutilating the dead) in Vietnam (17). In a study of parolees, violence was three times more likely if the parolee had been previously arrested for a violent offense (18). In a large cohort of all boys aged ten to eighteen who were born in Philadelphia, 70 percent of all violent acts committed by nonwhites were committed by young male chronic offenders, and 45 percent of all violent acts committed by whites were performed by boys with a chronic history of arrests (19).

Psychiatric Syndromes

An individual's lifetime risk of violence is significantly increased if he has one of several syndromes. The syndrome most closely associated with crime, and violent crime in particular, is sociopathy. Using Feighner's (20) criteria, Guze (1) found that 78 percent of male felons and 65 percent of female felons had sociopathy. Hare (21) reported that of 202 criminals, the majority were psychopaths. Virkkunen and Huttunen (22) wrote that of sixty violent offenders, thirty-two (53.3 percent) had antisocial personality disorder.

Other authors diagnosed sociopathy in a minority of felons, but still at a rate well in excess of that seen in the general population. Herjanic, Henn, and Vanderpohl (23) found sociopathy in 28 percent of male offenders and 13 percent of female offenders. Piotrowski, Losacco, and Guze (24) identified sociopathy in 24 percent of felons referred to psychiatrists for mental evaluations, and Schuckit (25) listed this diagnosis for 16 percent of 199 men arrested for their first felony. Swank and Winer (26) made the diagnosis of sociopathy in 13 percent of randomly selected county jail inmates.

In studies of violent offenders where research criteria were not used nor diagnoses employed, there is a high frequency of behaviors associated with sociopathy. A group of enlisted men court-martialed for exploding fragmentation grenades ("fragging") at hated officers often manifested "poor scholarship," "no viable marriages," and "previous incidents of antisocial behavior" (27). Yager's group of violent maladjusted combat veterans, as compared to nonviolent maladjusted combat veterans, contained significantly more individuals with histories of enuresis, fighting, arrests, fire-setting, and dropping out of school. A significant number of Macdonald's hundred homicide cases (28) manifested the triad of enuresis, fire-setting, and cruelty to animals. Finally, Hellman and Blackman (29) found the same triad, or part of the triad, in twenty-three (74%) of thirty-one people charged with aggressive crimes, making a diagnosis of "character disorder" in the majority.

Other psychiatric conditions were associated with violence. In the Guze study (1), 41 percent of female felons met criteria for Briquet's syndrome. To our knowledge, no other studies of female offenders checked for this diagnosis.

Taylor and Abrams (30) reported that 48.1 percent of patients during manic episodes manifested assaultive or threatening behavior. Falconer et al. (31) reported that 38 percent of patients with temporal lobe epilepsy had pathologic aggressiveness. Ounstead (32) found a history of outbursts of rage in thirty-six of one hundred epileptic patients, and Pincus (33) found an association between epilepsy and violence. However, not all researchers agree that there is a higher frequency of violence among epileptics (34, 35). Violence during partial complex seizures in psychomotor epileptics is rare; it is far more likely to occur at other times.

Intoxication with alcohol or drugs is extremely common at the time of violent crime. In one study (36) comparing 109 murderers with thirty-nine matched nonviolent criminals, the principal difference was that the murderers were far more likely (54 percent to 5 percent) to have been intoxicated with alcohol or drugs. In ten other studies of murderers, the percentage who had been drinking just prior to the homicide ranged from 19 to 83 percent, with a median of 54 percent (28). In five other such studies about 50 percent of the murderers had been drinking at the time of the crime (37). In the military, 87.5 percent of a group of "fraggers" were intoxicated with alcohol or drugs at the time of the "fragging." In one study of rapists 50 percent were intoxicated at the time of the rape (38).

No doubt in many cases the intoxicant diminishes inhibitions (and certain drugs, such as amphetamine taken in high doses [39], cause psychosis), but the exact contribution of the intoxicant, or of a diagnosis of alcohol or drug dependence, is less clear. For example, among a group of habitually violent adolescent offenders, it was well known that "reds [secobarbital] make you rowdy," and there was a preference for taking alcohol or secobarbital (40) in anticipation of perpetrating violence. Common characteristics of amphetamine abusers are armed robbery to support drug habits, conflicts over dealing in drugs, and carrying weapons (39).

The seemingly strong relationship between a diagnosis of alcoholism or drug dependence and violence is not as clear as might be expected. Guze found that 43 percent of male felons were definitely alcoholic and 11 percent probably so, and that 47 percent of female felons were alcoholic (1). Guze did not state the association of these diagnoses with violent crimes in particular, however, or take into account additional factors such as the concurrent presence of sociopathy. Thirty-five percent of Rada's sample of convicted rapists were alcoholics (38), but Rada did not take other possible contributing factors into account. In a 1973 review of the literature on homicide and alcohol Goodwin (37) stated that there was as yet no proved association between a diagnosis of alcoholism and the crime of homicide.

A 1944 study (41) showed that aggressiveness and EEG abnormalities could be induced by giving alcohol intravenously to people with histories of alcohol-related violence followed by amnesia. This finding, however, could not be replicated in a controlled double-blind study in a similar group of patients (42), casting serious doubt on the concept of pathologic intoxication, defined as a delirium-like aggressive psychosis induced by ingesting small amounts of alcohol and followed by sleep and amnesia for the event.

Although violence is more likely in patients with the above diagnoses than in the general population, violence can of course be precipitated by illness in patients with any diagnosis, regardless of whether the frequency of violence in patients with that diagnosis exceeds that of the general population. Violence has been reported in amphetamine psychosis (39), phencyclidine psychosis (43), LSD intoxication (44), cocaine intoxication (45), drug withdrawal (45), alcoholic hallucinosis (45), primary degenerative dementia (45), multi-infarct dementia (45), Huntington's chorea (45), brain tumor (45), intracranial tuberculoma (46), subdural hematoma (45), subarachnoid hemorrhage (45), late paraphrenia (47), and major depression

(45). In England, one-fourth of homicides are followed by suicide of the perpetrator (48), suggesting an association in some cases between homicide and depression.

A controversy exists regarding whether the frequency of crime in general, or violent crime in particular, is more common in people who have been hospitalized for psychiatric reasons than in the general population. Most studies (49–53) after 1961 show that the frequency is higher than in the general population. Most studies before then (54–57) showed a lower rate of arrests among former psychiatric patients. In one study (57), crimes by former patients were explained on the basis that the posthospital arrests occurred in people with prehospital criminality; this was not demonstrated in the other studies. The reasons for the increased posthospital arrest rates reported since 1961 are not known but could be related to shorter hospital stays, access of larger numbers of people with wider ranges of diagnoses (e.g. patients in substance abuse treatment programs) to more hospitals, or diminished use of electroconvulsive therapy.

ABNORMAL ELECTROENCEPHALOGRAM

There is a significant relationship between EEG abnormality and sociopathy, criminality, and violence. This association, which has been summarized by Stafford-Clark (58), appears in Table 13–3 (59–62). Williams (63) found that for habitually aggressive criminals, 56.9 percent had abnormal electroencephalograms, most typically slowing in the theta frequency in the anterior temporal and lateral frontal regions of the brain. He reports, as do

TABLE 13–3 The Relationship of Personality Disorder to the Incidence of Abnormal Electroencephalograms

CATEGORY	INCIDENCE OF ABNORMAL EEGS (PERCENT)	AUTHORITY
Flying personnel	5	Williams (1941) (59)
Royal Army Medical Corps personnel	10	Williams (1941) (59)
Mixed controls	15	Hill, Watterson (1942) (60)
Controls in prison	25	Stafford-Clark, Pond, Doust (1951) (61)
Mixed psychoneurotics	26	Williams (1941) (59)
Inadequate psychopaths	32	Hill, Watterson (1942) (60)
Aggressive psychopaths	65	Hill, Watterson (1942) (60)
Motiveless murderers	73	Stafford-Clark, Taylor (1949) (62)
Aggressive psychopaths in prison	83	Stafford-Clark, Pond, Doust (1951) (61)

SOURCE: D. Stafford-Clark, Table 9.1, p. 1199 in *British Medical Journal* 2 (December 5, 1959). Reproduced with permission from the Editor.

Gibbs, Bagchi, and Bloomberg (64), that with aging these abnormalities often diminish in degree, perhaps paralleling the decline in criminality as individuals become middle-aged.

Other Correlates of Violence

Other variables are correlated with violence. These include being male, being a teenager or young adult, being black, being separated or divorced, or having a history of observing (or being victim of) parental violence. Unfortunately the literature on these variables provides no compelling evidence to support a physician's concern that *because* a given patient is male, young, black, or separated or divorced, in the absence of such factors as prior violence or a diagnosis of sociopathy, he is violent. Nevertheless, physicians should be aware of these variables, whose relationship to violence awaits further clarification.

MALE GENDER

Although the frequency of violence by women is increasing, the ratio of male violence to female violence is 9:1 (14). For women who are violent, the violent behaviors are more likely to occur around the time of menstruation; 49 percent of all crimes committed by women occur during menstruation or during the four premenstrual days (65).

TEENAGER OR YOUNG ADULT

The Rand study found that habitual offenders committed a mean of 3.2 serious crimes per month as "juveniles," 1.5 per month as young adults, and 0.6 per month after that (66). In a 1975 study males between fifteen and twenty, who made up 8.5 percent of the American population, accounted for 35 percent of arrests for violent crimes (67). In a study of assaultive suicidal patients, patients under forty-five were more likely to assault other patients or staff while in the hospital (68).

The following is an example of the apparent diminution of a man's violence potential with age:

A thirty-seven-year-old unemployed psychiatrically disabled man of mixed Chicano and American Indian heritage was admitted to a psychiatric inpatient service because of an intensification of auditory hallucinations that were continually present for seventeen years despite numerous hospitalizations and high doses of various neuroleptic drugs. The voices usually told him to kill himself, but for years he had been able to resist them because "I don't agree with them." He had no other symptoms and lived congenially with his mother and sister-in-law. His reason for being hospitalized was "to make the voices go away," to which he added that he had not felt irritable or in danger of hurting anyone since he was imprisoned as a teenager. He described himself as having been a "wild" teenager, who fought frequently, drank heavily, and took multiple drugs. On one occasion while he was intoxicated, he was hearing voices and, thinking a friend was responsible for the voices, bludgeoned the friend to death. He was imprisoned for several years for this homicide. After he entered prison the voices remained, but he learned to tolerate them, and his fighting and drug-taking totally ceased. There was no family history of psychiatric illness.

He was a muscular, tattooed, friendly, and cooperative man whose physical (and mental status) examination was normal except for his complaint of hallucinations and moderate anxiety about having them. His diagnosis was drug-induced hallucinosis. As he had not engaged in any antisocial behavior for close to fifteen years, he was given no additional diagnosis. His hallucinations disappeared after six ECT, and he remained symptom-free for nearly a year after discharge.

History of Separation, Divorce, or Lack of Family Support and History of Parental Cruelty

Felons are more likely than the general population to be separated or divorced (1). It should also be noted that there is also an increased rate of divorce among sociopaths and alcoholics. The degree of support provided by the family of a recently discharged psychiatric patient is related to his ability to function in the community upon discharge (69).

Felons are also more likely to have been reared away from the home of their biological parents (e.g. reared in orphanages or foster homes or reared by friends) (1), to have divorced or separated parents (1), to have observed (or been victim of) parental violence (27, 70–73), or to have had parents who were criminals (1).

Black

Although the rate of suicide is significantly greater for whites than for blacks, the reverse is true for violent crimes. For example, in 1977 blacks constituted less than 12 percent of the American population but accounted for 46 percent of the arrests for violent crime (14). Unfortunately, statistics such as the latter do not control for such variables as diagnosis of sociopathy or being reared in a one-parent household. We have not found "blackness" to be a useful predictor of violence in our hospitalized patients.

Management

Measures to be taken as violence is occurring or is just about to occur are described in detail in Chapter 8. The best management of hospital violence, however, is its prevention.

Interviews should be conducted with respect, thoroughness, and empathy. Patients perceiving physicians to be making a sincere effort to provide excellent care are less likely to retaliate against them. Defensiveness and arguing should be avoided. Missed appointments and anticipated visits by other physicians should be discussed with the patient in advance.

Half of all episodes of violence in the hospital occur in the emergency room. The emergency room physician does not know the patient, and where there is some reason to anticipate violence, designated emergency room staff should be available at a moment's notice and be prepared to initiate immediately all appropriate measures. While greeting the patient, the physician should be accompanied by a staff member; based on the physician's impression of the patient's greeting behavior, a decision is made to lighten the vigilance, to have a staff member listen at the office door every five minutes or to attend the interview, or immediately to medicate the patient as described in Chapters 5 and 8.

Some emergency room offices are equipped with "panic button" buzzer systems, which notify the crisis team or hospital security personnel that a staff member in a certain room is in trouble. Almost all mentally ill patients thought to be imminently violent should be hospitalized. When a sociopath or alcoholic who was previously calm and has no treatable condition becomes angry at the emergency room physician for not admitting him or for not giving him medication (popular "sociopathic" requests are for narcotics, benzodiazepines, and mood-elevating substances), discharge home from the emergency room is usually still in order despite the anger. The hospital's security personnel should be called to escort the patient off the premises.

Many treatable violent patients are aware, and often afraid, of their potential for violence, and are glad or at least willing to admit themselves to the hospital (74). Frequently, however, the patient will need to be admitted involuntarily by certificate. In such cases, until the staff is prepared to restrain him, the patient should not be told that this is definitely going to happen. If the patient must be told something concerning admission, and the physician does not think the patient will become immediately violent or try to escape, the patient could be told, "I *think* you should be in the hospital and I'm going to try to *arrange* it," which is honest but doesn't usually have a confrontational quality. If the physician has reason to suspect that the patient might become immediately violent and must tell the patient something concerning admission, he might have to lie by saying he is not sure or even that the patient will not be admitted.

When violence is felt not to be imminent, the decision to admit should depend upon the treatability of the patient's condition and his willingness to be admitted. Despite an increased lifetime risk of violence, patients with sociopathy and no immediate homicide risk or superimposed treatable condition (e.g. drug-induced psychosis, major affective illness, adulthood MBD/hyperactivity syndrome) should be discharged with the explanation by the psychiatrist that he doesn't feel he is capable of changing the patient's life-style and behavior, and that the patient is responsible for his own actions. This frankness is appreciated by some patients who have abused the good will of physicians or have been naively assured by physicians that they can be helped. When sociopaths are admitted to psychiatric units, behavior disruptive of ward routine often ensues: "The manipulator and impulse disorder patient soon give up helpful participation in the therapeutic community and develop instead a rapacious subculture, preying on the relative helplessness of other patients on the psychiatric staff's tendency to 'treat patients rather than 'punish' them" (75).

When a violent patient is admitted to a psychiatric service, the physician should discuss this violence potential with the staff. If the violence is thought to be imminent after it is apparent that the prospect of admission is not sufficient to calm the patient, and an immediate definitive treatment (e.g. a barbiturate for sedative-hypnotic withdrawal, an anticonvulsant for epilepsy, physostigmine for anticholinergic delirium) is not identified, the patient should immediately receive either sodium amobarbital for sedation (see Chapter 8), or intramuscular haloperidol 20 mg. (dosage can be higher based on the patient's weight and general health), and this should be repeated at least once within twelve hours, with a minimum of four such doses given in the first forty-eight hours (see Chapter 5).

Once urgent matters are dealt with, the primary objective is the treatment of the condition for which the patient was admitted. These conditions and their treatments of choice have been discussed elsewhere in the book.

Money (76) and Berlin et al. (77) reported (uncontrolled) studies of the successful treatment of sex offenders (rapists, pedophiliacs, exhibitionists) with medroxyprogesterone, an antiandrogenic substance that lowers plasma testosterone levels and diminishes sex drive for deviant as well as normal sexual behavior. Understandably, impotence was a common side effect. These researchers reported that in many cases, even after the medication was discontinued, the deviant sexual behavior did not return. They also reported a high rate of patient discontinuation of the drug after several months.

Sheard (78, 79) performed a controlled study, and Tupin (80) an uncontrolled one, demonstrating the successful prescription of lithium in standard therapeutic doses for prisoners with a history of irritability and aggressive outbursts unassociated with other features of mania or melancholia. Unfortunately these studies did not take into account the possibility that the diminution of aggressive behavior in these patients was the product of a sedative effect of lithium. Despite the incompleteness of the data on this subject, we suggest a trial of lithium carbonate in patients who have no personal or family history of affective disorder and who manifest irritability associated with frequent feelings of being about to "explode" with little provocation. We have seen a significant calming effect in two instances, in both of which the patient had a diagnosis of antisocial personality disorder and had been a drug abuser. Yudofsky *et al.* (81) reported on the successful treatment with propanolol of rage and violent behavior in four patients with diffuse coarse brain disease. Such a treatment could be considered when other means are ineffectual in patients with diffuse coarse brain disease and associated with violent behavior, but experience with this treatment for this behavior is quite limited.

After the patient's condition on the unit is stabilized or improved, the subject of passes and discharge will arise. Discharge should be based upon the patient's having achieved maximum therapeutic benefit, being no longer imminently dangerous, and having taken measures (e.g. having a friend or relative sell weapons, arranging for outpatient follow-up, taking of appropriate medication, providing for treatment in event of emergency, taking of disulfiram by alcoholics) to decrease the probability of violence. All such efforts should be discussed with the patient (and usually with his family) and noted in the chart. The chart must also include a statement concerning the patient's short-term and long-term risk for violence, the measures to be taken to reduce it, and the extent to which it realistically can be reduced. Passes should be given almost exclusively under the same circumstances, as a means of testing the patient's capacity to function outside the hospital prior to discharge. If the patient wishes to leave prior to this time, he must be competent to sign out against medical advice, and he must be thought not to be a short-term suicide or homicide risk; if he is discharged, his relatives should be informed about the long-term risks of violence and the impossibility of holding the patient against his wishes based upon a long-term prediction.

References

1. Guze, S. B. *Criminality and Psychiatric Disorders*. New York: Oxford University Press, 1976.
2. Madden, D. J.; Lion, J. R.; Penna, M. W. Assaults on psychiatrists by patients. *Am. J. Psychiat.* 133(4): 422–25, 1976.

3. Whitman, R. M.; Armao, B. B.; Dent, O. B. Assault on the therapist. *Am. J. Psychiat. 133*(4): 426–29, 1976.

4. Wise, T. Where the public peril begins: A survey of psychotherapists to determine the effects of Tarasoff. *Stanford Law Rev. 31:* 165–90, 1978.

5. Tardiff, K. J. A survey of psychiatrists in Boston and their work with violent patients. *Am. J. Psychiat. 131:* (9): 1008–14, 1974.

6. U.S. Department of Justice, Federal Bureau of Investigation. *Uniform Crime Reports for the United States.* Washington, D.C.: GPO, 1980.

7. *Vital Statistics of the United States, 1975* vol. 2, *Mortality.* Washington, D.C.: U.S. Department of Health, Education, and Welfare National Center for Health Statistics, 1976.

8. Monahan, J. Prediction research and the emergency commitment of dangerous mentally ill persons: A reconsideration. *Am. J. Psychiat. 135*(2): 198–201, 1978.

9. Kozol, H.; Boucher, R.; Garofalo, R. The diagnosis and treatment of dangerousness. *Crime and Delinquency 18:* 371–91, 1972.

10. Steadman, H.; Cocozza, J. *Careers of the Criminally Insane.* Lexington, Mass.: Lexington Books, 1974.

11. Cocozza, J.; Steadman, H. The failure of psychiatric predictions of dangerousness: Clear and convincing evidence. *Rutgers Law Rev. 29:* 1084–1101, 1976.

12. Steadman, H. A new look at recidivism among Patuxent inmates. *Bull. Am. Acad. Psychiat. and the Law 5:* 200–209, 1977.

13. Thornberry, T.; Jacoby, J. *The Criminally Insane: A Community Follow-up of Mentally Ill Offenders.* Chicago: University of Chicago Press, 1979.

14. Monahan, J. *Predicting Violent Behavior: An Assessment of Clinical Techniques.* Beverly Hills: Sage, 1981.

15. Megargee, E. I. Methodological Problems in the Prediction of Violence. In Hays, J. R.; Roberts, T. K.; Solway, K. S. (eds.), *Violence and the Violent Individual.* New York: S.P. Medical and Scientific Books, 1981.

16. Kaplun, D.; Reich, R. The murdered child and his killers. *Am. J. Psychiat. 133*(7): 809–12, 1976.

17. Yager, J. Personal violence in infantry combat. *Arch. Gen. Psychiat. 32:* 257–61, 1975.

18. Wenk, E. A.; Robinson, J. O.; Smith, G. W. Can violence be predicted? *Crime and Delinquency 18:* 393–402, 1972.

19. Wolfgang, M. E. A Sociocultural Overview of Criminal Violence. In Hays, J. R.; Roberts, T. K.; Solway, K. S. (eds.), *Violence and the Violent Individual.* New York: SP Medical and Scientific Books, 1981.

20. Feighner, J.; Robins, E.; Guze, S.; *et al.* Diagnostic criteria for use in psychiatric research. *Arch. Gen. Psychiat. 26:* 56–63, 1972.

21. Hare, R. D. Psychopathy and Violence. In Hays, J. R.; Roberts, T. K.; Solway, K. S. (eds.), *Violence and the Violent Individual.* New York: SP Medical and Scientific Books, 1981.

22. Virkkunen, M. Reactive hypoglycemic tendency among habitually violent offenders. *Neuropsychobiology 8:* 35–40, 1982.

23. Herjanic, M.; Henn, F. A.; Vanderpearl, R. H. Forensic psychiatry: Female offenders. *Am. J. Psychiat. 134*(5): 556–58, 1977.

24. Piotrowski, K. W.; Losacco, D.; Guze, S. B. Psychiatric disorders and crime. *Dis. Nerv. Sys. 37:* 309–11, 1976.

25. Schuckit, M. A.; Herrman, O.; Schuckit, J. J. The importance of psychiatric illness in newly arrested prisoners. *J. Nerv. Ment. Dis. 165:* 118–25, 1977.

26. Swank, G. E.; Winer, D. Occurrence of psychiatric disorder in a county jail population. *Am. J. Psychiat. 133*(11): 1331–32, 1976.

27. Bond, T. C. The why of fragging. *Am. J. Psychiat. 133*(11): 1328–33, 1976.

28. Macdonald, J. M. *The Murderer and His Victim.* Springfield, Ill.: C. C. Thomas, 1961.

29. Hellman, D. S.; Blackman, N. Enuresis, firesetting and cruelty to animals: A triad predictive of adult crime. *Am. J. Psychiat. 123:* 1431–35, 1966.

30. Taylor, M.; Abrams, R. The phenomenology of mania. *Arch. Gen. Psychiat. 19:* 520–22, 1973.

31. Falconer, M. A. Clinical, Radiological, and EEG Correlations with Pathological Changes in Temporal Lobe Epilepsy and Their Significance in Surgical Treatment. In Baldwin, M.; Bailey, P. (eds.), *Temporal Lobe Epilepsy.* Springfield, Ill.: C. C. Thomas, 1958.

32. Ounstead, C. Aggression and epilepsy: Rage in children with temporal lobe epilepsy. *J. Psychsom. Res. 13:* 237–42, 1969.

33. Pincus, J. H. Can violence be a manifestation of epilepsy? *Neurology 24:* 629–36, 1974.

34. Stevens, J. R.; Hermann, B. P. Temporal lobe epilepsy, psychopathology and violence. *Neurology 31:* 1127–32, 1981.

35. International Workshop on Aggression and Epilepsy. The nature of aggression during epileptic seizures. *New Eng. J. Med. 305*(12): 711–16, 1981.

36. Langevin, R.; Paitich, D.; Orchard, B.; *et al.* The role of alcohol, drugs, suicide attempts and situational strains in homicide committed by offenders seen for psychiatric assessment: A controlled study. *Acta Psychiat. Scand. 66:* 229–42, 1982.

37. Goodwin, D. L. Alcohol in suicide and homicide. *Quart. J. Stud. Alc. 34:* 144–56, 1973.

38. Rada, R. T. Alcoholism and forcible rape. *Am. J. Psychiat. 132*(4): 444–46, 1975.

39. Ellinwood, E. H. Assault and homicide associated with amphetamine abuse. *Am. J. Psychiat. 127*(9): 1170–75, 1971.

40. Tinklenberg, J. R.; Murphy, P. L.; Murphy, P.; *et al.* Drug involvement in criminal assaults by adolescents. *Arch. Gen. Psychiat. 30:* 685–89, 1974.

41. Marinacci, A. A. Special type of temporal lobe (psychomotor) seizures following ingestion of alcohol. *Bull. L.A. Neurol. Soc. 28:* 241–50, 1963.

42. Bach-y-Rita, G.; Lion, J.; Ervin, F. R. Pathological intoxication: Clinical and electroencephalographic studies. *Am. J. Psychiat. 127*(5): 698–703, 1970.

43. Fauman, M. & B. J. Violence associated with phencyclidine abuse. *Am. J. Psychiat. 136*(12): 1584–86, 1979.

44. Reich, P.; Hepps, R. B. Homicide during a psychosis induced by LSD. *JAMA 219:* 869–71, 1972.

45. Atkinson, J. H. Managing the violent patient in the general hospital. *Postgrad. Med. 71*(1): 193–201, 1982.

46. Simon, R. H. Intracranial tuberculoma coexistent with uncinate seizures and violent behavior. *JAMA 245*(12): 1247–48, 1981.

47. Petrie, W. M.; Lawson, E. C.; Hollender, M. H. Violence in geriatric patients. *JAMA 248:* 443–44, 1982.

48. West, D. J. *Murder Followed by Suicide.* London: Heinemann, 1965.

49. Giovannoni, J. M.; Gurel, L. Socially disruptive behavior of ex-mental patients. *Arch. Gen. Psychiat. 17:* 146–53, 1967.

50. Zitrin, A.; Hardesty, A. S.; Burdock, E. I.; *et al.* Crime and violence among mental patients. *Am. J. Psychiat. 133*(2): 142–49, 1976.

51. Sosowsky, L. Explaining the increased arrest rate among mental patients: A cautionary note. *Am. J. Psychiat. 137*(12): 1602–4, 1980.

52. Greenberg, F.; Klinger, B. I.; Grumet, B. Homicide and deinstitutionalization of the mentally ill. *Am. J. Psychiat. 134*(6): 685–86, 1977.

53. Rappeport, J. R.; Lassen, G. Dangerousness-arrest rate comparisons of discharged patients and the general population. *Am. J. Psychiat. 121:* 776–83, 1965.

54. Ashley, M. C. Outcome of 1,000 cases paroled from the Middletown State Hospital. *N.Y. State Hosp. Quart. 8:* 64–70, 1922.

55. Pollock, H. M. Is the paroled patient a menace to the community? *Psychiat. Quart. 12:* 236–44, 1938.

56. Cohen, L. H.; Freeman, H. How dangerous to the community are state hospital patients? *Comm. Med. 9:* 697–700, 1945.

57. Brill, H.; Malzberg, B. Statistical report based on the arrest records of 5354 male ex-patients released from New York State mental hospitals during the period 1946–48. *Ment. Hosp. Serv. Suppl. 153,* Washington, D.C.: American Psychiatric Association, August 1962.

58. Stafford-Clark, D. The foundations of research in psychiatry. *Br. Med. J. 2:* 1199, 1959.

59. Williams, D. The significance of an abnormal electroencephalogram. *J. Neurol. Psychiat. 4:* 257–68, 1957.

60. Hill D.; Watterson, D. Electroencephalographic studies of psychopathic personalities. *J. Neurol. Psychiat. 5:* 47–65, 1942.

61. Stafford-Clark, D.; Pond, D.; Doust, J. W. L. The psychopath in prison: a preliminary report of a cooperative research. *Br. J. Delinq. 2:* 117–29, 1951.

62. Stafford-Clark, D.; Taylor, F. H. Clinical and electroencephalographic studies of prisoners charged with murder. *J. Neurol. Neurosurg. Psychiat. 12:* 325, 1949.

63. Williams, D. Neural factors related to habitual aggression. *Brain 92:* 503–20, 1969.

64. Gibbs, F. A.; Bagchi, B. K.; Bloomberg, W. Electroencephalographic study of criminals. *Am. J. Psychiat. 102:* 294–98, 1945.

65. Dalton, K. Menstruation and crime. *Br. Med. J. 2:* 1752–53, 1961.

66. Petersilia, J.; Greenwood, P.; Lavin, M. *Criminal Careers of Habitual Felons.* Santa Monica, Calif.: Rand Corporation, 1977.

67. Zimring, F. E. Background In Confronting Youth Crime. *Report of the Twentieth Century Fund Task Force in Sentencing Policy Toward Young Offenders.* New York: Holmes & Meier, 1978.

68. Tardiff, K. The risk of assaultive behavior in suicidal patients. *Acta Psychiat. Scand. 64:* 295–300, 1981.

69. Fairweather, G.; Sanders, D.; Tornatzky, L. *Creating Change in Mental Health Organizations.* New York: Pergamon, 1974.

70. Coleman, K. H.; Weinman, M. Conjugal violence: A comparative study in a psychiatric setting. In Hays, J. R.; Roberts, T. K.; Solway, K. S. (eds.), *Violence and the Violent Individual.* New York: SP Medical and Scientific Books, 1981.

71. Sendi, I. B.; Blomgren, P. G. A comparative study of predictive criteria in the predisposition of homicidal adolescents. *Am. J. Psychiat. 132*(4): 423–27, 1975.

72. Kempe, C. H.; Silverman, F. N.; Steele, B. F.; *et al.* The battered child syndrome. *JAMA 181:* 17, 1962.

73. Silver, L.; Dublin, D.; Lourie, R. Does violence breed violence? Contributions from a study of the child abuse syndrome. *Am. J. Psychiat. 126:* 152–55, 1969.

74. Lion, J.; Bach-y-Rita, G.; Ervin, F. R. The self-referred violent patient. *JAMA 205*(7): 91–93, 1968.

75. Liss, R.; Frances, A. Court-mandated treatment: Dilemmas for hospital psychiatry. *Am. J. Psychiat. 132*(9): 924–27, 1975.

76. Money, J. Use of an androgen-depleting hormone in the treatment of male sex offenders. *J. Sex. Res. 6*(3): 165–72, 1970.

77. Berlin, F. S.; Meinecke, C. F. Treatment of sex offenders with antiandrogenic medication: Conceptualization, review of treatment modalities, and preliminary findings. *Am. J. Psychiat. 138*(5): 601–7, 1981.

78. Sheard, M. H.; Marini, J. L.; Bridges, C. I.; *et al.* The effect of lithium on impulsive aggressive behavior in man. *Am. J. Psychiat. 133*(12): 1409–13, 1976.

79. Sheard, M. H. Effects of lithium on human aggression. *Nature 230:* 113–14, 1971.

80. Tupin, J. P.; Smith, D.; Clanon, T. L.; *et al.* The long-term use of lithium in aggressive prisoners. *Comp. Psychiat. 14*(4): 311–17, 1973.

81. Yudofsky, S.; Williams, D.; Gorman, J. Propanolol in the treatment of rage and violent behavior in patients with chronic brain syndromes. *Am. J. Psychiat. 138:* 218–20, 1981.

CHAPTER 14

The Catatonic Patient

Catatonia has long been recognized as a syndrome rather than a specific disease process (1, 2). It is characterized by specific motor behaviors and by periods of extreme hyperactivity and hypoactivity. Studies (2–4) show that 25 to 50 percent of individuals who exhibit catatonic features have affective disorder and that about 20 percent of patients with bipolar affective disorder exhibit one or more catatonic features (3). Those patients who have catatonia as part of their affective disease are indistinguishable from affectively disordered patients without catatonia in their demographic characteristics, psychopathology, and treatment response and in the prevalence and pattern of psychiatric illness in their first-degree relatives (3, 5–7). Although between 5 and 10 percent of catatonics satisfy criteria for the diagnosis of schizophrenia, catatonia generally has a favorable treatment response (3).

The traditional catatonic features are shown in Table 14–1. Mutism and stupor, although characteristic of catatonia, are not pathognomonic. Other motor behaviors should be present, and most patients have three or more features (3). There appears to be no relationship among any one feature or number of features and any one diagnosis or response to treatment (3). Thus the presence of one or two features has as much diagnostic and treatment significance as the presence of seven or eight features. Three features, mutism, negativism, and stupor, occur together more frequently than by

TABLE 14-1 Classical Catatonic Features

Mutism	Echolalia	Automatic obedience
Stupor	Stereotypy	Posturing
Echopraxia	Catalepsy	Gegenhalten (negativism)

chance (8) and correspond to the clinical syndrome of *negativistic stupor*, that is, akinetic mutism or coma vigil secondary to frontal lobe damage (9–11), third ventricle tumors (12), and lesions of the reticular activating system and caudal hypothalamus (13). Mutism, stereotypy, catalepsy, and automatic obedience also occur together more frequently than by chance (8), correspond to the classical description of catatonia (14), and are associated with the diagnosis of mania (2, 3, 8).

Luria (15) described several patients with catatonia-like symptoms following frontal lobe injury. Dogs with ablated frontal lobes also demonstrate many catatonic features (16, 17). The relationship between frontal lobe lesions and catatonia-like behaviors is not surprising, since the frontal lobe is intimately involved in the regulation of motor activity (15). The frontal lobe signs of *pathological inertia* (difficulty initiating motor acts or stopping them once started) and *stimulus bound behavior* (motor response to stimuli despite instructions to the contrary) may underlie all catatonic features.

Specific procedures to elicit catatonic signs is rarely part of the routine mental status examination. The examiner should, however, always test for catatonia when the following behaviors are observed: odd gaits inconsistent with known neurologic disease (e.g. tiptoe walking, hopping), standing in one place for prolonged periods, holding the arms up as if carrying something, shifting position when the examiner shifts positions, repeating most of the examiner's questions prior to answering, responding to most of the examiner's questions with the same question (e.g. *E:* "How old are you?" *Pt:* "How old are *you?*"), making odd hand or finger movements that are not typically dyskinetic, performing inconspicuous repetitive actions (e.g. making a series of clicking sounds before or after speaking, tapping or automatically touching objects while walking about), mutism, psychomotor retardation, speech that becomes progressively less voluble until it becomes an incomprehensible mumble (prosectic speech).

Patients displaying one or more of the above features while conversing with the examiner may allow themselves to be placed in odd postures, may be unable to resist when the examiner moves their arms despite instructions to the contrary, or may be unable to resist shaking the examiner's proffered hand despite instructions to the contrary (automatic obedience). Some patients with catatonic features will automatically obey the examiner's request to stick their tongues out despite being told they will be jabbed with a sharp needle.

Patients with classical catatonic features are often misdiagnosed because of the false expectation that they must be totally mute and immobile. In fact most patients with catatonic features speak and move about (2–4, 6, 7, 14). The following vignette illustrates this:

Mrs. H., a short, plump sixty-three-year-old, walked about the hospital on her tiptoes. When her doctor entered the inpatient unit, she would hop and skip up to him, give him a warm greeting, and then begin a long, detailed discourse of her experiences since last they met. Her speech was so rapid that at times she was incomprehensible. If interrupted, she became angry and accused her doctor of being unconcerned. She would, however, allow the doctor to place her in odd postures while she spoke. When she permitted him to speak and he told her he wanted her to resist his manipulations of her arms and hands, she would laugh and agree to "fight him off" but, nevertheless, still was unable to resist. When interviewed in the doctor's office, she could become extremely cooperative and carry out a prolonged "normal conversation" while sitting with her legs fully extended and raised above the floor. The doctor, thirty-one years her junior and in apparent better physical condition, was able to maintain the same posture for fewer than five minutes.

Because catatonia is a syndrome, treatment should generally be directed at the primary condition. During the interim between admission and the institution of definitive treatment, mobile patients with some catatonic features may not require any somatic intervention. Those who are agitated may require sodium amobarbital for sedation. Those who are immobile and mute (i.e., stuporous), and are unable to eat and becoming dehydrated, may be motorically disinhibited by intramuscular sodium amobarbital (approximately 250 mg.) administered forty-five minutes before meals, thus permitting them to eat and drink sufficient amounts until definitive treatment is begun. Intravenous sodium amobarbital, administered slowly, may also be used as a diagnostic procedure, as it may motorically disinhibit the stuporous patient, thus facilitating examination.

Although neuroleptics and lithium have each been used successfully in the treatment of patients with catatonic features, the initial use of ECT for the full catatonic syndrome is of particular importance. Catatonia is frequently complicated by malnutrition, dehydration, hyperpyrexia, and occasional outbursts of sudden violence or excited behavior (2, 3, 14, 18, 19). The mortality rate untreated can be as high as 50 percent (14, 18, 20, 21). In a series of reports, most catatonics were shown to be individuals with affective disorder who respond well to appropriate treatment (2, 3, 19, 22). Early workers (21, 23) wrote that catatonia was particularly responsive to ECT, with rapid improvement often occurring after one or two treatments. "Lethal" catatonia (18), associated with hyperpyrexia, violent outbursts, and self-mutilation, should be considered a medical emergency (24), and ECT has been reported to be lifesaving in this condition (25). Similar catatonic syndromes, secondary to typhoid fever (26), fever of unknown origin (27), and kidney transplant (28), have been reported to respond dramatically to ECT, following treatment failure with a variety of pharmacologic agents. Resolution of the catatonia then permitted appropriate management of the systemic condition. Considering the delayed antipsychotic effect of neuroleptics, their toxicity, the fact that they may themselves precipitate catatonic symptoms (29), and the rapid reversal of catatonia with induced seizures, ECT should be considered the treatment of choice for the catatonic patient.

References

1. Hearst, E. D.; Munoz, R. A.; Tuason, V. B. Catatonia: Its diagnostic validity. *Dis. Nerv. Syst. 32:* 453–56, 1971.

2. Abrams, R.; Taylor, M. A.. Catatonia: A prospective clinical study. *Arch. Gen. Psychiat. 33:* 579–81, 1976.

3. Taylor, M. A.; Abrams, R. Catatonia: Prevalence and importance in the manic phase of manic-depressive illness. *Arch. Gen. Psychiat. 34:* 1223–25, 1977.

4. Morrison, J. R. Catatonia: Retarded and excited types. *Arch. Gen. Psychiat. 28:* 39–41, 1973.

5. Morrison, J. R. Catatonia: Prediction of outcome. *Comp. Psychiat. 15:* 317–24, 1974.

6. Kirby, G. H. The catatonic syndrome and its relation to manic-depressive insanity. *J. Nerv. Ment. Dis. 40:* 694–704, 1913.

7. Bonner, C. A.; Kent, G. H. Overlapping symptoms in catatonic excitement and manic excitement. *Am. J. Psychiat. 92:* 1311–22, 1936.

8. Abrams, R.; Taylor, M. A.; Stolurow, K. A. C. Catatonia and mania: Patterns of cerebral dysfunction. *Biol. Psychiat. 14:* 111–17, 1979.

9. Pincus, J. H.; Tucker, G. J. *Behavioral Neurology.* 1st ed. New York: Oxford University Press, 1974, p. 103.

10. Benson, D. F. Disorders of Verbal Expression. In Benson, D. F.; Blumer D. (eds.), *Psychiatric Aspects of Neurological Disease*, vol. 1. New York: Grune & Stratton, 1975, p. 125.

11. Hecaen, H.; Albert, M. L. Disorders of Mental Functioning Related to Frontal Lobe Pathology. In Benson, D. F.; Blumer, D. (eds.), *Psychiatric Aspects of Neurological Disease*, vol. 1. New York: Grune & Stratton, 1975, p. 141.

12. Slater, E.; Roth, M. *Clinical Psychiatry.* Baltimore: Williams & Wilkins, 1969, p. 498.

13. Solomon, S. Clinical Neurology and Pathophysiology. In Freeman, A. M.; Kaplan, H. I.; Sadock, B. J. (eds.), *Comprehensive Textbook of Psychiatry*, vol. 1, 2d ed. Baltimore: Williams & Wilkins, 1975, p. 250.

14. Kahlbaum, K. L. *Catatonia.* Levij, Y.; Prider, T. (trans.). Baltimore: Johns Hopkins Press, 1973.

15. Luria, A. R. *The Working Brain.* New York: Basic Books, 1973, pp. 89, 187–225.

16. Pavlov, I. P. *Complete Collected Works,* vols. 1–3. Moscow and Leningrad: Izd. Akad. Nauk SSSR, 1949. Cited in Luria, A. R. *The Working Brain.* New York: Basic Books, 1973, pp. 89–90.

17. Anoklin, P. K. *Problems in Higher Nervous Activity.* Moscow: Izd. Akad. Med. Nauk SSSR, 1949. Cited in Luria, A. R. *The Working Brain.* New York: Basic Books, 1973, pp. 89–90.

18. Laskowska, D.; Urbaniak, K.; Jus, A. The relationship between catatonic delirious states and schizophrenia, in the light of a follow-up study (Stauder's Lethal Catatonia). *Br. J. Psychiat. 111:* 254–57, 1965.

19. Powers, P.; Douglas, S.; Waziri, R. Hyperpyrexia in catatonic states. *Dis. Nerv. Syst. 37:* 359–61, 1976.

20. Brussel, J. A.; Schneider, J. The B.E.S.T. in treatment and control of chronically disturbed mental patients. *Psychiat. Quart. 25:* 55–64, 1951.

21. Roubicek, J. Mutism and electric shock treatment. *Z Vlaslni Otisk Neurol. Psychiat. Cesk 10:* 1–9, 1948.

22. Abrams, R.; Taylor, M. A. Catatonia: Prediction of response to somatic treatment. *Am. J. Psychiat. 134:* 70–80, 1977.

23. Sargant, W.; Slater, E. *An Introduction to Physical Methods of Treatment in Psychiatry. 3d ed.* Baltimore: Williams & Wilkins, 1954.

24. Penn, H.; Racy, J.; Lapham, L.; *et al.* Catatonic behavior, viral encephalopathy and death. *Arch. Gen. Psychiat. 27:* 758–61, 1972.

25. Hamilton, M. *Fish's Schizophrenia.* Bristol, Eng.: John Wright & Sons, 1976.

26. Breakley, W. R.; Kala, A. K. Typhoid catatonia responsive to ECT. *Br. Med. J. 2:* 357–59, 1977.

27. O'Toole, J. K.; Dyck, G. Report of psychogenic fever in catatonia responding to electroconvulsive therapy. *Dis. Nerv. Syst. 38:* 852–53, 1977.

28. Bernstein, D. M.; Adzick, G. R. Electrotherapy and renal transplantation: Impediment to treatment. *Minnesota Med. 60:* 410–11, 1977.

29. Johnson, G. C., Manning, D. E. Neuroleptic-induced catatonia: Case report. *J. Clin. Psychiat. 44:* 310–12, 1983.

CHAPTER 15

Schizophrenia

Historical Review

In 1896, in the fifth edition of his *Textbook of Psychiatry* (1), Kraepelin presented both his classification of mental illness, in which dementia praecox and manic–depressive insanity were clearly differentiated, and his conceptualization and description of the two putative diseases. That textbook undoubtedly has had a more profound effect on twentieth-century psychiatry than any other single written work. Modern classification throughout the world is but a variation of that presented by Kraepelin.

The two principal forces influencing the development of Kraepelin's synthesis of mental illness were the ideas of Karl Kahlbaum (2) and Edmond Hecker (3) and Kraepelin's own training in experimental psychology (4).

Nineteenth-century psychological theory divided the mind into three functioning regions: *thinking, volition* or will, and feelings or *emotions* (5). Kraepelin's concepts of psychological disease were rooted in such a notion of a tripartite mind, and his cross-sectional criteria for dementia praecox included deficits in all three spheres (1, 6, 7). In contrast, he believed manic-depressive insanity to involve a disturbance in feeling, sparing the other two mind spheres.

The other important influence on Kraepelin's thinking was the work of Kahlbaum and Hecker, who delineated what they believed to be discrete illnesses: catatonia and hebephrenia. Kraepelin was thoroughly versed in their writings and considered the clinical criteria and course of illness established by Hecker for hebephrenia especially applicable to catatonia. As both disorders had an early onset, could result in chronic personality deterioration, and affected all three regions of the tripartite mind, Kraepelin felt justified in considering the two syndromes variants of a single disease process. In later writings (6) he included, along with catatonia and hebephrenia, dementia paranoides and other dementias under Morel's (8) term dementia praecox.

Although the modern notion is that Bleuler dramatically altered Kraepelin's concept of dementia praecox, on the contrary Bleuler actually reinforced many of Kraepelin's ideas (9). However, Bleuler believed the term dementia praecox to be too specific and not always fitting the clinical course, which he believed more variable than originally described. Nevertheless, he was in full agreement with Kraepelin that dementia praecox or, as he termed it, schizophrenia (split mind), affected the three regions of the tripartite mind (his "four A's" are a reworking of this concept); was "one or very few diseases, a single disease accounting for the vast majority of cases"; and always resulted in some residual deficit. That remains our present-day notion of the nature of schizophrenia, and modern diagnostic criteria—Feighner (10), RDC (11), DSM-III (12)—clearly encompass all the basic characteristics delineated by Kraepelin and Bleuler.

Today, among nonprofessionals, schizophrenia has become synonymous with psychosis. This misconception has developed, in large part, from past deficiencies in psychiatric diagnostic reliability and research methodology (13–15), which permitted an extraordinary overdiagnosis of schizophrenia (16, 17). A concurrent lack of adherence to basic Kraepelinian concepts of the syndrome also led to a broadening of the requirements for diagnosis (18), resulting in a clinical picture that would have been unrecognizable to Kraepelin and Bleuler.

To put the degree of overdiagnosis in perspective, federal and state statistics prior to the mid-1970s (19, 20) indicate that the national range of psychiatric admission prevalence of schizophrenia was 24 to 40 percent, that 30 percent of all first admissions to psychiatric hospitals were labeled schizophrenic, that 60 percent of all mental hospital beds were occupied by such individuals, and that, because of the relatively large number of state mental hospital beds compared with total beds of other specialties, 25 percent of all U.S. hospital beds regardless of specialty identification were occupied by individuals labeled schizophrenic. These figures are almost certainly fallacious.

In the 1960s the United States and the United Kingdom collaborated in a study of diagnostic patterns in the two countries (21). This project demonstrated (22–24) that U.S. psychiatrists overdiagnosed schizophrenia and underdiagnosed affective disorder and personality deviation. Affective disorder was actually diagnosed twenty times more frequently in England and Wales than in the United States, and project diagnosticians, using specific diagnostic criteria, were in general agreement with the U.K. psychiatrists, who diagnosed 50 percent less schizophrenia, three times as much depression, and nine times as much mania in the same patient sample as did the U.S. psychiatrists. Other studies (25, 26) comparing international patterns of diagnosis supported the U.S.-U.K. observation of the American psychiatrists' propensity to overdiagnose schizophrenia at the expense of affective disorder. Numerous additional studies (27–35) also demonstrated that patients labeled as acute, good-prognosis, paranoid, catatonic, and schizo-affective schizophrenia rarely satisfied research criteria for schizophrenia and most frequently satisfied research criteria for affective disorder. For example, Taylor et al. (27) examined twenty-six consecutive patients who had an admission diagnosis of acute schizophrenia and found only one who satisfied research criteria for schizophrenia. Many were found to have no psychiatric illness or personality deviation, and half satisfied research criteria for mania. These "acute schizophrenics," rediagnosed as manic, were then compared with two groups of patients, one group satisfying research criteria for schizophrenia, the other satisfying research criteria for mania. The "acute schizophrenics" rediagnosed as manic were no different from the research group of manics but were markedly different from the research group of schizophrenics on a variety of clinical, genetic, and treatment response variables. These investigators concluded that many patients receiving the diagnosis of acute schizophrenia actually suffer from affective illness. Table 15–1 shows the results of studies applying modern diagnostic criteria to samples of consecutive psychiatric admissions. The average prevalence of schizophrenia observed in these studies is less than 4 percent, whereas between one-quarter and one-third of most samples

TABLE 15–1 The Prevalence of Schizophrenia
in Psychiatry Patient Samples

STUDY	CRITERIA	N	% SCHIZOPHRENIA
Woodruff et al. (1972) (36)	Modified Wash. U.	500	4.4
Morrison et al. (1972) (37)	Wash. U.	3,800	5.3
Taylor et al. (1975) (38)	Taylor et al.	247	4.5
Nielsen and Nielson (1977) (39)	WHO	976	0.6
Helzer et al. (1977) (40)	Wash. U.	101	5.0
Strauss and Gift (1977) (41)	Wash. U.	272	3.5
	RDC	272	1.5
Weissman et al. (1978) (42)	RDC	511	0.4
Taylor and Abrams (1978) (16)	Taylor and Abrams	465	6.7
Ries et al. (1980) (43)	Modified Wash. U.	254	6.3

satisfied criteria for affective disorder. Pope and Lipinsky (17) estimate that at least 40 percent of patients previously diagnosed schizophrenic actually suffer from affective disorders. These figures represent a more than tenfold decrease in the observed hospital prevalence of schizophrenia. Population studies (44, 45) and family risk studies (45-49) also consistently find figures for schizophrenia lower than previously reported with old diagnostic methods and suggest that schizophrenia is a rare disorder, affecting between 0.3 and 0.6 percent of the population. This would come as no surprise to Kraepelin, the father of the schizophrenia disease concept, who made the diagnosis in only 5 percent of patients admitted to his Munich Clinic in 1893 (50).

The low figures for schizophrenia are a function of rigorous criteria and not a change in the true prevalence of schizophrenia. This is demonstrated in one study (41) in which the application of broad criteria led to a hospital admission prevalence for schizophrenia of 20 to 25 percent, whereas the application of research criteria to the same sample identified from 1.5 to 3.3 percent as schizophrenic. Data from several studies (51-53) demonstrate that failure to use rigorous criteria allows cultural sensitivity, theoretical bias, and availability of new treatments to influence unduly the frequency of diagnosis of schizophrenia.

Another factor leading to the overdiagnosis of schizophrenia, particularly at the expense of affective disorder, has been the misconception that certain psychopathological features are pathognomonic of schizophrenia. Kurt Schneider (54) was the first to suggest that in the absence of coarse brain disease, the presence of thought-broadcasting, complete auditory hallucinations, experiences of influence, experiences of alienation, and delusional perceptions were decisive in the diagnosis of schizophrenia. He termed these phenomena "first-rank" to indicate their specificity. Many of the items of the *Research Diagnostic Criteria* (RDC) displayed in Table 15-2 (A-1, A-2a, A-5, A-6) are descriptions of first-rank symptoms. Although they occur in a substantial proportion of schizophrenics, it is clear that these phenomena also occur in affective states, and their presence in mania or depression does not predict a poor treatment response or increased familial risk for schizophrenia (35, 55, 56).

Catatonic behaviors also have been mistakenly considered pathognomonic of schizophrenia. However, the literature (31, 32, 57-59) clearly demonstrates that catatonia is a syndrome associated with a variety of disease processess and that, whereas few catatonics satisfy research criteria for schizophrenia, many satisfy research criteria for affective disorder, respond well to treatment, and have a high risk for affective disorder among their first-degree relatives.

"Bizarre behavior" is frequently invoked to support a diagnosis of schizophrenia. However, manic patients also display a wide variety of exotic

TABLE 15-2 Research Diagnostic Criteria (RDC) for Schizophrenia
(A through C required)

A. At least two of the following in the absence of alcohol or drug abuse or withdrawal:
   1. The individual expresses (a) that his thoughts are escaping aloud from his head as if he were a radio; (b) alien thoughts are being inserted into his head; or (c) his thoughts are being pulled out of his head by an outside force.
   2. The individual expresses (a) experiencing being controlled by an alien force; (b) other bizarre delusions, or (c) multiple delusions.
   3. The individual expresses nonpersecutory or jealous delusions lasting at least one week.
   4. The individual experiences delusions of any type if accompanied by hallucinations of any type lasting at leat one week.
   5. The individual experiences auditory hallucinations in which either a voice keeps up a running commentary on the individual's behavior or thoughts, or two or more voices converse with each other (voices are experienced as coming from outside the "self" and are clearly perceived).
   6. The individual experiences hallucinations of any type throughout the day for several days or intermittently for at least one month.
   7. The individual experiences auditory hallucinations of voices having no apparent relation to depression or elation.
   8. The individual exhibits thought disorder (understandability of speech is impaired by distorted grammar, incomplete sentences, lack of logical connections, lack of readily understandable relationships between thoughts).
   9. Catatonic motor behavior (maintaining odd postures for prolonged periods, automatic repetitive movements).
B. A period of illness lasting at least two weeks.
C. At no time during the active period of illness does individual exhibit sufficient signs or symptoms to meet criteria for manic or depressive syndrome.

SOURCE: R. L. Spitzer, J. Endicott, and E. Robins, *Research Diagnostic Criteria for a Selected Group of Functional Disorders (RDC)*, 2d ed. New York: Biometrics Research, New York State Psychiatric Institute, 1975. Used by permission.

behaviors (57, 60–62). Table 15–3 shows the frequency of various symptoms exhibited by a group of fifty-two patients satisfying research criteria for mania. Only the most permissive observer would fail to classify as "bizarre" public nudity, sexual exposure, fecal smearing, and the decoration of one's head with bits and pieces of brightly colored debris. These and other pathological behaviors occur with such frequency in mania that they clearly cannot be considered specific to a diagnosis of schizophrenia.

Perhaps the gravest error leading to misdiagnosis is the notion that thought disorder is synonymous with schizophrenia (63, 64). Formal thought disorder (e.g. tangential speech, neologisms, driveling speech, word approximations) is observed in more than 40 percent of hospitalized schizophrenics (65). However, flight-of-ideas and clang associations, both characteristic of mania (57, 60, 61, 63), are often imprecisely labeled as schizophrenic thought disorder ("loosening of associations" or "incom-

TABLE 15-3 Frequency of Various Symptoms in Fifty-Two Manic Patients

SYMPTOMS	PERCENTAGE OF PATIENTS AFFECTED
Mood disorder	100.0%
Irritable	80.8
Expansive	65.5
Euphoric	30.8
Labile, with depression	28.8
Hyperactivity	100.0
Rapid/pressured speech	100.0
Flight-of-ideas	76.9
Grandiose delusions	59.6
Assaultive/threatening behavior	48.1
Incomplete auditory hallucinations	48.1
Persecutory delusions	42.3
Confusion	32.7
Singing/dancing	32.7
Head decoration	32.7
Autochthonous [sudden delusions] ideas	26.9
Visual hallucinations	26.9
Nudity/sexual exposure	23.1
Fecal incontinence/smearing	19.2
Olfactory hallucinations	15.4
Catatonia (posturing, catalepsy, mannerisms, stereotypies, automatic cooperation)	13.5
First-rank symptoms of Schneider	11.5

SOURCE: M. A. Taylor and R. Abrams, Table 2 in "The Phenomenology of Mania," *Archives of General Psychiatry* 29: 521 (October 1973). Copyright © 1970–73 by American Medical Association. Used by permission.

prehensible speech"), thereby satisyfing one criterion for schizophrenia in several sets of diagnostic criteria and increasing the probability of a false positive diagnosis. Thus, a clear understanding of the nonspecificity of first-rank symptoms, catatonic features, bizarre behavior, and thought disorder is essential for the accurate diagnosis of the major psychoses.

SCHIZOAFFECTIVE DISORDERS

The misconception that certain psychopathological features are path-ognomonic of schizophrenia and the observation that some patients exhibit these features during otherwise typical affective states have, in part, led to the formulation that a group of disorders exist (schizoaffective and allied conditions) intermediate between schizophrenia and affective disorder. Despite numerous studies of the diagnostic validity of schizoaffective psychosis or atypical psychosis, however, there is no reliable, operationally defined set of criteria generally accepted by researchers and clinicians.

When subjecting the schizoaffective and allied disorders concept to the process of diagnostic validation, the data suggest that (1) there is no generally accepted set of diagnostic criteria for schizoaffective and allied conditions and that symptoms thought to identify these patients occur with such frequency in manics and depressives that they are unhelpful in diagnosing schizoaffective states; (2) schizophrenic symptoms have no predictive value in the presence of sufficient signs and symptoms to satisfy criteria for affective disorder, and responsivity to short-term and prophylactic lithium treatment does not discriminate schizoaffectives from affectives but does discriminate them from schizophrenics; (3) long-term follow-up studies generally find schizoaffectives to have a benign outcome similar to typical affectives, but different from typical schizophrenics; and (4) family risk studies, supported by twin and adoption study data, demonstrate first-degree relatives of schizoaffectives to be at high risk for affective disorder and at a risk for schizophrenia that may be no greater than that for the general population. The conclusion generated by these data is that, although samples are somewhat heterogeneous, the vast majority of patients receiving the diagnosis schizoaffective or allied disorder have affective disease (35).

Diagnostic Criteria

The search for a satisfactory diagnostic system for schizophrenia remains unfulfilled. Several sets of research criteria have contributed to the present form of the official diagnostic manual of the American Psychiatric Association, but DSM-III contains several blind spots and loopholes, which permit frequent false identification of patients as schizophrenic. For example, DSM-III requires six criteria to be met to diagnose schizophrenia (Table 15–4). Criterion A requires any of six clinical features, none of which is pathognomonic of schizophrenia and several of which (2, 6c) suggest affective disorder. Criterion B could pertain equally to any psychosis (as could criteria E and F) and criterion C (perhaps the best discriminating feature) will not exclude the manic or depressive who is untreated or inadequately treated and thus remains symptomatic for the natural length of affective episodes, which average six months. Criterion D makes little sense, as the literature clearly demonstrates that "psychotic symptoms" are frequently observed in affective states. Thus, the clinician can use DSM-III accurately only as a reference point. To diagnose schizophrenia appropriately, he must be fully aware of all the specific behaviors and other clinical features associated with the disorder, identify those behaviors and features in his patients, and only then apply these to DSM-III.

TABLE 15-4 Diagnostic Criteria for Schizophrenic Disorder*

A. At least one of the following during a phase of the illness:
1. Bizarre delusions (content is patently absurd and has no possible basis in fact), such as delusions of being controlled, thought-broadcasting, thought insertion, or thought withdrawal
2. Somatic, grandiose, religion, nihilistic, or other delusions without persecutory or jealous content
3. Delusions with persecutory or jealous content accompanied by hallucinations of any type
4. Auditory hallucinations in which either a voice keeps up a running commentary on the individual's behavior or thoughts, or two or more voices converse with each other
5. Auditory hallucinations on several occasions with content of more than one or two words, having no apparent relation to depression or elation
6. Incoherence, marked loosening of associations, markedly illogical thinking, or marked poverty of content of speech if associated with at least one of the following:
   a. Blunted, flat or inappropriate affect
   b. Delusions or hallucinations
   c. Catatonic or other grossly disorganized behavior
B. Deterioration from a previous level of functioning in such areas as work, social relations, and self-care
C. Duration: Continuous signs of the illness for at least six months at some time during the person's life, with some signs of the illness at present. The six-month period must include an active phase during which there were symptoms from A, with or without a prodromal or reduced phase.
D. The full depressive or manic syndrome, if present, developed after any psychotic symptoms, or was brief in duration relative to the duration of the psychotic symptoms in A.
E. Onset of prodromal or active phase of the illness before age forty-five
F. Not due to any organic mental disorder or mental retardation

SOURCE: J. B. W. Williams (Ed.), *Diagnostic and Statistical Manual of Mental Disorders*, Third Edition (*DSM-III*), pp. 188–90. Washington, D.C.: American Psychiatric Association, 1980. Used by permission.

Behaviors

The description by nineteenth- and early-twentieth-century psychiatrists of behavior characteristic of what today we call schizophrenia cannot be surpassed, and the works of Haslam (66), Kahlbaum (2), Hammon (67), Spitzka (68), Peterson (69), Kraepelin (1, 6, 7), and Bleuler (9) are essential reading for anyone truly interested in the forms of psychopathology. We can only briefly present here the rich description they provide us.

Although the physical impression of schizophrenia today is often confounded by chronic exposure to neuroleptics, early workers in the predrug era described schizophrenics as physically awkward, gangly in appearance, and dyskinetic in their movement. Fine hand movements are particularly jerky in nature, poor sequential finger movement characteristic, and a tendency to grasp objects with an ulnar (primitive, using the palm) rather than radial (maturated, using index finger and thumb) dominance is often observed (9, 70, 71).

Schizophrenics also demonstrate poor motor regulation, varying from perseverative behavior (repetitive movements and actions) and motor inertia (difficulty starting motor actions and stopping them once started) to motor overflow (adventitious movements) and motor impersistence (inability to maintain a single motor task despite adequate motor and sensory function).

Emotional blunting has been considered a core feature of schizophrenia since the earliest descriptions of the syndrome. Recent studies (72, 73) have demonstrated that the assessment of emotional blunting can be made reliably (See Chapter 2, Table 2–4). Globally, patients with emotional blunting appear withdrawn and indifferent to their surroundings. They lack emotional spontaneity, and their moods are shallow. They are often apathetic or lazy, lack warmth and empathy, are vocally and facially expressionless, are indifferent to their family and friends, have little concern for their present situation, and have no plans, ambitions, desires, or drive.

Classically, this profound deficit in affect begins in the late teens or early twenties and progresses to a stage in which the sufferer is unable to maintain employment, has few or no friends, remains unmarried or separated from his spouse, and prefers to spend his time alone, at home, dependent on others. Such patients often end their days at the fringes of society, dirty and disheveled, living in the streets, hoarding garbage in rooming houses, or aimlessly wandering the grounds of state hospitals.

Thought disorder is the second core feature of the schizophrenic syndrome. However, it is somewhat of a misnomer, as classical workers used the term in referring primarily to abnormalities of language production (e.g. paraphasic speech, speech without content, neologisms) rather than to aberrant concept formation and abstraction (e.g. unable to recognize the basic category to which objects such as apples and pears belong), which also are observed in schizophrenics. Thus, schizophrenic language, phenomenologically, is not schizophrenic thought, though disturbances in the former often have been asserted to result from the latter. Formal thought disorder, by convention, refers to schizophrenic language production.

It long has been asserted (74, 75) that the language of schizophrenics shares phenomenologic similarities with aphasic speech. The data from several studies (63, 64, 75–78) suggest that although aphasics (particularly those with posterior language disorder) and schizophrenics do share similar elements of speech, the language productions of schizophrenics do not fit classical aphasic patterns associated with vascular disorders. These differences primarily reflect the schizophrenic's ability to use polysyllabic words (e.g. territorial imperative), while posterior aphasics have difficulty with such complex words and evidence a significant deficit in auditory comprehension resulting in frequent nonsequitive utterances. Both posterior aphasics and schizophrenics have fluent speech with reduced meaning and content words (e.g. nouns).

Approximately 40 percent of schizophrenics exhibit formal thought disorder (65). This language production is characterized by the use of words or phrases without precise meaning (word approximations), the use of nonsense words (neologisms) or real words with private meanings, driveling speech in which the syntax appears intact but the meaning (content) of the speech is lost, and responses that are nonsequitive or vague and beside the point (tangential). Schizophrenics often speak in a stilted, manneristic fashion, and the fluency of their speech often is disturbed, with paucity of speech, verbigeration (associations are repeated in a stereotyped manner), or perseveration (words or phrases are repetitively inserted in the flow of speech). Some examples of schizophrenic speech appear in Table 15-5.

Hallucinations and delusional phenomena often are observed in schizophrenia. The most dramatic are the first-rank symptoms of Schneider discussed earlier. Among schizophrenics, approximately 50–75 percent exhibit first-rank symptoms, 30–40 percent delusional ideas, and 40–60 percent hallucinations of one form or another (54–56, 79). The following case vignettes will illustrate the syndrome:

A twenty-six year old man was hospitalized after being found lying on a major highway. He had wandered away from home where he lived with his parents, who cared for him. The patient had one previous five-month hospitalization from which he was discharged home, where he remained for the next year and a half doing nothing but watching television and wandering about his neighborhood.

The patient's childhood was unremarkable, although he had to repeat the first grade. He finished high school with a B average, never used street drugs or abused alcohol. Except for consulting a psychologist at age fourteen because of "nerves," his past history was unremarkable. Prior to his illness he was a quiet, shy, bashful person. He had few friends and never married.

On examination he appeared unkempt and disheveled. He was quiet, cooperative, alert, and oriented with mild psychomotor retardation. There were no other features of depression. He exhibited profound emotional blunting and except for an occasional inappropriate smile rarely interacted with anyone, showed little emotion when his parents visited, and seemed not to care that he was in a hospital. He had no hallucinations, delusions, or first-rank symptoms. Despite the paucity of his speech he showed no formal thought disorder. There was no systemic or coarse neurologic explanation for his condition, which improved minimally with neuroleptics. He returned home.

A twenty-seven-year-old man was hospitalized following a family conflict. This was one of several hospitalizations, the first beginning at age twenty-five. His father stated

TABLE 15-5 Examples of Schizophrenic Speech
(Formal Thought Disorder)

TERM	EXAMPLE
1. Word approximation (paraphasia)	I have to go to the *buying place* (store); I need to get *writers* (pens).
2. Neologism	The *glob mander* is the one.
3. Private use of words	I *maturated* the sink because it was dirty.
4. Driveling speech	He may be it, but it won't be the way they wanted. I don't know, perhaps it can, but why not let him make up their minds?
5. Nonsequitive speech	Q. How old are you? A. I am a very healthy person.
6. Tangential speech	Q. What happened to get you into the hospital again? A. I've been living with my mother. Q. And what happened? A. She used to go there with me. Q. But why did she want you here now? A. She thought I should. Q. Why did she think that? Did you get sick? A. I have my own room there. Q. Well, that's good. By why did she think you should come back to the hospital? What was the matter? A. Some people might say I'm better off here.
7. Verbigeration	The univeral will is important. The universal will . . . the universal, universal . . . sal . . . sal, sal . . .
8. Perseverated speech (stock words)	The consequences of my actions requires immediate concern. Actions of family, actions of people, actions of government require concern. I am an active person and my actions need concerned attention.

the patient had stopped taking his medication, refused to look for work, and had become agitated, suspicious, angry, and aggressive.

His childhood was unremarkable, but in high school he was referred for psychiatric evaluation. At age nineteen he was rejected by the Army for a "nervous disorder." Prior to his illness he was a "loner" who in high school had increasing periods of truancy, finally dropping out at age sixteen. He never worked and had no friends.

On examintion the patient appeared slightly disheveled. He was neither hyperactive nor agitated. He was alert and irritable. He expressed fears of being touched, stepping on cracks between floor tiles, and touching his teeth. He showed profound emotional blunting. His speech was stilted, but he had no formal thought disorder. He said he spoke constantly with a "girl friend," whose voice he heard clearly coming from outside his room. He had no other hallucinations or delusional ideas, and there was no systemic or coarse neurologic explanation for his condition, which improved minimally with neuroleptics. He returned home.

A forty-three-year-old man was hospitalized at his family's request because he was found putting metal screws into his legs and for talking about cutting his tongue and penis. During the few weeks prior to hospitalization he had become progressively seclusive, began "chain smoking," took little care of his personal hygiene, and drank large quantities of coffee. He denied any pain from the screws in his legs and gave as his reason: "shorts . . . electronics."

This patient's illness began at age twenty-three, when over the course of a year he became seclusive and never came out of his room except to eat or go to the bathroom. During the subsequent twenty years he rarely spoke to his family, never called them by their first names, and showed not the slightest interest in them or anything else. On occasion he used to yell unintelligibly out of his window even though no one was outside.

On examination the patient appeared untidy but alert. He frequently closed his eyes in a ticlike fashion and scratched his body in a purposeless way. He showed no concern for his surroundings, his situation, or his family. His speech was mumbled, with periods of driveling. He said someone was telling him to put screws in his body and "electronics" were influencing him.

In the hospital he preferred to stay in bed with a blanket over his head. There was no systemic or coarse neurologic explanation for his condition, which improved minimally. He returned home.

The essential common feature of the three cases is the progressive and permanent deterioration in volition and affect, beginning in late adolescence or young adult life. This is the classical "Kraepelinian concept" of dementia praecox (6, 7), first described systematically by John Haslam, a British psychiatrist, in 1809 (66).

Diagnosis

Modern criteria for schizophrenia reflect the classical Kraepelinian concept and require the patient to exhibit one or more of the following psychopathologic phenomena:

1. Emotional blunting
2. First-rank symptoms
3. Formal thought disorder

However, the number and combination of psychopathological features that are required to satisfy different sets of criteria is arbitrary. Occasionally the core symptoms are combined with other clinical features, such as hallucinations and/or delusions.

Unlike Kraepelin and Bleuler, modern diagnosticians also require exclusion criteria, which must be met for the patient to be diagnosed schizophrenic. The following are generally required:

1. No evidence of a clouded or altered sensorium (which could indicate an acute intoxication, drug-induced syndrome, or acute neurologic disease)
2. No evidence of preexisting focal neurological disease (many of which can present with a schizophrenic psychosis)
3. No evidence of systemic illness, such as renal or heart disease, which can compromise brain function to the degree resulting in a schizophrenic-like psychosis.
4. No evidence of preexisting significant drug abuse (particularly hallucinogenic compounds) or alcoholism, which can each result in a schizophrenic-like psychosis
5. No evidence of signs or symptoms of affective disorder in sufficient numbers or degree to suggest the strong possibility of depression, mania, or a mixed affective state

The further subtyping of schizophrenia into such groups as "paranoid," "hebephrenic," "undifferentiated," and "catatonic" probably does not result in greater homogeneity when modern criteria initially are used to diagnose patients. Several studies (27–35) clearly demonstrate that patients labeled acute, paranoid, or catatonic schizophrenia by *DSM-II* criteria rarely have schizophrenia and in most instances satisfy modern criteria for affective disorder. However, it may be of benefit further to subdivide groups of patients satisfying modern criteria for schizophrenia by the presence or absence of emotional blunting, or other so-called negative symptoms (47, 80–82). The presence of such psychopathological features as delusions of persecution (paranoid), catatonic motor features (catatonia), or a silly mood (hebephrenia) have not been found helpful in discriminating subgroups of patients with differing treatment response, course, laboratory, or family history variables (83, 84).

There are, however, several clinical and laboratory features, which, when present, will increase the probability of the diagnosis of schizophrenia.

Diagnostically Helpful Variables

Age at Onset

The peak onset of schizophrenia typically occurs in late adolescence, between fifteen and twenty-five years of age (85). Any patient who develops a schizophrenic-like psychosis for the first time after age forty should be suspected of having coarse brain disease, no matter how "typical" the cross-sectional presentation. The clinician who is caring for such a "late-onset schizophrenic" patient should vigorously pursue this possibility, which may be more amenable to treatment.

ILLNESS COURSE

Long-term outcome studies (34, 85–88) in schizophrenia have failed to demonstrate a clear-cut course predicted by cross-sectional diagnostic criteria. Results indicate significant variability among schizophrenic samples. Nevertheless, several studies have clearly shown that schizophrenics have a poor outcome with progressive, nonepisodic deterioration when compared with affectively ill patients. Any patient with an episodic illness who has relatively intact interepisode functioning or has responded well to previous treatment should be considered nonschizophrenic until proven otherwise.

FAMILY HISTORY

Family history often provides a clue to a patient's diagnosis. Unfortunately the past deficiencies in psychiatric diagnostic practice that led to the over-diagnosis of schizophrenia has resulted in many patients with a family history of schizophrenia, where in fact the relatives in question do not satisfy criteria for schizophrenia and frequently do satisfy criteria for affective disorder. Virtually none of the genetic studies of schizophrenia conducted prior to 1972 employed criteria acceptable by present-day standards, and the patient samples investigated were almost certainly heterogeneous and probably included many individuals with affective disorder (49).

The reduced numbers of individuals satisfying modern criteria for schizophrenia is also observed in recent family studies (45–49) in which the morbidity risk (MR) for schizophrenia in first-degree relatives of schizophrenic patients is much lower than the 10–15 percent previously reported. For example, Winokur and associates (47) found a MR for schizophrenia of only 2.75 percent. Among the first-degree relatives of paranoid patients the MR was only 0.83 percent. Karlsson (48), in an Icelandic study of the first-degree relatives of "process" schizophrenics, found an MR for schizophrenia of 2.70 percent, whereas a recent study by Tsuang et al. (45) and one by Abrams and Taylor (49) found the first-degree relatives of schizophrenics to have MRs for schizophrenia of 3.2 and 1.61 percent, respectively.

Other genetic studies (49) report figures that are in general agreement with those detailed above. The mean first-degree relative MR for schizophrenia reported in these studies is between 3 and 4 percent, and about 10 percent of schizophrenic patients had a positive family history for schizophrenia. These figures contrast sharply with the 15 percent MR for affective disorder in first-degree relatives of affectively ill patients and the 30 percent positive family history for affective disorder among these patients. Thus, among schizophrenics a negative family history generally is to be expected. A positive family history of psychiatric disorder should alert the clinician to diagnostic possibilities other than schizophrenia.

EVIDENCE OF BRAIN DYSFUNCTION

There is increasing evidence for brain dysfunction in patients with schizophrenia who otherwise have no history suggestive of neurologic disease. Studies examining for soft neurologic signs (89, 90), electroencephalographic (91–93) and computer-enhanced tomographic abnormalities (94–96), and neuropsychological deficits (97) have demonstrated that on each of these measures schizophrenics differ significantly from normal controls and from patients with other psychiatric disorders. Once the exclusion criteria have been met and focal neurologic and other coarse brain disorders have been ruled out, a diagnostic evaluation employing the above measures can be helpful in identifying schizophrenics.

Soft neurologic signs (adventitious motor overflow, motor impersistence, double-simultaneous discrimination, Gegenhalten, grasp reflex, snout reflex, palmomental reflex, arm drift), when observed in adults, are usually pathological, although not specifically localizing. Psychiatric patients frequently exhibit one or more of these clinical phenomena, and approximately 50 to 75 percent of schizophrenics exhibit at least one feature.

Studies employing visual electroencephalographic analysis of psychiatric patients report that approximately 30 percent of consecutive acute admissions will demonstrate some abnormality. One-fourth of patients with affective disorder have abnormal electroencephalographic findings, and 50 percent of schizophrenics have abnormal electroencephalograms. The abnormalities are not epileptic and are characterized by nonspecific slowing, which, when asymmetrical, lateralize to the left parasylvian areas. Research electroencephalographic studies, using computer-analyzed evoked responses and power spectral analysis, also find schizophrenics to differ from normals and other psychiatric patients.

Computer-enhanced tomography during the past decade has dramatically demonstrated structural abnormalities in the brains of some schizophrenics. Studies in England and the United States reveal 30 to 50 percent of schizophrenics to have mild, diffuse cortical atrophy and/or independent enlargement of their lateral ventricles. Approximately 20 percent have cerebellar vermis atrophy. These findings appear to be independent of duration of illness or treatments received and have been correlated with diffuse cognitive impairment and chronicity.

The evaluation of higher cortical (cognitive) function in patients with major psychoses using standardized test batteries (e.g. Halstead–Reitan, Luria–Nebraska), as well as research instrumentation and strategies, has revealed 50 to 75 percent of schizophrenics to have marked diffuse impairment. In some studies the cognitive impairment observed in schizophrenics is indistinguishable in degree and pattern from that of demented patients.

Several investigators (97) have further observed schizophrenics specifically to have asymmetrical cognitive impairment with more pronounced deficits in the dominant hemisphere. The degree and pattern of this impairment have been contrasted with that observed in patients with affective disorder, who globally have less deficit and whose deficits when asymmetrical are more pronounced in the nondominant hemisphere. Patients with schizophrenia or affective disorder also have been categorized correctly into diagnostic groups solely on the basis of cognitive impairment patterns independent of psychopathology or other clinical information.

Thus, when the patient's global behaviors and psychopathology are ambiguous or insufficient to provide for a definitive diagnosis, supporting demographic, clinical, and laboratory information can be used to enhance diagnostic accuracy. "Typical" schizophrenia, then, is associated with the following:

Illness onset before forty
Chronic course
Negative family history
Presence of soft neurologic signs
Nonspecific electroencephalographic abnormality
Mild, diffuse cortical atrophy on CT scan
Diffuse cognitive impairment on neuropsychological testing

Treatment

The vast majority of patients satisfying modern criteria for schizophrenia will require periodic hospitalization. Most will eventually require long-term institutionalization or placement in a structured community setting such as a halfway house or hostel. Day treatment centers and day hospitals can also be of benefit in the continuing care of schizophrenics, although the cost-effectiveness of these facilities has not been established.

The primary goal of hospitalization of a schizophrenic is to provide a structured setting in which a proper diagnostic evaluation can be accomplished and a treatment plan developed and carried out. As schizophrenia is most likely to be a syndrome representing several pathophysiologic processes, treatment must be individualized. Neuroleptic administration, however, remains the primary therapeutic modality (98).

Treatment goals should be directed at the reduction of the symptoms that led to hospitalization and the commencement of social and vocational rehabilitation. Although 50 to 60 percent of patients ill less than three years who receive pharmacotherapy have a social recovery, it is the rare patient who has a complete remission. The degree of outcome is extremely variable at first, with most patients having a deteriorating course with permanent social and industrial impairment (99).

Neuroleptic Management

Pre-1970 studies of the efficacy of neuroleptics in the treatment of schizophrenia concluded that daily doses below 400 mg. of chlorpromazine or its equivalent were not effective (100). These studies were undoubtedly contaminated by the inclusion for study of a significant number of manic patients in varying states of excitement, suggesting that for rigorously diagnosed schizophrenics, who are rarely excited, doses can be considerably less. Reports from England in the 1950s and 1960s recommending lower doses for schizophrenia than those used in the United States probably reflected the narrow British concept of the disorder and its elimination of many manic patients from drug trials (101, 102). In our experience chlorpromazine, or its equivalent, in daily doses of 200 to 600 mg. will suffice for controlling symptoms in the majority of schizophrenics satisfying modern diagnostic criteria.

Once the patient is ready for discharge, the dose should be maintained for a minimum of eight months, as discontinuation prior to that time results in relapse in from 50 to 75 percent of patients. Treatment beyond one year, however, without a drug holiday to evaluate the need for further neuroleptic treatment, is not warranted, as the risk for tardive dyskinesia in these patients is great. It is unclear how many patients require futher treatment (98, 99).

The automatic use of additional medications during the acute hospitalization phase of illness is not justified. Antiparkinsonism drugs are not without risk and should be withheld until sufficient extrapyramidal symptoms develop to warrant treatment (98–100). Once employed and an effective dose schedule is established, antiparkinsonisms should be continued for three to four months, at which time they should be gradually stopped, as only one-third of patients require further treatment with these compounds (103, 104). Details of this management are discussed in the chapter on neuroleptics.

Other Acute Treatments

The use of other drugs or electroconvulsive treatment in schizophrenia must be determined on an individual basis. It is likely that subgroups of patients will have differential responses to different compounds. Propranolol (105), diphenylhydantoin (106, 107), and naloxone (108, 109) have each been tried with anecdotal success. In patients labeled schizophrenic by pre-1970 diagnostic criteria or who have the "schizoaffective" or catatonic syndromes, ECT, lithium, and tricyclic antidepressants can be of benefit (34, 35, 60, 110).

Behavioral Approaches

Most schizophrenics have significant cognitive impairment, which in degree and extent is similar to that observed in some demented patients (97). Elaborate psychotherapeutic interventions demanding high-level abstraction and comprehension are therefore inappropriate for these patients. The intense interpersonal nature and inherent ambiguity of psychotherapeutic interactions can only exacerbate the schizophrenic's already significant confusion and anxiety. Direct, reality-oriented, concrete comments best serve these patients. A calm, reassuring, caring manner is also helpful in reducing anxiety and in gaining the patient's cooperation for needed tests and compliance with medication and retraining strategies.

A structured inpatient setting, with formalized reinforcers (e.g. off-ward privileges, special foods) of positive social behaviors can also reduce the frequency of objectionable "management problem" behaviors. The interpersonally intense therapeutic community setting does not benefit these patients, and the long-term residential psychoanalytic institute is anachronistic and without the slightest evidentiary support of its therapeutic effectiveness (111, 112).

Discharge Planning

Appropriate discharge planning must consider (1) the degree to which the symptoms leading to hospitalization have been ameliorated, (2) the degree to which the patient's family or guardian has accepted the treatment plan, and

(3) available community resources for bed, board, and industrial training and placement.

The need to educate and counsel the family, to gain their understanding and support, is obviously critical for the success of the discharge plan. This is true whether the patient returns home or is placed in a community care program. This family educational process should begin early in hospitalization and should involve the family in discussions with any placement or "aftercare" programs.

Any retraining, placement, or behavioral intervention aftercare programming also must consider the cognitive strengths and weaknesses and residual psychopathology of the individual patient. Neuropsychological assessment of higher cortical functions and vocational assessment of industrial skills are essential aids in any meaningful discharge plan. For example, a patient who has significant fine motor dysregulation will most probably fail if given training involving the use of machinery, whereas the same patient might do well in a job requiring only heavy lifting (primarily involving axial muscles) and other unskilled movement.

Management Problems

Because of their deficits in volition and emotional spontaneity, schizophrenics are usually easily managed in a hospital setting. They virtually do nothing and bother no one.

On the other hand most of the management problems they do present also result from their lack of drive and loss of social graces. These problems include not keeping clean and properly dressed, lying on the floor in hallways, constantly smoking in the rooms and often burning bedding and furniture, not taking medication, and doing nothing on a unit in which the nursing staff takes great pride in its structured activities program. These problems can usually be avoided or controlled by (1) the appropriate pharmocotherapeutic and interpersonal strategies described above, (2) the education of staff concerning the nature of the patient's illness, and (3) providing a formal structured reinforcement program for rewarding positive social behaviors. An essential component to this program is a set of clear, easily understood unit rules and regulations that are unambiguously enforced and a set of precise privileges and rewards associated with the adherence to the unit rules and the maintenance of acceptable behaviors.

Less commonly, schizophrenics will be irritable and agitated and will become socially disruptive or uncooperative (e.g. refusing to follow unit rules, refusing to take medication or cooperate with diagnostic tests). Violence, however, is uncommon and usually stereotyped (e.g. automatically striking out at someone without provocation). When a schizophrenic becomes violent, it usually is against a background of emotional blunting, making it difficult to predict. Occasionally a schizophrenic will be menacing, staring hostilely at staff, speaking in a threatening manner, and/or exhibiting aggressive behaviors such as punching walls or angrily shouting. These behaviors should be treated as emergency situations and are discussed in detail in Chapters 5 and 9.

References

1. Kraepelin, E. *Psychiatrie: Ein Lehrbuch fur Studierende und Arzte.* 5th ed. Leipzig: Barth, 1896.

2. Kahlbaum, K. L. *Clinische Abhandlungen linige Psychische Krankheiten I: Katatonia oder das Spannungsuresein.* Berlin: Springer, 1874.

3. Hecker, E. Die häbephrenie. *Arch. Pathol. Anat. Physiol. Clin. Med. 52:* 394–429, 1871.

4. Kolle, K. *Grosse Nervenaerzte: Emil Kraepelin.* vol. 1. Stuttgart: Thieme, 1956.

5. Heinroth, J. C. *Textbook of Disturbances of Mental Life,* vol. 1., *Theory.* Schmorak, J. (trans.). Baltimore: Johns Hopkins University Press, 1975.

6. Kraepelin, E. *Dementia Praecox and Paraphrenia.* Barclay, R. M. (trans.) Huntington, N.Y.: Robert E. Krieger, 1971 (facsimile of 1919 ed.).

7. Kraepelin, E. *Lectures on Clinical Psychiatry.* Johnstone, T. (trans.). New York: Hafner, 1968 (facsimile of 1904 ed.).

8. Morel, B. A. *Traite des Maladies Mentales.* Paris: Victor Masson, 1860.

9. Bleuler, E. *Dementia Praecox or the Group of Schizophrenias.* Zinkin, (trans). New York: International Universities Press, 1950.

10. Feighner, J. P.; Robins, E.; Guze, S. B.; *et al.* Diagnostic criteria for use in psychiatric research. *Arch. Gen. Psychiat. 26:* 57–63, 1972.

11. Spitzer, R. L.; Endicott, J.; Robins, E. *Research Diagnostic Criteria for a Selected Group of Functional Disorders (RDC).* 2d ed. New York: Biometrics Research, New York State Psychiatric Institute, 1975.

12. APA Committee on Nomenclature. *Diagnostic and Statistical Manual of Mental Disorders.* 3d ed., *(DSM-III)* Washington, D.C.: American Psychiatric Association, 1980.

13. Ennis, B. J.; Litwash, T. R. Psychiatry and the presumption of expertise: Flipping coins in the courtroom. *Calif. Law Rev. 62:* 693–752, 1974.

14. Spitzer, R. L.; Fleiss, J. L. A re-analysis of the reliability of psychiatric diagnoses. *Br. J. Psychiat. 125:* 341–47, 1974.

15. Beck, A. T. Reliability of psychiatric diagnosis: 1. A critique of systematic studies. *Am. J. Psychiat. 119:* 210–16, 1962.

16. Taylor, M. A.; Abrams, R. The prevalence of schizophrenia: A reassessment using modern diagnostic criteria. *Am. J. Psychiat. 135:* 945–48, 1978.

17. Pope, H. G.; Lipinski, J. F. Diagnosis in schizophrenia and manic-depressive ill-

ness: A reassessment of the specificity of "schizophrenic" symptoms in light of current research. *Arch. Gen. Psychiat. 35:* 811–28, 1978.

18. APA Committee on Nomenclature. *Diagnostic and Statistical Manual of Mental Disorders.* 2d ed., *(DSM-II).* Washington, D.C.: American Psychiatric Association, 1968.

19. U.S. Department of Health, Education, and Welfare; National Institute of Mental Health. *Mental Health Statistical Note 138.* Washington D.C.: U.S. Government Printing Office, 1977.

20. Yolles, S. F., Kramer, M. Vital Statistics. In Bellack, L.; Loeb, L. (eds.), *The Schizophrenia Syndrome.* New York: Grune & Stratton, 1969, pp. 66–113.

21. Kramer, M. Cross-national study of diagnosis of the mental disorders: Origin of the problem. *Am. J. Psychiat. 125* (suppl.): 1–11, 1969.

22. Cooper, J. E.; Kendell, R. E.; Gurland, B. J.; *et al. Psychiatric Diagnoses in New York and London: Maudsley Monograph, no. 20.* London: Oxford University Press, 1972.

23. Sandifer, M.G.; Hordern, A.; Timburg, G. C.; *et al.* Similarities and differences in patient evaluation by U.S. and U.K. psychiatrists. *Am. J. Psychiat. 126:* 206–12, 1969.

24. Leff, J. International variations in the diagnosis of psychiatric illness. *Br. J. Psychiat. 131:* 329–38, 1977.

25. Rawnsley, K. An International Diagnostic Exercise. In *Proceedings of the Fourth World Congress of Psychiatry,* vol. 4. Amsterdam: Excerpta Medica Foundation, 1968.

26. Sharpe, S.; Gurland, B. J.; Fleiss J. L.; *et al.* Comparisons of American, Canadian and British psychiatrists in their diagnostic concepts. *Can. Psychiat. Assoc. J. 19:* 235–45, 1974.

27. Taylor, M. A.; Gaztanaga, P.; Abrams, R. Manic-depressive illness and acute schizophrenia: A clinical, family history and treatment response study. *Am. J. Psychiat. 131:* 678–82, 1974.

28. Taylor, M. A.; Abrams, R. Manic-depressive illness and good prognosis schizophrenia. *Am. J. Psychiat. 132:* 741–42, 1975.

29. Fowler, R. C.; McCabe, M. S.; Cadoret, R. J.; *et al.* The validity of good prognosis schizophrenia. *Arch. Gen. Psychiat. 26:* 182–85, 1972.

30. Abrams, R.; Taylor, M. A.; Gaztanaga, P. Manic-depressive illness and paranoid schizophrenia: A phenomenologic, family history and treatment response study. *Arch. Gen. Psychiat. 31:* 640–42, 1974.

31. Morrison, J. R. Catatonia: Retarded and excited types. *Arch. Gen. Psychiat. 28:* 39–41, 1973.

32. Abrams, R.; Taylor, M. A. Catatonia: A prospective clinical study. *Arch. Gen. Psychiat. 33:* 579–81, 1976.

33. Rosenthal, N. E.; Rosenthal, L. N.; Stallone, F.; *et al.* Toward the validation of RDC schizo-affective disorder. *Arch. Gen. Psychiat. 37:* 804–10, 1980.

34. Pope, H. G., Jr.; Lipinski, J. F.; Cohen, B. M.; *et al.* Schizo-affective disorder: An

invalid diagnosis? A comparison of schizo-affective disorder, schizophrenia and affective disorder. *Am. J. Psychiat. 137:* 921-27, 1980.

35. Taylor, M. A.: Schizo-affective and Allied Disorders. In Post, R. M.; Ballenger, J. C. (eds.), *The Neurobiology of Manic Depressive Illness.* Baltimore: Williams & Wilkins, 1984, pp. 136-56.

36. Woodruff, R. A. J.; Clayton, P. J.; Guze S. B. Suicide attempts and psychiatric diagnosis. *Dis. Nerv. Syst. 33:* 617-21, 1972.

37. Morrison, J.; Clancy, J.; Crowe, R.; *et al.* The Iowa 500: 1. Diagnostic validity in mania, depression and schizophrenia. *Arch. Gen. Psychiat. 27:* 457-61, 1972.

38. Taylor, M. A.; Abrams, R.; Gaztanaga, P. Manic-depressive illness and schizophrenia: A partial validation of research diagnostic criteria utilizing neuropsychological testing. *Comp. Psychiat. 16:* 91-96, 1975.

39. Nielson, J. & J. A. Eighteen years of community psychiatric service in the Island of Samso. *Br. J. Psychiat. 131:* 41-48,, 1977.

40. Helzer, J. E.; Clayton, P. J.; Pambakian, R.; *et al.* Reliability of psychiatric diagnosis: 2. The test-retest reliability of diagnostic classification. *Arch. Gen. Psychiat. 34:* 136-41, 1977.

41. Strauss, J. S.; Gift, T. E. Choosing an approach for diagnosing schizophrenia. *Arch. Gen. Psychiat. 34:* 1248-53, 1977.

42. Weissman, M. M.; Myers, J. K.; Harding, P. A. Psychiatric disorders in a U.S. urban community 1975-1976. *Am. J. Psychiat. 135:* 945-48, 1978.

43. Ries, R.; Bokan, J.; Schuckit, M. C. Modern diagnosis of schizophrenia in hospitalized psychiatric patients. *Am. J. Psychiat. 137:* 1419-21, 1980.

44. Nielson, J. & J. A. A census study of mental illness in Samso. *Psychol. Med. 7:* 491-503, 1977.

45. Tsuang, M. T.; Winokur, G.; Crowe, R. R. Morbidity risks of schizophrenia and affective disorders among first-degree relatives of patients which schizophrenia, mania, depression and surgical conditions. *Am. J. Psychiat. 137:* 497-504, 1980.

46. Kety, S. S; Rosenthal, D.; Wender, P. H.; *et al.* The Types and Prevalence of Mental Illness in the Biological and Adoptive Families of Adopted Schizophrenics. In Rosenthal, D.; Kety, S. S. (eds.), *The Transmission of Schizophrenia.* Oxford: Pergamon Press, 1968, pp. 345-62.

47. Winokur, G.; Morrison, J.; Clancy, J.; *et al.* The Iowa 500: The clinical and genetic distinction of hebephrenia and paranoid schizophrenia. *J. Nerv. Ment. Dis. 159:* 12-19, 1974.

48. Karlsson, J. L. An Icelandic family study of schizophrenia. *Br. J. Psychiat. 123:* 549-54, 1973.

49. Abrams, R.; Taylor, M. A. The genetics of schizophrenia: A reassessment using modern diagnostic criteria. *Am. J. Psychiat. 140:* 171-75, 1983.

50. Kraepelin, E. *Psychiatrie.* Leipzig: Weiner, 1893.

51. Kendell, R. E.; Cooper, J. E.; Gourley, A. J.; *et al.* Diagnostic criteria of American and British psychiatrists. *Arch. Gen. Psychiat. 25:* 123-30, 1971.

52. Baldessarini, R. Frequency of diagnosis of schizophrenia versus affective disorder from 1944 to 1968. *Am. J. Psychiat. 127:* 759-63, 1970.

53. Kurionsky, J. B.; Gurland, B. J.; Spitzer, R. L.; *et al.* Trends in the frequency of schizophrenia by different diagnostic criteria. *Am. J. Psychiat. 134:* 631–36, 1977.

54. Schneider, K. *Clinical Psychopathology.* New York: Grune & Stratton, 1959.

55. Carpenter, W. T., Jr.; Strauss, J. S.; Muleh, S. Are there pathognomonic symptoms in schizophrenia? *Arch. Gen. Psychiat. 28:* 847–52, 1973.

56. Abrams, R.; Taylor, M. A. The importance of schizophrenic symptoms in the diagnosis of mania. *Am. J. Psychiat. 138:* 658–61, 1981.

57. Kraepelin, E. *Manic-Depressive Insanity and Paranoia.* Barclay R. M. (trans.), Robertson, G. M. (ed.). New York: Arno Press, 1976, reprinted from 1921 Livingstone ed.).

58. Hearst, E. D.; Munoz, R. A.; Tuason, V. B. Catatonia: Its diagnostic validity. *Dis. Nerv. Syst. 32:* 453–56, 1971.

59. Taylor, M. A.; Abrams, R. The prevalence and importance of catatonia in the manic phase of manic-depressive illness. *Arch. Gen. Psychiat. 34:* 1223–25, 1977.

60. Taylor, M. A.; Abrams, R. The phenomenology of mania: A new look at some old patients. *Arch. Gen. Psychiat. 29:* 520–22, 1973.

61. Carlson, G. A.; Goodwin, F. K. The stages of mania. *Arch. Gen. Psychiat. 28:* 221–28, 1973.

62. Lipkin, K. M.; Dyrud, J.; Meyer, G. G. The many faces of mania. *Arch. Gen. Psychiat. 22:* 262–67, 1970.

63. Andreasen, N. C.; Grove, W. The Relationship Between Schizophrenic Language, Manic Language, and Aphasia. In Gruzelier, J.; Flor-Henry, P. (eds.), *Hemisphere Asymmetries of Function in Psychopathology.* Amsterdam: Elsevier/North Holland Biomedical Press, 1979, pp. 373–90.

64. Andreasen, N. C. Thought, language and communication disorders: 2. Diagnostic significance. *Arch. Gen. Psychiat. 36:* 1325–30, 1979.

65. Taylor, M. A.; Greenspan, R.; Abrams, R. Lateralized neuropsychological dysfunction in affective disorder and schizophrenia. *Am. J. Psychiat. 136:* 1031–34, 1979.

66. Haslam, J. *Observations on Madness and Melancholy.* New York: Arno Press, 1976.

67. Hammond, W. A. *A Treatise on Insanity in Its Medical Relations.* In series, Mental Illness and Social Policy: The American Experience. New York: Arno Press, 1973.

68. Spitzka, E. C. *Insanity: Its Classification, Diagnosis and Treatment.* In series, Mental Illness and Social Policy: The American Experience. New York: Arno Press, 1973.

69. Church, A.; Peterson, F. *Nervous and Mental Diseases.* 2d ed. Philadelphia: W. B. Saunders, 1900.

70. Chapman, J. The early symptoms of schizophrenia. *Br. J. Psychiat. 112:* 225–51, 1966.

71. Kleist, K. *Untersuchungen zur Kenntnis der Psychomotrischen Bewegungsstorungen bei Geisteskranken.* Leipzig: Klinkhart, 1908.

72. Abrams, R.; Taylor, M. A. A rating scale for emotional blunting. *Am. J. Psychiat.* 135: 225–29, 1978.

73. Andreasen, N. C. Affective flattening and the criteria for schizophrenia. *Am. J. Psychiat.* 136: 944–47, 1979.

74. Chaika, E. A linguist looks at "schizophrenic" language. *Brain and Language 1:* 257–76, 1974.

75. Kleist, K. Schizophrenic symptoms and cerebral pathology. *J. Ment. Sci.* 106: 246–55, 1960.

76. Horsfall, G. H. An investigation of selected language performance in adult schizophrenic subjects. Doctoral dissertation, University of Florida, Gainesville, 1972. *Dissertation Abstracts International 34:* 425B–453B, University Microfilms 73–15, 507, 1973.

77. Faber, R.; Reichstein, M. B. Language dysfunction in schizophrenia. *Br. J. Psychiat.* 139: 519–22, 1981.

78. Faber, R.; Abrams, R.; Taylor, M. A.; *et al.* Comparison of schizophrenic patients with formal thought disorder and neurologically impaired patients with aphasia. *Am. J. Psychiat.* 140: 1348–51, 1983.

79. Hamilton, M. (ed). *Fish's Clinical Psychopathology: Signs and Symptoms in Psychiatry.* Rev. repr. Bristol: John Wright & Sons, 1974.

80. Andreasen, N. C. Negative symptoms in schizophrenia: Definition and reliability. *Arch. Gen. Psychiat.* 39: 784–88, 1982.

81. Andreasen, N. C.; Olsen, S. Negative versus positive schizophrenia: Definition and validation. *Arch. Gen. Psychiat.* 39: 789–94, 1982.

82. Crow, T. J. Molecular pathology of schizophrenia: More than one disease? *Br. Med. J.* 280: 66–68, 1980.

83. Brill, N.; Glass, J. Hebephrenic schizophrenia reactions. *Arch. Gen. Psychiat.* 12: 545–51, 1965.

84. Goodwin, D. W.; Alderson, P.; Rosenthal, R. Clinical significance of hallucinations in psychiatric disorders. *Arch. Gen. Psychiat.* 24: 76–80, 1971.

85. Pfohl, B.; Winokur, G. Schizophrenia: Course and Outcome. In Henn, F. A.; Nasrallah, H. A. (eds.), *Schizophrenia as a Brain Disease.* New York: Oxford University Press, 1982, pp. 26–39.

86. Tsuang, M. T.; Woolson, R. F.; Fleming, J. A. Long-term outcome of major psychosis: 1. Schizophrenia—Affective disorders compared with psychiatrically symptom-free surgical conditions. *Arch. Gen. Psychiat.* 36: 1295–1301, 1979.

87. Strauss, J. S.; Carpenter, W. T. The prediction of outcome in schizophrenia: 2. Relationships between predictor and outcome variables—A report from the WHO International Pilot Study of Schizophrenia. *Arch. Gen. Psychiat.* 31: 37–42, 1974.

88. Strauss, J.; Carpenter, W. T. Characteristic symptoms and outcome in schizophrenia. *Arch. Gen. Psychiat.* 30: 429–34, 1974.

89. Cox, S. M.; Ludwig, A. M. Neurological soft signs and psychopathology: 1. Findings in schizophrenia. *J. Nerv. Ment. Dis.* 167: 161–65, 1979.

90. Quitkin, F.; Rifkin, A.; Klein, D. F. Neurologic soft signs in schizophrenia and character disorders. *Arch. Gen. Psychiat. 33:* 845–53, 1979.

91. Abrams, R.; Taylor, M. A. Differential EEG patterns in affective disorder and schizophrenia. *Arch. Gen. Psychiat. 36:* 1355–58, 1979.

92. Vianna, U. The Electroencephalogram in Schizophrenia. In Lader, M. H. (ed.), *Studies of Schizophrenia. Br. J. Psychiat.* Special pub., ser. no. 10. Kent, Eng.: Headley Bros., 1975, pp. 54–58.

93. Tucker, G. J.; Detre, T.; Harrow, M.; *et al.* Behavior and symptoms of psychiatric patients and the electroencephalogram. *Arch. Gen. Psychiat. 12:* 278–86, 1965.

94. Nasrallah, H. A.; Jacoby, C. C.; McCalley-Whitters, M.; *et al.*, Cerebral ventricular enlargement in subtypes of chronic schizophrenia. *Arch. Gen. Psychiat. 39:* 774–77, 1982.

95. Frangos, E.; Athanassenos, G. Differences in lateral brain ventricular size among various types of chronic schizophrenics: Evidence based on a CT scan study. *Acta Psychiat. Scand. 66:* 459–63, 1982.

96. Golden, L. J.; Graber, B.; Coffman, J.; *et al.* Structural brain deficits in schizophrenia: Identification by computed tomographic scan density measurements. *Arch. Gen. Psychiat. 38:* 1014–17, 1981.

97. Taylor, M. A.; Abrams, R. Cognitive impairment in schizophrenia. *Am. J. Psychiat. 141:* 196–201, 1984.

98. Davis, J. M. Recent developments in the drug treatment of schizophrenia. *Am. J. Psychiat. 133:* 208–14, 1976.

99. Baldessarini, R. J. Drugs and the Treatment of Psychiatric Disorders. In Gilman, A. G.; Goodman, L. S.; Gilman, A. (eds.) *The Pharmacological Basis of Therapeutics.* 6th ed. New York: Macmillan, 1980.

100. Klein, D. F.; Davis, J. M. *Diagnosis and Drug Treatment of Psychiatric Disorders.* Baltimore: Williams & Wilkins, 1969.

101. Klein, D. F. Importance of psychiatric diagnosis in prediction of clinical drug effects. *Arch. Gen. Psychiat. 16:* 118–26, 1967.

102. Dransfield, G. A. A clinical trial comparing prochlorperazine ("stemitil") with chlorpromazine ("largactil") in the treatment of chronic psychotic patients. *J. Ment. Sci. 104:* 1183–89, 1958.

103. Orlov, P.; Kasparian, G.; Di Mascio, A.; *et al.* Withdrawal of antiparkinson drugs. *Arch. Gen. Psychiat. 25:* 410–12, 1971.

104. Klett, C. J.; Caffey, E. Evaluating the long-term need for antiparkinson drugs by chronic schizophrenics. *Arch. Gen. Psychiat. 26:* 374–79, 1972.

105. Atsmon, A.; Blum, I.; Wijsenbeck, H.; *et al.* The short-term effects of adrenergic–blocking agents in a small group of psychotic patients. *Psychiat. Neurol. Neurochirugia 74:* 251–58, 1971.

106. Kalinowsky, L. B.; Putnam, T. J. Attempts at treatment of schizophrenia and other nonepileptic psychoses with dilantin. *Arch. Neurol. Psychiat. 49:* 414–20, 1943.

107. Freyhan, F. A. Effectivness of diphenylhydantoin in management of nonepileptic psychomotor excitement states. *Arch. Neurol. Psychiat. 53:* 370–74, 1945.

108. Davis, G. C.; Post, R. M.; Wyatt, R. J. Intravenous naloxone administration in schizophrenia and affective illness. *Science 197:* 74–77, 199.

109. Gunne, L. M.; Lindstrom, L.; Terenius, L. Naloxone induced reversal of schizophrenic hallucinations. *J. Neurol. Trans. 40:* 13–19, 1977.

110. Taylor, M. A. Indications for Electroconvulsive Treatment. In Abrams, R.; Essman, W. B. (eds.), *Electroconvulsive Therapy in Theory and Practice.* New York: SP Medical and Scientific Books, 1982, pp. 7–39.

111. May, P. R. A. *Treatment of Schizophrenia: A Comparative Study of Five Treatment Methods.* New York: Science House, 1968.

112. Simpson, G. M.; May, P. R. A. Schizophrenic Disorders. In Greist, J. H.; Jefferson, J. W.; Spitzer, R. L. (eds.), *Treatment of Mental Disorders.* New York: Oxford University Press, 1982, pp. 143–83.

CHAPTER 16

Delusional Disorder

The currently used term "delusional disorder" represents the latest development in the conceptualization of paranoia. Originally a lay term for insanity, paranoia (beside one's self) was first conceived by Heinroth (1) as delusional ideas secondary to affective disturbances. Kahlbaum (2) next defined paranoia as a distinct disease entity similar in many respects to Esquirol's monomania (3), which denoted a disorder characterized by a single overwhelming delusional idea, but without personality or intellectual deterioration. Kraepelin (4, 5), who ultimately incorporated paranoia into his concept of dementia praecox, initially used the term to describe a chronic disorder of unshakable delusional ideas with an insidious onset and little deterioration of personality. Kraepelin later coined the term paraphrenia to denote milder delusional syndromes, distinct from dementia praecox, which developed in middle and late life (dementia praecox having an early onset) with little subsequent deterioration. Roth's (6) late paraphrenia and the paranoid reactive psychoses of Scandinavian psychiatry (termed paranoid states in the United States) (7) are variations of Kraepelin's paraphrenia concept. Paranoid personality, characterized by hypersensitivity, rigidity, suspiciousness, feelings of envy and jealousy, excessive self-importance, and a tendency to blame others, has been proposed as the trait underlying paranoid states (8, 9). The validity of this notion is unknown (10). The term delusional disorder was suggested by Winokur (11) to avoid the confusion resulting from the diverse concepts of paranoia and from the ambiguity of the term, which has been used to denote insanity, suspiciousness, persecutory or grandiose delusions, schizophrenia, and a specific disease entity distinct from other psychoses.

Delusional disorder (or simple delusional disorder if hallucinations are absent) as currently defined phenomenologically is characterized by systematized delusional ideas, no prominent affective features, no first-rank symptoms or formal thought disorder, and little, if any, emotional blunting or personality deterioration. No predisposing personality has been established as an antecedent of this disorder. More than half of these patients are male, and more than half are married at the time of onset, which is in the fourth or early fifth decade. The disorder occurs particularly frequently among immigrants (11, 12).

Follow-up data suggest that few of these patients develop schizophrenia and that about 25 to 40 percent become chronically ill (compared with 90 to 100 percent of schizophrenics) (11, 13, 14). Family studies (10, 11, 15) indicate little increased risk for schizophrenia or affective disorder and a low risk for delusional disorder. The population prevalence of delusional disorder is unknown but is probably less than 1 percent, making it a rare condition. Etiology is unknown, and treatment remains symptomatic. It appears to be a psychosis distinct from schizophrenia and affective disorder.

The following patient illustrates the condition:

A thirty-four-year-old unmarried white woman sought hospitalization because she wished to prove that she did not have a brain disease and that her conviction that her employer was trying to kill her was fact, not fancy. She requested an EEG, a CT scan, and a neuropsychiatric and neurologic evaluation. Although she recognized the possibility that she might be mentally ill, she thought this "unlikely" and systematically provided details to support her contention of a plot against her.

Approximately two years earlier, she became convinced that her employer at that time was covering up a scandal about nuclear material and that the employer had begun spying on her and ultimately tried to kill her when she found out about the scandal and tried to make it public. She was fired from that job.

Upon learning of the firing, her mother, whom she had not seen for six months, traveled to see her. Her mother described her as cool and distant (no longer hugging and kissing her as she had when they were last together). The mother stated that other than having this lack of warmth and of full emotional spontaneity, her daughter was the same as always. She had been a good student in high school, had a year of business training following school, and had been a popular person and a "good" daughter. She never had a serious illness or a head injury, never used street drugs, and used alcohol only in appropriate social circumstances, never to excess. There was no family history of psychiatric illness.

On examination, the patient was precisely groomed, was well-spoken, and appeared extremely efficient—a no-nonsense, cool, unemotional individual. She dispassionately related her beliefs about her past employer and stated that her present employers had also been trying to kill her since she began learning of their unethical business practices. Her beliefs involved elaborate details about events, people involved, and motivations for the plot. Some of the details were clearly shown to be false and others exaggerated. Most of her interpretations were clearly arbitrary, such as "I am sure the person who moved in across the street is a spy because that house has been unoccupied for almost a year and suddenly he moved in!" She exhibited no other psychopathology.

All laboratory results and psychological tests were within normal limits. Nevertheless, she agreed to treatment. Full consecutive courses of lithium, carbamazepine, haloperidol, ECT, and monoamine oxidase inhibitors were tried without success. Following discharge she quickly obtained employment as a bookkeeper with another firm.

Management

The above case illustrates the relative unresponsivity of these patients to standard treatment. Treatment response studies (16–19) are unhelpful as they are anecdotal or without adequate scientific design. We suggest a pragmatic approach, with ECT or neuroleptics as probably the most efficacious treatments.

References

1. Heinroth, J. C. *Textbook of Disturbances of Marital Life*, vols. 1 and 2. Baltimore: Johns Hopkins Press, 1975 (from the 1818 text).

2. Kahlbaum, K. Gruppierung der psychischen Krankheiten. Danzig: Kafemann, 1863.

3. Esquirol, E. *Des Maladies Mentales*. 1838. Three vols. in two. History of Medicine Series, New York Academy of Medicine. New York: Hafner Publishing, 1965 (facsimile of 1845 English ed. with Introduction by Saussure, R. D. E.).

4. Kraepelin, E. *Dementia Praecox and Paraphrenia*. Barclay, R. M. (trans.). Huntington, N.Y.: Robert E. Krieger Publishing Co., 1971 (facsimile of 1919 ed.).

5. Kraepelin, E. Manic-depressive Insanity and Paranoia. Barclay, R. M. (trans.). New York: Arno Press, 1976, (facsimile of 1921 ed.).

6. Roth, M. The natural history of mental disorder in old age. *J. Ment. Sci. 101:* 281–301, 1955.

7. McCabe, M. S. Reactive psychoses. *Acta Psychiat. Scand. 259,* 1975. (Suppl.)

8. Kay, K. W. K.; Roth, M. Environmental and hereditary factors in the schizophrenia of old age ("late paraphrenia"), and their bearing on the general problem of causation in schizophrenia. *J. Ment. Sci. 107:* 649–86, 1961.

9. Herbert, M.; Jacobson, S. Late paraphrenia. *Br. J. Psychiat. 113:* 461–69, 1967.

10. Watt, J. A. G.; Hall, D. J.; Olley, P. C.; *et al.* Paranoid states of middle life: Familial occurrence and relationship to schizophrenia. *Acta Psychiat. Scand. 61:* 413–26, 1980.

11. Winokur, G. Delusional disorder (paranoia). *Comp. Psychiat. 18:* 511–21, 1977.

12. Kendler, K. S. The nosologic validity of paranoia (simple delusional disorder): A review. *Arch. Gen. Psychiat. 37:* 699–706, 1980.

13. Retterstol, N. *Paranoid and Paranoic Psychoses.* Springfield, Ill.: C. C. Thomas, 1966.

14. Retterstol, N. *Prognosis in Paranoid Psychoses.* Springfield, Ill.: C. C. Thomas, 1970.

15. Kendler, K. S.; Hays, P. Paranoid psychosis (delusional disorder) and schizophrenia: A family history. *Arch. Gen. Psychiat. 38:* 547–51, 1981.

16. Bilikiewicz, T.; Sulestrowski, W.; Wdowiak, L. Les results der treatment de la paranoia et de la paraphrenie par le largactul. *Année Medico–Psychol 115:* 52–69, 1957.

17. Blanc, M.; Borenstein, P.; Brion, S.; *et al.* Étude comparative de l'activité de deux neuroleptiques. *Encephale 59:* 97–161, 1970.

18. Ey, H.; Bohard, F. Results d'une therapeutique medicomenteuse dans les delires chroniques. *Evolution Psychiatrique 35:* 251–95, 1970.

19. Riding, J.; Munro, A. Pimozide in the treatment of monosymptomatic hypochondriacal psychosis. *Acta Psychiat. Scand. 52:* 23–30, 1975.

CHAPTER 17

Puerperal Psychoses

Women are at greatest risk for psychiatric illness during the first several weeks after childbirth. This risk is about ten times that for women at other times in their lives but represents only about one per 1,000 births. The incidence of nonpsychotic disorders does not increase during parturition (1). The majority of postpartum psychoses begins within the first seven to ten days following childbirth. A second, much smaller peak occurs around the sixth to eighth week and appears associated with the first postpartum menses (2, 3). The onset frequency curve mirrors falling serum progesterone levels, and the massive hormonal changes occurring after childbirth have been implicated in the pathophysiology of postpartum states (4). Although the risk for psychopathology among women is lowest during pregnancy (4), women who develop postpartum psychoses usually exhibit some symptoms late in pregnancy (3), and the presence of psychopathology, however mild, during the third trimester suggests the likelihood of a psychosis developing after childbirth. Unfortunately, except for a previous episode of postpartum psychosis, there are no long-term predictors of the condition (1, 5). Two-thirds of patients develop the condition following their first pregnancy (2). There is no association between postpartum psychosis and premenstrual syndromes (6).

Prior to modern advances in obstetrical care, the majority of postpartum states were toxic in character, associated with fever and confusion, and were often fatal (2). Today affective disorder is the most frequently observed postpartum syndrome (3, 6), and depression the most frequent postpartum affective state (3, 6). Mania, however, is also an extremely common postpartum state, accounting for 10 to 15 percent of cases (2, 3, 6).

Postpartum psychosis is not a distinct disease. Phenomenologic, genetic, and treatment response data (1–3, 5, 6) suggest that puerperal states are heterogeneous and that the type of postpartum syndrome observed is essentially the same illness as its nonpuerperal counterpart. Nevertheless, postpartum psychotics are younger than nonpuerperal controls, and there is some evidence that, compared with the nonpuerperal affective illnesses, postpartum manics are more often disoriented, are unable to concentrate, and complain that "things are going too fast," whereas postpartum depressives are more likely to be delusional and to experience hallucinations. The data also suggest that postpartum psychoses are extremely responsive to treatment, particularly ECT (1–3), a procedure considered lifesaving for this condition in the 1940s (2). As postpartum manics are often confused and may become more so with neuroleptics or lithium, and postpartum depressives are often delusional and thus less likely to respond to antidepressant drugs (7, 8), we consider ECT to be the treatment of choice for this disorder. In general significant psychiatric illness during pregnancy should also be considered a clear clinical indication for ECT (9).

References

1. Nott, P. N. Psychiatric illness following childbirth: A case register study. *Psychol. Med.* 12: 557–61, 1982.

2. Protherol, C. Puerperal Psychoses: A long-term study 1927–1961. *Br. J. Psychiat.* 115: 9–30, 1969.

3. Dean, C.; Kendell, R. E. The symptomatology of puerperal illness. *Br. J. Psychiat.* 139: 128–33, 1981.

4. Taylor, M. A.; Levine, R. Puerperal schizophrenia: A physiological interaction between mother and fetus. *Biol. Psychiat.* 1: 97–101, 1969.

5. Katona, C. L. E. Puerperal mental illness: Comparisons with non-puerperal controls. *Br. J. Psychiat.* 141: 447–52, 1982.

6. Brockington, I. F.; Cernik, K. P.; Schofield, E. M.; et al. Puerperal psychosis: Phenomena and diagnosis. *Arch. Gen. Psychiat.* 38: 829–33, 1981.

7. Glassman, A. H.; Kantor, S. J.; Shostak, M. Depression, delusions and drug response. *Am. J. Psychiat.* 132: 716–19, 1975.

8. Davidson, J. C. T.; McLeod, M. N.; Kurland, A. A.; et al. Anti-depressant drug therapy in psychotic depression. *Br. J. Psychiat.* 131: 493–96, 1977.

9. Taylor, M. A. Indications for Electroconvulsive Treatment. In Abrams, R.; Essman, W. B. (eds.), *Electroconvulsive Therapy.* New York: SP Medical and Scientific Books, 1982, pp. 7–39.

CHAPTER 18

Behavioral Neurologic Disease

The history of psychiatry is punctuated by psychiatrists' yielding to neurologists and general physicians responsibility for the treatment of patients for whom a specific treatment has been developed or whose illness etiology has been established. The reclassification of epilepsy and syphilis as "nonpsychiatric" disorders are the most striking examples of this shift in responsibility. However, with the reemergence of interest in psychiatric diagnosis and in the biological processes of behavior the attitudes of psychiatrists are changing, and the understanding and treatment of brain disease are once again becoming part of the mainstream of psychiatric practice.

The relatively young field of behavioral neurology has developed, in part, from this shift in attitude and the clinical and research need to bridge the gap between traditional neurology with its emphasis on structural lesions and motor/sensory signs, and traditional psychiatry with its focus on behavior. Behavioral neurology relates behavior to structure. Its basic science is the field of neuropsychology (1–3).

Since all behavior, normal and abnormal, in its final common path reflects brain function, all behavioral syndromes (e.g. phobias, anxiety states, psychoses, personality deviations) can be considered behavioral neurologic conditions. This chapter, however, will focus on those conditions in which the neuropathology is more firmly established and the evidence is clear that brain pathological processes underlie the observable behavioral phenomena. The focus will also be limited to conditions likely to be observed in an active psychiatric hospital practice.

The Epilepsies

The association between seizure disorders and abnormal behavior has been known since the earliest Greek medical writers (4). Modern surveys (4–6) suggest that three-quarters of epileptics will develop behavioral difficulties and/or intellectual deficits in association with their seizure disorder and that nearly 50 percent will have interictal psychiatric symptoms effecting social functioning and ability to work. Epileptics comprise approximately 10 percent of psychiatric admissions. Psychiatrists must be prepared to recognize and treat these patients, whose behaviors make them inappropriate patients on most neurologic services.

The prevalence of seizure disorders is about 6 per 1,000. The etiology in most cases is unknown, and there are no reported differences among social classes (5, 7). Follow-up studies (1, 5, 8) indicate the course in many cases is poor, with the prognosis being worse for early onset cases. Seizure disorders are classified into

1. *Generalized* (the initial electrical discharge is generalized, originating from all or most centrencephalic structures)
2. *Partial* (the initial electrical discharge is focal, cortical, or subcortical in origin and may or may not become generalized)
3. *Mixed* forms

Generalized seizures are primary (unrecognizable etiology), whereas partial and mixed forms are assumed to be acquired. The observable manifestations of seizure disorders are also classified. Generalized seizures include the following types: petit mal, myoclonic, infantile spasms, clonic, tonic, tonic–clonic (grand mal), atonic, and akinetic. Partial seizures include simple (attacks without significant impairment of consciousness, accompanied by motor and sensory symptoms) and complex (attacks with significant impairment of consciousness, accompanied by behavioral, cognitive, and affective phenomena) (9–11).

Behavioral changes associated with epilepsy can directly relate to the seizure itself (the ictal state), the prodromal (hours to weeks preceding the seizure), or postictal (hours to days subsequent to the seizure) periods, or to the interictal period. Since the seizure itself rarely lasts more than fifteen minutes and is most often less than a minute, the behaviors that lead to psychiatric hospitalization or treatment are typically nonictal.

Prodromal symptoms usually develop a few hours or days prior to the fit. Irritability and dysphoria are most common, although psychosis can occur. Prodromal syndromes usually improve following the seizure. Observation of this relationship contributed to the development of induced seizures for the treatment of psychiatric disorders (12, 13).

Ictal phenomena requiring psychiatric treatment are most commonly seen in patients with complex partial seizures. Another term used to identify these syndromes is psychomotor epilepsy. Temporal lobe epilepsy (TLE) is the most common type of psychomotor epilepsy. Epilepsy in other cortical areas, particularly the frontal lobes, can also produce complex psychomotor phenomena. Petit mal status has also been reported to produce a confusional psychosis, which can last for days or weeks. However, any chronic generalized seizure disorder can eventually result in psychosis (12, 14–16).

Psychomotor, or complex partial seizure, syndromes are associated with some alteration in consciousness. The alteration can be an extremely subtle one during which the patient may appear only slightly hesitant or somewhat distracted in his responses. Perplexity, oneiroid states, syndromes characterized by disorientation and agitation, and complex behavior patterns during which the patient is unresponsive to all but the most intense stimulation (e.g. shouting, physical restraints) can also occur. Absence phenomena are also observed, but these tend to be longer and less frequent than those of petit mal and more gradual in onset and termination. Psychomotor episodes tend to be short in duration, frequent, and, for a given patient, similar in form and content from one episode to another (10–12, 14–17).

Virtually every type of psychopathology has been reported during psychomotor states. The *classical psychomotor ictal* presentation is that of temporal lobe epilepsy and is characterized by automatic, repetitive behaviors termed *automatisms*, which can take the form of complicated acts. Some reported automatisms are laughing, weeping, sobbing, raging, screaming, lip-smacking, chewing, swallowing, rubbing, scratching, grimacing, assuming odd postures, dressing and undressing, continual repetition of the same phrases, getting something to eat or drink, fugue states, and violent behavior. Other repetitive ictal behaviors are coughing, sneezing, yawning, hiccupping, gagging, vomiting, and belching.

During the fit the patient may appear unblinking, wide-eyed, expressionless, staring ahead or to one side. Partial or complete loss of posture may occur, as well as pupillary dilation, pallor or flushing, perioral cyanosis, salivation, sweating, tachycardia, hypertension, gastrointestinal motility changes, incontinence of urine (rarely of feces), respiratory rate changes, and gasping or even apnea.

Associated experiences include alteration in mood, forced thinking, feeling of impending doom and anxiety, sensations of false familiarity (déjà vu) or unfamiliarity (jamais vu), depersonalization and derealization, oneiroid states, visual distortions (macropsia, micropsia), hallucinations (pleasant and unpleasant) in any sensory modality (particularly visual, olfactory, and gustatory), autoscopic phenomena (hallucinating oneself), and abdominal pains or a feeling of abdominal emptiness (hollowness), which "rushes" up into the subcostal area (sometimes through the chest and into the head). These episodes are usually short in duration and are always followed by some degree of amnesia for the event and some postictal fatigue, sleepiness, confusion, or depression (10–12, 14–17). Although most ictal phenomena are not lateralizable to the side of the seizure focus, several studies (18–21) have demonstrated that sudden, transient, shallow expressions of sadness or tearfulness are associated with nondominant hemisphere lesions, whereas sudden, transient, shallow expressions of euphoria or laughter are associated with dominant hemisphere lesions.

Other ictal syndromes include:

1. A parietal lobe syndrome characterized by feelings that body parts are unusually heavy, dead, as if made of metal; painful tingling similar to electrical shocks; unpleasant coldness or burning feelings; feelings that an arm or leg is moving on its own; experiences of body parts in new locations (e.g. a hand in one's abdomen); and altered attitude towards pain (painful stimuli become pleasant so that self-inflicted painful injuries may result). These experiences may lead to secondary delusional ideas of being possessed, being controlled by an outside force, or being dead (22).

2. A frontal lobe syndrome characterized by speech arrest, periods of shallow euphoria and depression, irritable outbursts, dysphoria, posturing, diminished wakefulness, hyperactivity, disorientation, uncontrollable confabulations, and lack of self-control (23–27).

Postictal Behavior

Postictal behaviors usually last only a few minutes but can extend to several hours or days. These behaviors are more variable and complex than most ictal phenomena. They include confusion, orienting behaviors (looking about, walking around, "absent-minded" talking, straightening up one's clothes), sleepiness, irritability (including violent "rage" behavior), sexual arousal, sexual behaviors that are usually socially inappropriate, and undressing. Confusional or delirious states lasting hours or days can occur, usually after grand mal seizures. Hallucinations and delusions can also occur. These postictal psychoses characteristically fluctuate in severity from day to day or from hour to hour. Although they are occasionally mistaken for schizophrenic psychoses, a history of seizure-like phenomena or episodes, an alteration in consciousness, and fluctuation of symptom severity should alert the clinician. The postictal period EEG in these patients usually will be abnormal, characterized by diffuse slow activity (10–12, 14–17).

Patients with petit mal epilepsy may also experience a prolonged subacute delirious state with altered consciousness, termed petit mal status. These episodes, lasting from hours to several weeks, are characterized by confusion or perplexity, hallucinations, vague delusional ideas, rambling speech, and agitation. The EEG characteristically shows a spike-wave pattern (28–30).

INTERICTAL BEHAVIOR

Interictal behavioral changes are varied (10–12, 16, 17, 31) and do not predict location of lesion or type of seizure disorder. Many nonepileptic psychiatric patients also exhibit these behaviors. Some 40 to 60 percent of epileptics experience these interictal behavioral changes. Excluding behaviors associated with mental retardation or developmental lag, the most common behavioral changes are those of personality. These personality changes associated with chronic epilepsy usually take a decade or more to develop. Several types have been described; the most common of them are termed "adhesive" or "viscous."

Patients with an "adhesive" personality are verbose, circumstantial, and perseverative. They are slow in thinking and speak in a pedantic manner. They lose sight of basic concepts and themes and focus on minutiae. Nothing is trivial; every detail must be considered ad nauseaum, mulled over, and digested in a humorless fashion. These patients lack spontaneity and use common expressions of speech and trite sayings almost to the exclusion of original word sequencing.

A second interictal personality is characterized by a profound deepening of the patient's emotional responses. These patients tend to overrespond to provocative stimuli. They have explosive rages, followed by hearty good-naturedness. They are emotionally labile, rash, suggestible, and excitable. They may develop a heightened sense of justice, morality, or religious conviction. For these patients, mundane, petty events assume cosmic significance. Detailed, perseverative, and trite written records may be kept, filling page after page of notebooks and scraps of paper with "universal truths." On occasion these patients become suspicious and develop vague delusional ideas. An interictal personality syndrome has been specifically described in temporal lobe epileptics (32). It is unlikely that these behaviors (hypergraphia, global hyposexuality, circumstantiality, and pseudo-abstractness) are specific (33). Other interictal syndromes, in decreasing prevalence, are anxiety states, depression, and neurasthenia. Deviant sexual behavior can also occur, and all late-onset (thirty-five years of age or older) major changes in sexual behavior (e.g. transvestism, fetishism, homosexuality) should be suspect as manifestations of a seizure disorder (10–12, 16, 17, 31.)

Psychosis and Epilepsy

The association between epilepsy and psychosis has been known for centuries (34). It is unclear whether these psychoses are consequences of seizure phenomena or a late-onset manifestation of the same pathophysiological process that caused the seizures. In any case these psychoses become manifest, on the average, ten to fifteen years after the first clinical seizure (10, 11, 14–17).

Psychosis in epileptics probably is most prevalent in those patients with other behavioral changes (e.g. interictal personality changes). Studies also suggest that the frequency of psychotic episodes is inversely related to the number of observable clinical seizures. Although temporal lobe foci have been most prominent in discussions of psychoses and epilepsy, these psychoses can occur with any type of major seizure disorder.

"Schizophrenia-like" conditions have been most commonly described in epileptics, particularly those with temporal lobe foci. However, the degree of interest in schizophrenia and epilepsy results in part from the misconception that persecutory and grandiose delusions, auditory hallucinations, and catatonic behavior (all observed in the psychoses associated with epilepsy) are specific for schizophrenia, rather than clinical phenomena observable in any psychosis. Nevertheless, epileptics, particularly those with bilateral fronto-temporal discharges, can present with nonaffective psychoses consistent with modern criteria for schizophrenia. These conditions have been referred to as symptomatic or secondary schizophrenias and may differ from the idiopathic variety in (1) preservation of affect with the ability to maintain good rapport and express warm feelings, (2) lack of significant personality deterioration despite years of illness, (3) the frequent presence of psychomotor phenomena such as autoscopy, déjà vu/jamais vu phenomena, dysmegalopsia, perceptual experiences of being possessed, episodes of dreamlike states, and somatic psychomotor features (e.g. abdominal rushes, paroxysmal sensory phenomena such as sudden feelings of heat, skin tightness, parasthesias), and (4) a greater likelihood of being married and of having a productive school and employment record. Psychotic features commonly observed include delusional ideas, auditory and visual hallucinations, catatonic features (particularly stereotypies and posturing of the hands about the head and face), and thought disorder.

Affective-like syndromes can also occur in epileptics. As these are typically episodic, are associated with reasonable interepisode functioning, and may present with typical depressive or manic features, differentiation from primary affective disorder is often difficult and requires an especially thorough behavioral neurologic evaluation.

Atypical psychoses may also be associated with epilepsy. A safe clinical rule is to consider seriously coarse brain disease in any patient whose presentation, course, or demographic characteristics are unusual. By atypical, we do not refer to the so-called schizo-affective patient but rather to any patient whose illness significantly deviates from the classical pattern. Some examples are (1) the patient with insomnia, appetite disturbance, psychomotor retardation, and loss of interest but no significant dysphoria or sadness; (2) the patient with complete auditory hallucinations (or any first-rank symptom of Schneider) and virtually no other psychopathology; (3) the patient who develops a schizophrenic syndrome after age forty; and (4) the patient with a mood disorder that is chronic rather than episodic.

The following clinical vignettes illustrate the psychoses associated with epilepsy:

Case 1

A thirty-eight-year-old irritable and suspicious man was hospitalized because he attempted to shoot himself in the chest. He denied all features of depression but stated that he was trying to kill a demon that was invading his body. He described the demon as a shadowy figure that either suddenly appeared next to him or approached from a distance, becoming bigger and bigger as it got closer. When next to him the demon would try to "push" its way into him, beginning on his right side. The patient stated he could feel the demon enter his body. The demon also occasionally said things to him from afar and always made him extremely anxious when it approached. When describing his attempt to shoot himself, he said he was only trying to kill the demon, insisting that he would not have been hurt and that only the demon would have been killed. He said these "possessions" had occurred about six times daily for the past seven years.

The patient also had a history of periodic irritability during which he occasionally destroyed property and threatened his wife. At the time of admission she was preparing to leave him. During the seven years of his illness he was functioning well at work, first as a sergeant in the Air Force and then in civilian life. Prior to the shooting attempt he was having some problems at work because of increasing irritability.

The patient's family stated that he was a warm, pleasant person prior to his illness, which apparently started after he fell from a helicopter and struck the back of his head, rendering him unconscious for several days. Following discharge from the Air Force he had several psychiatric hospitalizations, received the diagnosis of schizophrenia on each occasion, and was given neuroleptics with little therapeutic effect.

His EEG revealed left temporal spike discharges. He was treated with carbamazepine and made a full recovery.

Case 2

A fifty-four-year-old man was hospitalized because of assaultive behavior. The admitting physician found him to be hyperactive, irritable, and expansive in mood with rapid and pressured speech and flight-of-ideas. He was not delusional and had no first-rank symptoms of Schneider or perceptual dysfunction. During the month prior to admission he was sleeping less and was involving himself in numerous projects, none of which he completed. He was becoming a neighborhood nuisance because of intrusive behavior, which included arguing and fighting with passers-by. He had a twenty-year history of similar episodes interspersed with depressions.

During his late twenties and early thirties the patient was a successful animation cartoonist. Following a head injury he began having grand mal and partial complex seizures, and his ability to work deteriorated. His partial complex seizures were characterized by brief but frequent episodes of staring, perceptual distortion in several sensory modalities, and paresis of the left arm.

After ten years, during which his seizures were only moderately controlled, he began experiencing depressions and then alternating depressions and manias. Interepisode functioning decreased somewhat, and he developed interictal behavioral changes including hyposexuality, adhesiveness of personality, circumstantiality, and hypergraphia (notably drawings). As his psychoses became more frequent, his fits decreased in frequency, although he experienced more complex fitlike episodes, which were felt by his physicians to be "hysterical." This patient responded moderately well to a combination of carbamazepine and lithium carbonate.

Pseudo-Seizures

Pseudo-seizures, that is, clinical seizure-like behaviors without concomitant paroxysmal electrical discharges, occur most frequently in epileptics. It is important to be able to identify pseudo-seizures in order to monitor properly the control of seizures in epileptics and to treat adequately the nonepileptic who exhibits these phenomena.

The individual exhibiting exclusively pseudo-seizures will be most likely to have a preexisting psychiatric diagnosis (most commonly somatization disorder, hypochondriasis, histrionic personality, conversion symptom, sociopathy, or factitious syndrome). Seizure-like episodes will tend to occur following a precipitating stress event and where the episode will have the greatest impact on the observers. During these episodes, which may vary widely in form and content, little, if any, alteration in consciousness is reported or observed, and communication with the patient may be possible.

Pseudo-seizure episodes are characterized by little if any memory loss. Corneal reflexes are intact, and plantar reflexes are flexor. There is no associated incontinence, post-episode drowsiness, or depression of either stretch reflexes or the oculovestibular (caloric) response during grand mal–like episodes. During grand mal–like episodes the tongue is rarely bitten, the patient is generally not injured, and the EEG is normal (35).

The individual exhibiting true epileptic seizures will be most likely to have a normal premorbid personality, interictal personality changes, and episodes that are more random in occurrence and influenced primarily by diurnal and sleep patterns, sleep deprivation, menses, strong visceral stimuli (e.g. eating a large meal, coitus), or occasionally by specific sensory stimulation, such as flashing lights or music. True epileptic seizures tend to be stereotyped and repetitive within the same patient. Episodes are associated with alterations in consciousness, some memory loss, and unresponsiveness to all but the strongest stimuli. In grand mal–like attacks tongue biting and injury, absent corneal reflexes and extensor plantar reflexes, incontinence and postictal drowsiness and depression of stretch reflexes or oculovestibular (caloric) response are observed. The EEG, particularly if properly (utilizing the highest yielding montages, nasopharyngeal leads, hyperventilation, strobe light stimulation, and sleep tracing) and serially performed, is usually abnormal (35). One study (36) suggests that prolactin levels rise significantly after true seizures but not after pseudo-seizures. Obtaining a serum prolactin level during a "nonseizure" period and again thirty minutes after an episode may prove diagnostically helpful. In patients who have been drug-free for seventy-two hours or more, a postepisode prolactin level of 50 ng./ml. or more strongly suggests a true seizure disorder (37).

Other investigators suggest using intravenous saline plus suggestion (e.g.: "This medication may induce some of your symptoms.") as a provocative test for pseudo-seizures while recording the EEG. In one study of fifty-seven patients, forty-eight had pseudo-attacks to this provocation (38). The investigators also observed that 37 percent had an abnormal EEG, but only 12 percent had spike or spike-and-wave discharges.

Treatment

Proper treatment of the behavioral changes associated with epilepsy cannot be separated from the proper management of seizures. Seizure control is essential and must be based on (1) reliable and valid recording of seizure frequency, (2) accurate record-keeping of anticonvulsant drug consumption, (3) periodic anticonvulsant drug level monitoring, and (4) regular follow-up clinical assessments. Sustained pharmacotherapy, however, should not be instituted unless the patient has a history of two to three grand mal fits without an obvious provocative cause or a history of frequent partial complex fits that interfere with social function and ability to work (39, 40).

In general, once the decision to treat has been made, one of the drugs of choice should be selected and initially administered in the lowest possible therapeutic dose to minimize adverse side effects (see Table 18-1). Sufficient time should be allowed for serum steady state levels to be reached before the dose is increased. Increases should be gradual and monitored by serum drug levels. If side effects become unacceptable before seizure control is achieved, a gradual change to another drug should be made, tapering off the first drug while slowly introducing the second drug. Should the alternate also be of limited benefit, specific combinations of two drugs (see Chapter 5) may be tried (39–42). It should be emphasized, however, that routine polypharmacy (e.g. two or more drugs, each in low doses) generally leads to increased adverse reactions without offering any additive antiepileptic effect (43, 44). The clinician should also be sensitive to the fact that adverse behavioral change is a side effect of anticonvulsant medication. Should the patient begin to manifest novel psychopathology during treatment, *decreasing* rather than increasing the dose may be required (39–45). Indeed, in one study (46) the reduction to a single anticonvulsant (successful in 72 percent of forty chronic patients) not only resulted in improvement in alertness, concentration, mood, behavior, and sociability but also improved seizure control in 55 percent of the sample. Table 18-1 summarizes some of the general characteristics and indications of the more common anticonvulsants (39–45).

Should pharmacotreatment be successful, the patient should be maintained from two to four years free of attacks before discontinuation of treatment is considered. Stopping medication should be gradual over a six- to twelve-month period. A long history of seizures prior to control, the presence of structural brain damage, and the occurrence of partial complex fits of more than one seizure type are poor prognostic signs, which suggest that a relapse is more likely should therapy be stopped (39–45).

Standard psychotropic medications are of limited effectiveness for severe prodromal syndromes, prolonged postictal phenomena, and psychoses associated with epilepsy (47). Carbamazepine is probably the drug of choice for these conditions (48–50), whereas ECT may be the treatment of choice as its effect is rapid, with significant improvement often occurring after a single induced seizure (51). Should ECT be prescribed, the patient receiving a neuroleptics can be rapidly withdrawn from this, whereas the patient receiving an anticonvulsant will need a longer withdrawal period to avoid a spontaneous, uncontrolled seizure. Unfortunately there is no known effective treatment for interictal behavior changes.

Delirium

Delirium is a syndrome characterized by altered consciousness and diffuse cognitive impairment of acute onset. Virtually all delirious processes

TABLE 18-1 Profile of Commonly Used Anticonvulsants in Adult Epileptics with Psychiatric Syndromes

CHARACTERISTIC	PHENYTOIN	CARBAMAZEPINE	SODIUM VALPROATE	PHENOBARBITONE
Starting dose (mg.)	100 BID	100 BID	200 BID	30 HS
Daily dose range (mg.)	150–600	400–1,800	600–3,000	30–240
Minimal daily frequency	Once	Twice	Once	Once
Time to peak serum level (hours)	4–12	4–24	1–4	1–6
Percent bound to plasma	90	75	92	45
Half-life (hours)	9–140	10–30	8–20	50–160
Time from start to steady state (days)	7–21	10	4	Up to 30
Therapeutic serum level (ng./ml.)	10–20 / 20–30 (severe cases only)	5–12	25–80 / 80–160 (severe cases)	10–25 / 25–40 (severe cases)
Group	Hydantoin	Tricyclic	2-chain fatty acid	Barbiturate
Dose/serum relationship (free and bound)	Linear	Linear	Nonlinear	Linear
Primary indication(s) (in order of preference)	Tonic–clonic seizures / Partial–complex seizures	Partial–complex seizures / Tonic–clonic seizures	Tonic–clonic seizures / Petit-mal absences / Myoclonic seizures / Akinetic seizures / Partial–complex seizures	Tonic–clonic seizures

resolve; however, some (particularly associated with encephalitis or structural lesions) may terminate in a chronic, static defect state (52).

The classical delirious patient is perplexed, disoriented, anxious, and agitated. Tremulousness, tachycardia, sweating, and vasoconstriction resulting in cold, clammy skin and circumoral pallor are common. These patients are "fitful," are unable to understand events taking place around them, are fearful of staff and other patients, and may become irritable and assaultive. The last occurs particularly at night (the "sundown" syndrome), when reduced lighting and fewer staff ministrations exacerbate already impaired information processing.

These patients often have perceptual dysfunction. Affect-laden illusions and visual hallucinations are common. A delusional mood and delusional ideas, usually with persecutory content, can occur. Random, non-goal-directed associations are typical. Cognitive impairment, although diffuse, characteristically is most striking in the areas of memory (immediate recall, recent memory, and long-term memory may each be affected), orientation, and concentration. Motor coordination also is often impaired (52–55).

Most commonly the clinical presentation will be nonspecific, and the determination of etiology will require careful historical and laboratory investigation. The latter should include determinations of blood glucose; urea nitrogen and electrolytes; liver function; arterial PO_2 and PCO_2 and drug levels; urine glucose, acetone, and cells; and EKG (54, 56). The pattern of symptoms and associated systemic findings of some deliria, however, are typical for specific etiologies. These include drug-induced anticholinergic delirium, Wernicke's encephalopathy, and alcohol withdrawal states, which are discussed elsewhere in the text. Other common causes of deliria are epilepsy, head trauma, central nervous system infection, drug overdoses and urinary tract disease, pulmonary and cardiovascular dysfunction, and systemic infection (52–55).

Severe delirium is rarely misdiagnosed. Mild or subacute delirious processes often are unrecognized, particularly on acute medical/surgical services. Whereas 10 percent of acute medical/surgical patients are diagnosed as delirious, another 15 to 20 percent have unrecognized diffuse cognitive impairment (57). Subacute delirium should be suspected in patients whose systemic condition and treatments cannot account for their behavior. These patients will be unexpectedly lethargic and easily fatigued. They will have difficulty feeding, washing, or dressing themselves and will be unable to understand simple and clearly stated self-care instructions or administer other simple self-care procedures. They will appear uncertain, hesitant, or perplexed when faced with simple hospital chores or activities routinely expected of many patients (e.g. going to the bathroom, finding one's way from the visitor's room to bed) (52–55).

TREATMENT OF DELIRIUM

The obvious first steps in the management of the delirious patient are behavioral control (see Chapter 7) and identifying specific etiology. Treatment should then be directed toward resolving the primary disease process. If the causes of the delirious episode are not yet known, initial treatment should be directed at potential life-threatening conditions or conditions that if untreated can lead to permanent brain damage. Hypoglycemia, hyperthermia, and hypoxia are the most common situations requiring rapid intervention. All patients with deliria of unknown etiology should receive intravenous dextrose (50 ml. of a 50 percent solution) and be immediately examined for hyperthermia, hypotension, myocardial infarction and cardiac arrhythmia (frequently resulting in deliria in the elderly), pulmonary disease, and anemia.

The delirious patient is best managed in a quiet, calm, structured setting. A softly lighted hospital room with constant observation by familiar people and staff who clearly identify themselves and what they are doing help to reduce the patient's anxiety and agitation. When medication is required, anxiolytics are the drugs of choice. Further discussion of the treatment of deliria can be found in the Chapters 8, 10, and 19, on emergency psychiatry, consultation/liaison psychiatry, and substance abuse (52, 58).

Dementia

Dementia can occur at any age. It is, however, particularly common among the elderly, affecting 5 percent of people over age sixty-five and 20 percent or more of those over age eighty. It is not, however, a normal variant of the aging process. Dementia is a syndrome characterized by diffuse cognitive impairment, usually of slow onset. Although some dementing processes can resolve (e.g. those secondary to normal pressure hydrocephalus, myxedema, depression in the aged), most terminate in a chronic defect state. As theoretically defined, delirium implies a physiologic or biochemical dysfunctional state, whereas dementia implies loss of nervous tissue (neurons). In clinical practice neither implication is absolute (59–61).

Behaviorally, the classical demented patient is deteriorated in personality, often confused, amnestic, and occasionally psychotic. These patients may develop a coarsening of their personality, becoming tactless, cruel, ill-mannered, and ill-groomed. Their speech is perseverative, cliché-ridden, and stereotyped. They are often restless (rubbing, tapping, and folding hand movements are common) and occasionally severely agitated. Emotional lability (sudden shifts in mood), Witzelsucht (a shallow, silly, fatuous mood), emotional blunting, or emotional incontinence (sudden and unexpected brief outbursts of laughter or crying) can be observed. Neurologically, they display multiple soft neurologic signs, changes in muscle tone (often weakness and rigidity without cogwheeling), a puppet-like gait, nystagmus, the Kluver–Bucy syndrome (oral ingestive behavior, lack of sexual inhibition, placidity, visual agnosia), seizures of all types, urinary incontinence, and pupillary changes. Frontal, temporal, and parietal lobe cognitive syndromes can all be present. In the late stages of many dementing processes seizures may occur (59, 62, 63).

In the latter stages of a dementing process, the profound memory deficit, disorientation and readily observed nonbehavioral neurologic features facilitate diagnosis. In the early stages of dementia, signs and symptoms often are ambiguous and behavioral changes may be most prominent. Patients are often misdiagnosed as suffering from major depression, dysthmia or schizophrenia (59, 62, 63). Careful neurologic, behavioral neurologic, and mental status examinations are essential in early identification of these patients, so that those with resolvable disorders can receive appropriate care without exposure to unnecessary psychiatric treatments. Once a dementia is identified clinically, a basic diagnostic evaluation should include a complete blood count, thyroid studies, serum B_{12} and folate determinations, metabolic screening assessment, CT scanning, chest x-ray, and urinalysis (56, 59–63).

During the early stages of dementias with insidious onset (e.g. Alzheimer's type) frequent complaints include fatigue, mild sadness, headache, poor concentration, and loss of efficiency. Patients will frequently show a decline in their general activities and will lose interest in sports and hobbies. They may report a vague difficulty using words (particularly the expression of polysyllabic words) and in word finding. They may become lost in familiar places and lose efficiency in previously learned skills (e.g. cooking meals, typing, driving in heavy traffic). Denial of illness is commonly observed, and patients may offer absurd excuses for their poor performance of simple cognitive tasks. A general lack of spontaneity and mild recent memory problems are commonly observed. As women are at greater risk than men for most non-alcohol-related and noncardiovascular dementias, and as many dementing processes begin in the sixth decade or later, the early stage of dementia is most commonly confused with major depression (59–64). Such patients may even have a mild or transient improvement with antidepressant medication or ECT (51).

These secondary depressions may be identified clinically, as patients appear more apathetic than profoundly sad, and soft neurologic signs may be present. These patients tend to have no prior history of depressive illness and no family history of psychiatric disorder. EEG and CT-scan studies at this stage may reveal few, if any, abnormalities. Dexamethasone challenge is unhelpful, as a significant proportion of demented patients without depressive features will be nonsuppressors (65). Neuropsychological testing is often the most sensitive instrument for revealing the coarse nature of the condition (66).

Table 18-2 lists some of the more common dementing disorders encountered on a busy psychiatric service and displays some characteristics of each condition. As some dementing processes can be specifically treated, diagnosis should not end with classifying the patient as "demented." The clinician's goal should be to reach a specific diagnosis. In addition to a careful history and systemic, neurologic, behavioral neurologic, and mental status examination, diagnostic evaluation for dementia may include specific laboratory studies (hemogram, serum B_{12} and folic acid levels, VDRL, serum protein studies, BUN, serum glucose, thyroid studies, serum enzymes, serum calcium, serum copper and ceruloplasmin, serum electrolytes, urinalysis and urinary protein, copper and porphobilinogen, blood gas studies, and serum and urine screens for toxic substances), skeletal x-ray studies, spinal fluid studies for protein and VDRL, EEG and CT-scan evaluations, and neuropsychological testing. Angiography and blood and spinal fluid flow studies may also be required.

Treatment for Dementia

The treatment of dementia is rarely specific. Specific treatments include D-penicillamine for Wilson's disease, vitamin and hormonal replacement for nutritional and endocrine disorders, ventricular shunting for normal pressure hydrocephalus, penicillin for CNS syphillis, and surgery for vascular malformations and subdural hematoma (59-64, 67).

Nonspecific pharmacologic treatment includes low-dose neuroleptics for psychosis and anticonvulsants for seizures. The type of seizures will determine the choice of anticonvulsant. We prefer haloperidol for psychosis because of its high potency, relatively mild anticholinergic and hypotensive side effects, and availability in intramuscular form. Electroconvulsive treatment for psychoses secondary to dementia also can be effective particularly when depressive or manic features predominate (51). Despite claims (68) of novel treatments having significant beneficial effects on the cognitive functions of demented patients, unequivocal efficacy for a variety of strategies has not been established (69).

Hospital management must be structured. As demented patients often are negligent about their self-care and food intake, careful attention should be paid to maintaining their hygiene and providing them with an adequate diet. Maintaining their physical activity in structured exercise, sports, and socialization programs can delay deterioration and significantly enrich the patient's life. Family members and friends should be encouraged to visit often and participate in these activities. Physicians and ward staff often

TABLE 18–2 Dementing Disorders Commonly Seen Among Psychiatric Patients

IRREVERSIBLE CONDITIONS	TYPICAL CLINICAL FEATURES	TREATMENT	COMMENTS
Alzheimer's/Senile Dementia	More common in women Gross disorientation early Marked personality deterioration Neurologic signs and abnormal EEG late features Two onset peaks in 50s and 60s respectively	Symptomatic	Familial Identical neuropathology Early stages may be confused with depression Nucleus basalis (in basal forebrain) may be involved Associated with Down's syndrome and leukemia
Atherosclerotic/Multi-Infarct Dementia	More common in men Gross disorientation late Seizures Rarely develops before age 65 Sudden onset and focal neurologic signs common	Symptomatic	Other evidence of cardiovascular disease must be established to confirm diagnosis
Huntington's Chorea	Prominent frontal lobe cognitive features Dysarthria, gait disturbances, motor overflow features Multiple onset peaks, typically 35–45 CT scan diagnostic Psychosis can be first expression of the illness	Symptomatic (haloperidol may have specific GABA effect reducing choreiform movements)	Autosomal dominant gene transmission Possible GABA deficit

(Continued)

TABLE 18-2 (Continued)

IRREVERSIBLE CONDITIONS	TYPICAL CLINICAL FEATURES	TREATMENT	COMMENTS
Parkinson's Disease	More common in women Prominent frontal lobe cognitive features Extrapyramidal signs prominent Onset 50–60	L-DOPA of little benefit for behavioral and cognitive features Symptomatic behavioral treatment	Occurs in 20%–40% of Parkinsonian patients May see similar pattern in patients with tardive dyskinesia
Korsakoff's Syndrome	More common in males Gross disorientation Gross memory impairment Opthalmoplegias, peripheral neuropathies, cerebellar ataxia Infrequent seizures Typical onset in late 50s	Thiamine Multivitamins Symptomatic behavioral treatment	Confabulation need not be present 90% of cases alcoholics Possible genetic predisposition to low thiamine levels
Pick's Disease	More common in females (less so than Alzheimer's) Lobar syndromes predominate: frontal convexity, dominant temporal and parietal lobe Early (40) and late (50) onset peaks EEG, CT scan abnormal, but nonspecific Spinal fluid may show increased globulins	Symptomatic	Early onset cases confused with schizophrenia
Normal pressure hydrocephalus	Prominent frontal lobe features Ataxia Urinary incontinence CT-scan diagnostic	Ventricular shunting works best in patients with alteration of consciousness or early ataxic signs	10% are alcoholics

Wilson's Disease	Prominent frontal lobe cognitive features Prominent motor features (facial bradykinesia, tremors, limb rigidity dysarthria, "wing-beating," choreoathetosis Seizures Hepatolentricular degeneration Onset peak 15–25	D-penicillamine	Kayser–Fleischer rings not always present
Drug-induced dementia	More common in the elderly Sudden onset Gross disorientation EEG usually abnormal but nonspecific, often reversible	Stop all medications not essential to life	Common offending agents include digitalis, propranolol, phenacetin, bromides, anticholinergic medications, barbiturates, psychotropics
Dementias caused by metabolic disorder	Lethargy and disorientation most common Onset slow Symptoms of depression may be reversible	Correction of metabolic imbalance Symptomatic	Thyroid dysfunction (hypo- and hyper-) most common etiology; also hypo- and hyperparathyroidism, hypercalcemia, liver disease, Cushing's disease, uremia, hypernatremia, dehydration, and carcinoma
Dementias caused by deficiency states	Lethargy and confusion common Onset slow Symptoms of depression may be reversible	Replacement treatment Symptomatic	B_{12}, folate, general malnutrition
Dementias caused by other systemic conditions	Lethargy and confusion Onset slow May be reversible	Symptomatic Correction of systemic disorder	Common conditions include myocardial infarction, dysrhythmias, bilateral carotid artery disease, lupus, Pickwickian syndrome

underestimate the capabilities of demented patients. The patient's cognitive, behavioral, and physical abilities should be quickly assessed, and the patients should be expected and encouraged to participate in activities to the level of these abilities. The elderly and the demented patient should not be treated as a child. The use of first names, "we" instead of "you," and such childish terms as "tummy" are inappropriate. The mere fact that a patient is disoriented does not mean he likes to play with mud pies, and the content of any activity program should be of interest to adults. Further management details are described in Chapter 20.

Postconcussion Syndrome

A significant but unknown number of patients will have persistent symptoms following a mild head injury despite little if any clinical evidence of neuronal damage. The injury sustained usually results in a brief or mild disturbance in consciousness followed by headache, dizziness, hypersensitivity to sound or light, fatigue, poor concentration, and, rarely, irritability. Mild depressive features and physiologic signs of anxiety are commonly observed. Most postconcussion syndromes resolve within a few days or weeks of injury, but some will persist, resulting in significant deficits in social function and in ability to work (70–73).

Several studies (74, 75) have demonstrated that the majority of these patients are not malingering and had no preexisting neurotic traits. These patients may exhibit abnormal caloric testing (76) and many exhibit unequivocal vestibular dysfunction by electronystagmography and abnormal brain stem auditory evoked potentials (77). In one study (77) only 21 percent of patients were normal on both measures. Gronwall and Wrightson (78), reporting the clinical course of such patients, who were monitored with serial psychological testing, concluded that persistent cognitive dysfunction was the main factor in the syndrome. This has been our experience, and patients with prolonged postconcussion syndromes should receive careful neuropsychological evaluation. Patients with evidence of mild cognitive impairment (often nondominant hemisphere and frontal in pattern) may respond to amphetamines or monoamine oxidase inhibitors (MAOIs) in standard doses. Patients, particularly in the initial phase of the syndrome, who are irritable and become assaultive, have been shown to respond to propranolol in doses as high as 320 mg. daily.

We have also seen patients who developed a "postconcussion-like" syndrome following a viral infection. Mononucleosis, viral hepatitis, and influenza were the most common viral syndromes observed. These were followed by prolonged behavior changes without recognizable encephalitis, although direct brain involvement appeared to be the most likely etiology. These patients may also respond to amphetamines and MAOIs.

Localized Frontal, Parietal, Temporal Coarse Brain Syndromes

In any busy psychiatric service the clinician can expect his diagnostic and therapeutic skills to be challenged by the phenomenologically atypical patient, who does not have the profound diffuse cognitive impairment of dementia or the episodic paroxysmal behaviors of epilepsy but does appear to be "organic" in some vague indescribable manner.

Phenomenologically these patients may have well-formed delusions and hallucinations, as well as language difficulties. Their behavior is often "odd." Most have signs suggestive of coarse brain dysfunction, which can be substantiated by a thorough diagnostic evaluation. Although soft neurologic signs are common in these patients, focal nonbehavioral neurologic features are rare. In our experience 10 percent of acute psychiatric admissions fall into this category.

Although within this patient group somatic treatment is rather nonspecific, discrimination of syndrome subgroups can be helpful in rehabilitation and disposition planning and in simply reducing the ambiguity of clinic practice.

Nevertheless, the delineation of these syndromes as discrete diseases or pathological entities has never been demonstrated. It is likely that each syndrome can result from multiple causes. In our experience head trauma, viral infections (including influenza, mononucleosis), and gestational–obstetrical problems are the most frequently identifiable premorbid events likely to be causally related to these syndromes. For the majority of patients, however, no likely etiological event can be discerned. Vascular accidents and slow-growing tumors can also produce these syndromes, but such patients are likely to be identified early in their illness course as "neurological." Vascular malformations are also observed in this group of patients.

FRONTAL LOBE SYNDROMES

Two principal frontal lobe syndromes have been described in association with massive frontal lobe injury: the convexity syndrome and the medial-orbital syndrome (12, 23-27, 79-87).

The convexity syndrome, related to lesions within or near the lateral surface of the frontal lobes, is characterized by "negative symptoms." These patients are apathetic, indifferent to their surroundings, and emotionally unresponsive. They appear to have lost all drive and ambition. Loss of social graces is common, and they frequently appear disheveled and dirty. Their movements are slow and reduced in frequency (motor inertia). Occasionally they may remain in positions for prolonged periods (catalepsy) and may posture. A slight flexion at the waist, knees, and elbows is a typical body position of these patients. They occasionally move with a floppy, shuffling gait, progressively picking up steam, only to slow down gradually to a stop (glissando/deglissando gait). Unlike patients with Parkinson's disease, muscle tone is decreased and "pill rolling" is not present. These patients have difficulty attending to tasks but do respond to irrelevant, particularly intense stimuli. They will tend to walk next to walls (just touching them), rather than in the middle of the hallway and may even follow architectural contours rather than take a direct route across open space.

If convexity syndrome is due to dominant hemisphere pathology, it is also associated with a deficit in language and in verbal thinking. Impoverished thinking (vague and without detail) is almost always present; verbal fluency is significantly impaired; speech is often stereotyped with perseverative and verbigerated utterances; and Broca's or transcortical aphasia may be present. Most frontal lobe cognitive and soft neurologic signs (see Chapter 3) can be observed in these patients who may also be dyspraxic (gait, bucco–linguo–facial, ideomotor) and incontinent of urine.

A second frontal lobe syndrome is associated with dysfunction in the orbito–medial areas of the frontal lobes. Some patients may be asthenic and easily fatigued, bland, akinetic, aphonic, withdrawn, and fearful. They may have diminished wakefulness, be in an oneiroid state, or even be stuperous. Other patients may have an intense affect, expressing euphoria, irritability, or extreme lability of affect with rapid mood shifts or mixed and cycling mood states. Witzelsucht is common. These affectively intense patients are hyperactive and overresponsive to stimuli. They rapidly terminate one incomplete goal-directed behavior only to start another and may appear frenetic as they run about from one activity to another, never completing a task. These patients lose their inhibitions and become reckless. They are impulsive and may engage in buying sprees or other high-risk behaviors. They lack foresight, cannot make decisions, are unable to persevere, and have uncontrollable associations. They are strongly stimulus bound, distractable, intrusive, and importunate. They will interrupt conversations and will mimic the examiner's movements and comments. These are the patients who, despite repeated injunctions, will continually enter a room in which a group of people are in conference or who will pull fire alarms or change channels continually on television sets, simply because they see them. These patients may have uncontrollable, often fantastic confabulations and, when prevented from doing as they please, may have violent outbursts.

The obvious similarity in behaviors between these patients and patients with bipolar affective disorder requires particularly careful diagnostic evaluation. Localized CT-scan and EEG abnormalities, neurologic (particularly soft) signs, the shallowness of affect, a prolonged and insidious onset, a chronic nonepisodic course, and a negative family history for affective disorder would suggest coarse disease.

PARIETAL LOBE SYNDROMES

Coarse lesions of the parietal lobes can be associated with significant psychopathology (e.g. delusional ideas, experiences of alienation), which can lead to misdiagnosis and inappropriate treatment for a "functional" disorder (3, 9, 22, 86, 88). For example:

A fifty-five-year-old woman without previous psychiatric illness was hospitalized as "psychotic" because during the two days prior to admission she began accusing her daughter of being an impostor and of spying upon her. The patient was mildly dysphoric and said "things looked confused." A consultant's behavioral neurologic examination revealed her to have constructional difficulties and left-sided spatial neglect suggestive of right parietal lobe dysfunction. Computer-enhanced tomography confirmed a recent right posterior–inferior parietal infarct. The patient recovered fully without somatic treatment.

Two general patterns of symptoms have been observed in patients with parietal lobe lesions. Lesions of the dominant parietal lobe usually are associated with disorders of language (dyslexia, word-finding problems, conduction aphasia), problems with calculation, dyspraxias (ideomotor, kinesthetic), difficulties in abstraction, and contralateral sensory (graphanesthesia, astereognosis) and motor (hypotonia, posturing, paucity of movement) deficits. The best-known dominant parietal syndrome is the controversial Gerstmann's syndrome (dysgraphia, dyscalculia, right–left disorientation, finger agnosia), putatively involving a lesion in the posterior–inferior aspect (angular gyrus) of the dominant parietal lobe. Although the validity of the syndrome has been questioned by some authors, it has been reported (89) in more than 20 percent of chronic psychiatric patients.

Lesions of the nondominant parietal lobe are associated with profound (occasionally delusional) denial of illness (anosognosia), left-sided spatial neglect, constructional difficulties, problems getting dressed, and contralateral sensory and motor deficits. Capgras' syndrome (delusional ideas that close friends or relatives are impostors) and the first-rank symptom of experience of alienation (body parts or thoughts not belonging to one) have been described in patients with nondominant parietal lesions. These patients also may have difficulties orienting themselves in their environment. They complain that "things look confused" or "jumbled." They say they cannot find their way along previously familiar routes and that they can no longer drive a car because they lose track of the other vehicles around them. They may complain that their body is somehow different; that an arm or leg feels heavy or bigger than usual or that they are not always sure of the location of an arm or leg.

TEMPORAL LOBE SYNDROMES

Some patients without temporal lobe epilepsy will nevertheless have temporal lobe lesions. Patients with stroke, head injury, viral disease (particularly herpes), vascular malformations, and degenerative disease involving the temporal lobes can present with delusions, hallucinations (particularly auditory and visual), and mood disturbances. Patients with posterior (temporo–parietal) aphasia and patients with formal thought disorder share many of the same elements of language dysfunction. There is a strong association between temporal lobe dysfunction and psychopathology, and the absence of a classical epileptic picture and course is not sufficient to eliminate a temporal lobe etiology from the differential diagnosis of a psychotic patient (3, 12, 17, 90).

Disturbances in language and memory are most commonly observed in psychiatric patients suffering from temporal lobe dysfunction. When the dysfunction is in the dominant temporal lobe, euphoria, auditory hallucinations (often "complete" voices), formal thought disorder, and primary delusional ideas will be the likely psychopathology. These clinical phenomena will be associated with such cognitive deficits as decreased learning and retention of verbal material (read or heard), poor speech comprehension, and poor reading comprehension. When the dysfunction is in the nondominant temporal lobe, dysphoria, irritability, depression, and loss of emotional expression (aprosodia) will be the likely psychopathology. These clinical phenomena will be associated with such cognitive deficits as decreased recognition and recall of visual and auditory nonverbal material, amusia (loss of ability to repeat musical sounds), poor visual memory, decreased auditory discrimination and comprehension of tonal patterns, and decreased ability to learn and recognize nonsense figures and geometric shapes. Bilateral temporal lobe involvement is usually associated with dementia (9, 59–64).

TREATMENT OF LOCALIZED COARSE BRAIN SYNDROMES

Treatment of localized coarse brain syndromes centers on the specific neurologic condition underlying the psychopathology and is essentially symptomatic. The psychopathology will often resolve at the same rate and to the same degree as the cognitive impairment and any neurologic signs. In many cases, where there is spontaneous remission, no somatic treatment is necessary. When psychopathology is severe, it can be managed best by trying to fit the patient's clinical features to standard psychopathological syndromes (e.g. mania, depression, schizophrenia, dysthymic disorder) and then apply specific treatment. Thus maniform syndromes can respond to neuroleptics, lithium carbonate, carbamazepine, or ECT; depressive syndromes can respond to ECT and occasionally to lithium ion (in our experience, tricyclic antidepressants are rarely effective); schizophrenia-like features may respond to neuroleptics; and dysthymic disorders may respond to MAOIs or amphetamines. Doses for neuroleptics tend to be lower than those required for cases without coarse disease.

Psychological treatment, rehabilitation, and disposition must take into account the specific cognitive impairment of each case. Thus it would be inappropriate to expect a patient with dominant temporal lobe dysfunction to do well in a psychotherapeutic setting for which good language and thinking skills are required, to send a patient with significant nondominant parietal lobe dysfunction for training in a job requiring good motor perceptual coordination, or to expect a patient with a frontal lobe convexity syndrome to live alone and care for himself. Periodic neuropsychological assessment can help establish each patient's cognitive strengths and weaknesses, thus providing guidelines for ongoing care.

Headache

Most patients complaining of headache do not have coarse brain disease. Headaches that are dull, described as "a pressure feeling," generalized, and constant for several consecutive days rarely are associated with brain disease. Headaches that are of sudden onset, awaken a patient from sleep, or are unilateral are usually associated with pathology. Cervical osteoarthritis, eye pathology or visual acuity problems, dental pathology, sinusitis, temporomandibular joint problems (including the temopromandibular syndrome of unilateral, deep-seated pain in the side of the face due to jaw muscle spasms), and hypertension must all be considered in any diagnostic evaluation of headache (91-94).

Headaches caused by brain tumors result from increased intracranial pressure and rarely from traction of the tumor on pain-sensitive intracranial structures. Headaches from brain tumors have no characteristic pattern, may be similar to tension headaches, and may be mild, dull, bilateral, and fluctuating in severity. Their only distinguishing feature is their onset, which is usually within a few weeks of seeking medical attention (91, 93, 94).

Migraine headaches are throbbing and severe. They last for several hours, are associated with nausea and vomiting, and are exhausting or even prostrating. Migraines are usually, but not always, unilateral. They are usually preceded by ischemic symptoms such as flashing lights, scintillating scotomata, or sensory or motor symptoms. Patients with migraine tend to be young and female, and have a family history of migraine. Onset is rarely after age thirty. Ergot-containing preparations and propranolol are usually effective if begun during the early phases of an attack (94).

TREATMENTS

Infrequent "tension" headaches respond to analgesics. However, analgesics, anxiolytics, and sedatives are usually ineffective in the treatment of headaches for which a neurologic basis cannot be established. When the condition is chronic, tricyclic antidepressants are often effective. When the headache is associated with significant features of depression, tricyclic antidepressants, MAOIs, lithium ion (particularly good for cluster headaches), and ECT have been reported of benefit (51, 95).

References

1. Pincus, J. H.; Tucker, G. J. *Behavioral Neurology*. 2d ed. New York: Oxford University Press, 1978.
2. Kolb, B.; Whitshaw, I. Q. *Fundamentals of Human Neuropsychology*. San Francisco: W. H. Freeman, 1980.
3. Heilman, K. M.; Valenstein, E. (eds.). *Clinical Neuropsychology*. New York: Oxford University Press, 1979.
4. Reynolds, E. H.; Trimble, M. R. (eds.). *Epilepsy and Psychiatry*. Edinburgh: Churchill Livingstone, 1981.
5. Epilepsy Foundation of America. *Basic Statistics on the Epilepsies*. Philadelphia: F. A. Davis, 1975.
6. Pond, D. Epidemiology of the Psychiatric Disorders of Epilepsy. In Reynolds, E. H.; Trimble, M. R. (eds.), *Epilepsy and Psychiatry*. Edinburgh: Churchill Livingstone, 1981, pp. 27–32.
7. Burden, G. Social Aspects of Epilepsy. In Reynolds, E. H.; Trimble, M. R. (eds.), *Epilepsy and Psychiatry*. Edinburgh: Churchill Livingstone, 1981, pp. 296–305.
8. Ounsted, C.; Lindsay, F. The Long-term Outcome of Temporal Lobe Epilepsy. In Reynolds, E. H.; Trimble, M. R. (eds.), *Epilepsy and Psychiatry*. Edinburgh: Churchill Livingstone, 1981, pp. 185–215.
9. Strub, R. L.; Black, F. W. *Organic Brain Syndromes: An Introduction to Neurobehavioral Disorders*. Philadelphia: F. A. Davis, 1981, pp. 335–68.
10. Benson, D. F.; Blumer, D. Psychiatric Manifestations of Epilepsy. In Benson, D.

F.; Blumer D. (eds.), *Psychiatric Aspects of Neurologic Disease*, vol. 2. New York: Grune & Stratton, 1982, pp. 25–47.

11. Fenton, G. W. Psychiatric Disorders of Epilepsy: Classification and Phenomenology. In Reynolds, E. H.; Trimble, M. R. (eds.), *Epilepsy and Psychiatry*. Edinburgh: Churchill Livingstone, 1981, pp. 12–26.

12. Trimble, M. R. The Interictal Psychoses of Epilepsy. In Benson, D. F.; Blumer, D. (eds.), *Psychiatric Aspects of Neurologic Disease*, vol. 2. New York: Grune & Stratton, 1982, pp. 75–88.

13. Meduna, L. J. General discussion of the cardiazol therapy. *Am. J. Psychiat. Suppl. 94:* 40–50, 1938.

14. Toone, B. Psychoses of Epilepsy. In Reynolds, E. H.; Trimble, M. R. (eds.), *Epilepsy and Psychiatry*. Edinburgh: Churchill Livingstone, 1981, pp. 113–37.

15. Beard, A. W.; Slater, E. The schizophrenic–like psychoses of epilepsy. *Pro. Roy. Soc. Med. 55:* 311–16, 1962.

16. Davidson, K.; Bagley, C. R. Schizophrenia-like psychoses associated with organic disorders of the central nervous system: A review of the literature, in "Current Problems in Neuropsychiatry." *Br. J. Psychiat.* Special pub. no. 4, 1969, pp. 113–84.

17. Koella, W. P.; Trimble, M. R. (eds.). Temporal Lobe Epilepsy, Mania, and Schizophrenia and the Limbic System, *Advances in Biological Psychiatry*, vol. 8. Basel: S. Kruger, 1982.

18. Sackeim, H. A.; Greenberg, M. S.; Weiman, A. L.; *et al.* Hemispheric asymmetry in the expression of positive and negative emotions: Neurologic evidence. *Arch. Gen. Psychiat. 39:* 210–18, 1982.

19. Ahern, G. L.; Schwartz, G. E. Differential lateralization for positive versus negative emotion. *Neuropsychologia 17:* 693–98, 1979.

20. Gainotti, G. Emotional behavior and hemispheric side of the lesion. *Cortex 8:* 41–55, 1972.

21. Hecaen, H. Clinical Symptomatology in Right and Left Hemispheric Lesions. In Mountcastle, V. B. (ed.), *Interhemispheric Relations and Cerebral Dominance*. Baltimore: Johns Hopkins University Press, 1962, pp. 215–43.

22. Critchley, M. *The Parietal Lobes*. New York: Hafner Press, 1953.

23. Damascio, A. The Frontal Lobes. In Heilman, K. M.; Valenstein, E. (eds.), *Clinical Neuropsychology*. New York: Oxford University Press, 1979, pp. 360–412.

24. Hecaen, H.; Albert, M. L. Disorders of Mental Functioning Related to Frontal Lobe Pathology. In Benson, D. F.; Blumer, D. (eds.), *Psychiatric Aspects of Neurologic Disease*, vol. 1. New York: Grune & Stratton, 1975, pp. 137–69.

25. Luria, A. R. Frontal Lobe Syndromes. In Vinken, P. J.; Bruyn, G. W. (eds.), *Handbook of Clinical Neurology*, vol. 2, *Localization in Clinical Neurology*. New York: Elsevier/North Holland, 1969, pp. 725–75.

26. Lishman, W. A. *Organic Psychiatry*. London: Blackwell Scientific, 1978.

27. Teuber, H. L. The Riddle of Frontal Lobe Function in Man. In Warren, J. M.; Akert, K. (eds.), *The Frontal Granular Cortex and Behavior*. New York: McGraw-Hill, 1964, pp. 410–44.

28. Marsden, C. D.; Reynolds, E. H. Neurology. In Laidlaw, J.; Richens, A. (eds.), *A Textbook of Epilepsy*. 2d ed. Edinburgh: Churchill Livingstone, 1982, pp. 97–146.

29. Roger, J.; Lob, H.; Tassinari, C. A. Generalized Status Epilepticus as a Confusional State (Petit Mal Status or Absence Status Epilepticus). In Vinken, P. J.; Bruyn, G. W. (eds.), *Handbook of Clinical Neurology 15*. Amsterdam: North Holland, 1974, pp. 145–82.

30. Ellis, J. M.; Lee, S. I. Acute prolonged confusion in later life as an ictal state. *Epilepsia 19:* 119–28, 1978.

31. Fenton, G. W. Personality and Behavioral Disorders in Adults with Epilepsy. In Reynolds, E. H.; Trimble, M. R. (eds.), *Epilepsy and Psychiatry*. Edinburgh: Churchill Livingstone, 1981, pp. 77–91.

32. Bear, D. M.; Fedio, P. Quantitative analysis of interictal behavior in temporal lobe epilepsy. *Arch. Neurol. 34:* 454–567, 1977.

33. Mungas, D. Interictal behavior abnormality in temporal lobe epilepsy: A specific syndrome or non-specific psychopathology? *Arch. Gen. Psychiat. 39:* 108–11, 1982.

34. Hill, D. Historical Review. In Reynolds, E. H.; Trimble, M. R. (eds.), *Epilepsy and Psychiatry*. Edinburgh: Churchill Livingstone, 1981, pp. 1–11.

35. Riley, T. L.; Roy, A. (eds.). *Pseudoseizures*. Baltimore: Williams & Wilkins, 1982.

36. Trimble, M. Serum prolactin in epilepsy and hysteria. *Br. Med. J.* 2(6153): 1682, 1978.

37. Collins, W. C. J.; Lanigan, O.; Callaghan, N. Plasma prolactin concentrations following epileptic and pseudoseizures. *J. Neurol. Neurosurg. Psychiat. 46:* 505–8, 1983.

38. Cohen, R. J.; Suter, C. Hysterical seizures: Suggestion as a provocative EEG test. *Ann. Neurol. 11:* 391–95, 1982.

39. Reynolds, E. H. The Management of Seizures Associated with Psychological Disorders. In Reynolds, E. H.; Trimble, M. R. (eds.), *Epilepsy and Psychiatry*. Edinburgh: Churchill Livingstone, 1981, pp. 322–36.

40. Richens, A. Clinical Pharmacology and Medical Treatment. In Laidlow, J.; Richens, A. (eds.), *A Textbook of Epilepsy*. 2d ed. Edinburgh: Churchill Livingstone, 1982, pp. 292–348.

41. Delgado–Escueta, A. V.; Treiman, D. M.; Walsh, G. O. The treatable epilepsies, part 1. *New Eng. J. Med. 308:* 1508–14, 1983.

42. Delgado–Escueta, A. V.; Treiman, D. M.; Walsh, G. O. The treatable epilepsies, part 2. *New Eng. J. Med. 308:* 1576–84, 1983.

43. Perucca, E. Drug Interactions. In Laidlaw, J.; Richens, A. (eds.), *A Textbook of Epilepsy*. 2d ed. Edinburgh: Churchill Livingstone, 1982, pp. 358–71.

44. Rivinus, T. M. Psychiatric effects of the anti-convulsant regimens. *J. Clin. Psychopharm. 2:* 165–92, 1982.

45. Dam, M. Adverse Reactions to Anti-Epileptic Drugs. In Laidlaw, J.; Richens, A.

(eds.), *A Textbook of Epilepsy*. 2d ed. Edinburgh: Churchill Livingstone, 1982, pp. 348-58.

46. Shorvon, S. D.; Reynolds, E. H. Reduction of polypharmacy for epilepsy. *Br. Med. J. 2:* 1023-25, 1979.

47. Trimble, M. R. Psychotropic Drugs in the Management of Epilepsy. In Reynolds, E. H.; Trimble, M. R. (eds.), *Epilepsy and Psychiatry*. Edinburgh: Churchill Livingstone, 1981, pp. 337-46.

48. Dalby, M. A. Anti-epileptic and psychotropic aspects of carbamazepine ("Tegretol") in the treatment of psychomotor epilepsy. *Epilepsia 12:* 325-34, 1971.

49. Dalby, M. A. Behavioral Effects of Carbamazepine. In Penny, J. K.; Daly, D. D. (eds.), *Complex Partial Seizures*, vol. 2, *Neurology*. New York: Raven Press, 1975, pp. 331-44.

50. Folks, D. G.; King, D.; Dowdy, S. B.; *et al.* Carbamazepine treatment of selected affectively disordered inpatients. *Am. J. Psychiat. 139:* 115-17, 1982.

51. Taylor, M. A. Indications for Electroconvulsive Treatment. In Abrams, R.; Essman, W. B. (eds.), *Electroconvulsive Therapy in Theory and Practice*. New York: Spectrum, 1982, pp. 7-39.

52. Strub, R. L.; Black, F. W. *Organic Brain Syndromes: An Introduction to Neurobehavioral Disorders*. Philadelphia: F. A. Davis, 1981, pp. 89-118.

53. Adams, R. D.; Victor, M. Delirium and Other Confusional States. In Wintrobe, M. M.; Thorn, G. W.; Adams, R. D.; *et al.* (eds.), *Harrison's Principles of Internal Medicine*. New York: McGraw-Hill, 1974, pp. 149-56.

54. Plum, P.; Posner, J. B. *Diagnosis of Stupor and Coma*. 2d ed. Philadelphia: F. A. Davis, 1972.

55. Lipowski, Z. J. Delirium, clouding of consciousness and confusion. *J. Nerv. Ment. Dis. 145:* 227-55, 1967.

56. Peterson, G. C. Organic Brain Syndrome: Differential Diagnosis and Investigative Procedures in Adults. In Hendrie, H. C. (ed.), *Psychiatric Clinics of North America*, vol. 1/1, *Brain Disorders: Clinical Diagnosis and Management*. Philadelphia: W. B. Saunders, 1978, pp. 21-36.

57. Sierles, F. Behavioral Medicine. In Sierles, F. (ed.), *Clinical Behavioral Science*. New York: SP Medical and Scientific Books, 1982, pp. 159-77.

58. Varsamis, J. Clinical Management of Delirium. In Hendrie, H. C. (ed.), *Psychiatric Clinics of North America*, vol. 1/1, *Brain Disorders: Clinical Diagnosis and Management*. Philadelphia: W. B. Saunders, 1978; pp. 71-80.

59. Slaby, A. E.; Wyatt, R. J. *Dementia in the Presenium*. Springfield, Ill.: C. C. Thomas, 1974.

60. Torack, R. M. *The Pathologic Physiology of Dementia: With Indications for Diagnosis and Treatment*. Berlin: Springer-Verlag, 1978.

61. Benson, D. F. The Treatable Dementias. In Benson, D. F.; Blumer, D. (eds.), *Psychiatric Aspects of Neurologic Disease*, vol. 2. New York: Grune & Stratton, 1982, pp. 123-48.

62. Strub, R. L.; Black, F. W. *Organic Brain Syndromes: An Introduction to Neurobehavioral Disorders.* Philadelphia: F. A. Davis, 1981, pp. 119–212.

63. Cummings, J. L. Cortical Dementias. In Benson, D. F.; Blumer, D. (eds.), *Psychiatric Aspects of Neurologic Disease,* vol. 2. New York: Grune & Stratton, 1982, pp. 93–121.

64. Wells, C. E. Diagnostic Evaluation and Treatment in Dementia. In Wells, C. E. (ed.), *Dementia.* 2d ed. Philadelphia: F. A. Davis, 1977, pp. 247–76.

65. Spar, J. E.; Gerner, R. Does the dexamethasone suppression test distinguish dementia from depression? *Am. J. Psychiat. 139:* 238–40, 1982.

66. Fitzhugh–Bell, K. B. Neuropsychological Evaluation in the Management of Brain Disorders. In Hendrie, H. C. (ed.), *Psychiatric Clinics of North America,* vol. 1/1, *Brain Disorders: Clinical Diagnosis and Management.* Philadelphia: W. B. Saunders, 1978, pp. 37–50.

67. Roth, M. The Management of Dementia. In Hendrie, H. C. (ed.), *Psychiatric Clinics of North America,* vol. 1/1, *Brain Disorders: Clinical Diagnosis and Management.* Philadelphia: W. B. Saunders, 1978, pp. 81–99.

68. Yesavage, J. A.; Tinklenberg, J. R.; Hollister, L. E.; *et al.* Vasodilators in senile dementia. *Arch. Gen. Psychiat. 36:* 220–23, 1979.

69. Reisberg, B.; Ferris, S. H.; Gershon, S. An overview of pharmacologic treatment of cognitive decline in the aged. *Am. J. Psychiat. 138:* 593–600, 1981.

70. Strub, R. L.; Black, F. W. *Organic Brain Syndromes: An Introduction to Neurobehavioral Disorders.* Philadelphia: F. A. Davis, 1981, pp. 269–97.

71. Sisler, G. C. Psychiatric Disorder Associated with Head Injury. In Hendrie, H. C. (ed.), *Psychiatric Clinics of North America,* vol. 1/1 *Brain Disorders: Clinical Diagnosis and Management.* Philadelphia: W. B. Saunders, 1978, pp. 137–52.

72. Alexander, M. P. Traumatic Brain Injury. In Benson, D. F.; Blumer, D. (eds.), *Psychiatric Aspects of Neurologic Disease,* vol. 2. New York: Grune & Stratton, 1982, pp. 219–48.

73. Merskey, H.; Woodforde, J. M. Psychiatric sequelae of minor head injury. *Brain 95:* 521–28, 1972.

74. Lidvall, H. F.; Linderoth, B.; Norlin, B. Causes of the post-concussional syndrome. *Acta Neurol. Scand. Suppl. 56,* vol. 50, 1974.

75. Taylor, A. R. Post-concussional sequelae. *Br. Med. J. 3:* 67–71, 1967.

76. Harrison, M. S. Notes on the clinical features and pathology of post-concussional vertigo with special reference to positional nystagmus. *Brain 79:* 474–82, 1956.

77. Rowe, M. J.; Carlson, C. Brainstem auditory evoked potentials in post-concussional dizziness. *Arch. Neurol. 37:* 679–83, 1980.

78. Gronwall, D.; Wrightson, P. Delayed recovery of intellectual function after minor head injury. *Lancet 2:* 605–9, 1974.

79. Luria, A. R. *Higher Cortical Functions in Man.* New York: Basic Books, 1966.

80. Milner, B. Residual Intellectual and Memory Deficits After Head Injury. In Walker, A. E.; Caveness, W. F.; Critchley, M. (eds.), *The Late Effects of Head Injury.* Springfield, Ill.: C. C. Thomas, 1969, pp. 84–89.

81. Milner, B. Interhemispheric differences in the localization of psychological processes in man. *Br. Med. Bull. 27:* 272–77, 1971.

82. Black, W. F. Use of the MMPI with patients with recent war-related head injury. *J. Clin. Psychol. 30:* 571–73, 1974.

83. Levin, H. S.; Grossman, R. G. Behavioral sequelae of closed head injury: A qualitative study. *Arch. Neurol. 35:* 720–27, 1978.

84. Lishman, W. A. The psychiatric sequelae of head injury: A review. *Psychol. Med. 3:* 304–18, 1973.

85. Miller, E. The long-term consequences of head injury: A discussion of the evidence with special reference to the preparation of legal reports. *Br. J. Soc. Clin. Psychol. 18:* 87–98, 1979.

86. Pincus, J. H.; Tucker, G. J. *Behavioral Neurology.* 2d ed. New York: Oxford University Press, 1978, pp. 135–37.

87. Luria, A. R. *The Working Brain.* New York: Basic Books, 1973, pp. 187–225.

88. Luria, A. R. *The Working Brain.* New York: Basic Books, 1973, pp. 147–68.

89. Birkett, D. P. Gerstmann's syndrome. *Br. J. Psychiat. 113:* 801, 1967.

90. Luria, A. R. *The Working Brain.* New York: Basic Books, 1973, pp. 128–46.

91. Wolff, H.; Dalessio, D. J. *Headache and Other Head Pain.* 2d ed. New York: Oxford University Press, 1972.

92. Pincus, J. H.; Tucker, G. J. *Behavioral Neurology.* 2d ed. New York: Oxford University Press, 1978, pp. 258–63.

93. Wells, C. E.; Duncan, G. W. *Neurology for Psychiatrists.* Philadelphia: F. A. Davis, 1980, pp. 97–114.

94. Walton, J. N. *Essentials of Neurology.* 3d ed. Philadelphia: Lippincott, 1971, pp. 71–83.

95. Scheinberg, P. *Modern Practical Neurology: An Introduction to Diagnosis and Management of Common Neurologic Disorders.* 2d ed. New York: Raven Press, 1981, pp. 177–86.

CHAPTER 19

Substance Abuse

Alcohol-Related Syndromes

An alcoholic is someone whose use of alcohol directly results in medical, social, occupational, or legal problems. The alcoholic is often overtly intoxicated (more than twice monthly) and usually suffers a progressive deteriorating course despite periods of abstinence (1). Alcoholism is best defined by its consequences rather than the amount of alcohol consumed, although there is a rough correlation between duration and degree of alcohol consumption and its adverse results. Thus, a heavy drinker—an individual who drinks more than the average person, i.e., two to three drinks daily, and is occasionally intoxicated—is not by definition a problem drinker. Probably 10 to 20 percent of the population are heavy drinkers, and 3 to 5 percent of men and 1 percent of women are alcoholics (2, 3). Alcoholism is more prevalent among males, non-Baptists, blacks, urbanites, sociopaths, the affectively ill, waiters, bartenders, longshoremen, musicians, and writers (4-6). The onset for men is in the late teens or twenties, whereas for women the onset is more variable (7). Alcoholism is familial (8, 9) and apparently is specifically transmitted from parent to child whether or not the child is exposed to the alcoholic parent (10, 11).

It is a misconception to think of an alcoholic only as someone who has cirrhosis, withdrawal episodes, and gin for breakfast. These are features of chronic drinking. In the early stages of the disorder the alcoholic is more likely to experience family objections to his "drinking too much," the loss of friends because of drinking, and periods of self-doubt about drinking too much. Continued drinking will usually lead to trouble at work or loss of a job, arrests for drunk driving or disturbing the peace, fights when drinking, and unsuccessful attempts at abstinence before the alcoholic begins drinking before breakfast, experiences loss of memory when drinking, or suffers from physical deterioration from alcohol (12, 13). Testing for the presence of high blood levels of alpha-amino-n-butyric acid (AANB) (an amino acid released from liver cellular damage) relative to leucine and gamma glutamyl transpeptidase (GGTP) may be helpful in clinically ambiguous cases as there is some evidence (14, 15) that this test (see Table 19-1) indicates active alcoholism before there are social or medical features of the illness.

Approximately 10 percent of admissions to short-term psychiatric treatment units in general hospitals are alcohol-related (16). Alcoholics who are acutely intoxicated, withdrawing from alcohol, or suffering from Wernicke–Korsakoff syndrome generally should not be admitted to such a unit. When such patients are admitted, it is usually because of antisocial behavior secondary to sociopathy or because of odd or suicidal behavior associated with affective disorder (13, 17–19). As there is no known effective treatment for sociopathy (17) and the treatments of primary alcoholism are of questionable efficacy (13, 20), the best strategy in dealing with the heavy-drinking sociopath is immediate discharge from the unit to prevent the patient from disrupting the care of others. Should the patient be motivated, referral to Alcoholics Anonymous, an alcohol rehabilitation program, or a disulfiram maintenance program may be of benefit (13, 20).

TABLE 19-1   Laboratory Test for Chronic Alcohol Consumption

1. NPO after midnight
2. Blood drawn at 8 A.M. and stored for amino acid analysis
3. Levels of plasma AANB and leucine determined (in μM) by amino acid analyzer, e.g. Beckman 119
4. Abnormal results (M)

IF LEUCINE IS	THEN 85% ALCOHOLICS/HEAVY DRINKERS HAVE AANB LEVEL
20	5–8
40	10
60	15
80	20
100	25
120	30
140	33
160	35

As between 25 and 30 percent of manic-depressives are problem drinkers (19, 21), it is likely that a large number of patients with concomitant affective disorder and alcoholism will be hospitalized. In our experience the majority of these patients will be bipolar. These patients are particularly difficult to treat, for as soon as the clinician gains the upper hand on one disorder, the other rears its ugly head. Nevertheless, two double-blind studies (22, 23) found lithium carbonate to be superior to placebo in patients who suffered from alcoholism and affective disorder. However, as the dropout rate in both studies was high, the number of those patients likely to respond to lithium is unclear. Maintenance treatment is also complicated by the likelihood of relapse of one or the other condition and the sometimes dogmatic opposition of Alcoholics Anonymous to support patients' receiving any medication. ECT for the acute affective episode followed by maintenance ECT to prevent future manic or depressive episodes is a practical and efficacious alternative treatment plan (24).

Disulfiram, which interfaces with the metabolism of alcohol by blocking the action of acetaldehyde dehydrogenase, thus resulting in a buildup of acetaldehyde, is helpful for some alcoholics (13, 20). Unfortunately, many patients are unmotivated to continue treatment and need only discontinue the drug to begin drinking again. Psychotherapy, aversive conditioning techniques, and a variety of pharmacologic approaches for alcoholics have been tried without demonstrated success (13, 20).

ALCOHOL INTOXICATION

Acute alcohol intoxication is characterized by facial flushing, slurred speech, ataxia, nystagmus, mild diffuse cognitive impairment, loquacity, circumstantial and rambling speech, euphoria (initially), irritability, sadness, and emotional lability. Intoxication is directly related to the blood alcohol level, which is dependent on the amount and rate of alcohol consumed and the individual's body weight (see Table 19-2). Psychiatric intervention is usually sought because of combative or suicidal behavior (17-19).

Management focuses on controlling self-destructive or dangerous behavior. A calm, firm, and reassuring manner is sufficient to manage the majority of patients. Restraints and benzodiazepine sedation (little potentiation occurs, and doses as high as 50 to 100 mg. chlordiazepoxide have been given successfully) (25) occasionally may be required. Vital signs should be monitored, blood alcohol levels obtained, and the patient carefully observed to prevent aspiration from vomiting. If blood levels are above 300 mg. percent (usually producing stupor or coma), high doses of intravenous fructose will significantly lower the blood level. As alcohol is metabolized at a rate of about 1 ounce per hour, the acutely intoxicated but otherwise healthy individual will recover spontaneously in a short time (26).

TABLE 19-2   Alcohol Intoxication[a]

CONSUMPTION[b]	BLOOD LEVEL	BEHAVIOR
1-2 drinks[c]	75 mg. %	Decreased inhibitions Slightly delayed reaction time
3 drinks	75-100 mg. %	Delayed reaction time Slight dysarthria and fine motor ataxia
4 drinks	100-150 mg. %	Intoxication
5 drinks	150 mg. %	Sleepiness, truncal ataxia

[a] For individuals between 140 and 175 pounds.
[b] Rate of one drink per thirty minutes.
[c] One drink equals 1 oz. of 100 proof alcohol, 4 oz. of wine, 12 oz. of beer.

Death from acute alcohol intoxication usually follows the concomitant ingestion of sedatives or CNS depressants (13). A general screening for drugs should thus always be obtained. Diabetic acidosis or hypoglycemia (best treated with intravenous glucose) or alcohol–disulfiram reactions (flushing, tachycardia, hypotension, headache and dizziness, nausea and vomiting, best treated with pressor agents, ascorbic acid, and antihistamines) are life-threatening conditions, which may masquerade as simple alcohol intoxication and must also be ruled out (26).

Alcohol Withdrawal

The alcohol withdrawal syndrome is associated with a sudden and precipitous drop in the consumption of alcohol. Most commonly, however, the patient continues to drink but switches from high- to low-alcohol-containing beverages. The syndrome is characterized by coarse tremors of the hand, tongue, and eyelids; nausea and vomiting; general weakness and malaise; tachycardia; sweating; hypertension and/or orthostatic hypotension; dysphoria and irritability; and, when severe, some alteration in consciousness, diffuse cognitive impairment, insomnia, agitation, and at times extreme excitement (27). Severity of withdrawal is positively correlated with the degree and duration of alcohol consumption and inversely related to the patient's general physical health (e.g. a severe syndrome is more often observed in association with pancreatitis, infection, hepatic insufficiency, subdural hematoma, fractures, or vitamin deficiencies) (27, 28). In most cases withdrawal is benign and short-lived (27). When severe (about 5 percent of cases develop delirium tremens), the patient exhibits an alteration in consciousness and may experience illusions and hallucinations in any sensory modality. These patients commonly have visual hallucinations, although auditory hallucinations are by no means rare (27).

Initial emergency treatment may require temporary restraints. Prolonged restraints are contraindicated, as patients with alcohol withdrawal delirium may struggle against restraints until dangerously exhausted. Rapid sedation is essential. Anxiolytics are the primary pharmacologic choices. Doses must be titrated against the patient's initial response, with mild sedation being the goal. An initial 50- to 100-mg. dose of chlordiazepoxide or 15 to 20 mg. of diazepam intravenously should temporarily control the typical withdrawal delirium and provide an indication (based upon the patient's sedative response) for a definitive withdrawal drug schedule, which may be as high as 600 mg. of chlordiazepoxide daily. Some clinicians prefer 10 to 15 ml. of fresh intramuscular paraldehyde to initially control withdrawal agitation. Anxiolytics, however, have advantages over paraldehyde in that intramuscular paraldehyde is painful, whereas intravenous anxiolytics (particularly diazepam) have anticonvulsant properties and are not excreted through the lungs as is paraldehyde (which produces a horrendous olfactory barrier to further interactions with the patient) (20). As spontaneous seizures during withdrawal are not uncommon, 100 mg. oral or intravenous diphenylhydantoin (poorly absorbed intramuscularly) may also be administered during emergency treatment and maintained at a daily dose of 400 mg. PO during the detoxification period. Administration of anticonvulsants beyond this period is not justified (27, 29, 30). Hospitalization is always required. Additional treatment with intramuscular thiamine, 100 mg. twice daily (alcoholics often have a mild malabsorption syndrome), and multivitamins (particularly B complex and C) is essential and may prevent a Wernicke–Korsakoff syndrome (31). Magnesium sulfate to prevent seizures secondary to hypomagnesemia is of questionable benefit (32), and fluid and electrolyte administration is rarely needed unless the patient's hematocrit is elevated and he exhibits other signs of dehydration. Most alcoholics are overhydrated, and seizures may be induced with unnecessary intravenous fluid administration (33). Intravenous glucose should also be avoided, as thiamine is a cofactor in carbohydrate metabolism, and a heavy carbohydrate load may further deplete thiamine stores (26, 34).

Neuroleptics are contraindicated. They have no cross-tolerance properties with alcohol, suppress the immune system (already compromised in many alcoholics), lower the seizure threshold, tax hepatic metabolic processes, and increase the morbidity and mortality rate. Barbiturates, used in some centers, are generally not recommended as they are myocardial irritants, and alcoholics in withdrawal often have cardiac arrhythmias (35, 36).

When hallucinations persist after all signs of delirium have abated, the patient is said to have alcoholic hallucinosis (37). The etiology of this disorder is unclear. Several studies, however, fail to demonstrate a relation-ship to schizophrenia in either outcome (90 percent recover by six months) or family history (low for schizophrenia, high for alcoholism) (38). As these pa-tients have not responded to benzodiazepines during the acute phase of their disorder, neuroleptics or ECT may be of benefit.

WERNICKE'S SYNDROME

Wernicke's syndrome, a delirious state, is characterized by sudden onset of opthalmoplegia (most often abducens nerve/external rectus muscle paralysis), nystagmus (almost always present), ataxia, memory loss, altered consciousness, and diffuse cognitive impairment. Signs of peripheral neuropathy and myocarditis may also be present, and a history of Korsakoff syndrome (see Chapter 18) is typical. Wernicke's syndrome is most com-monly observed in alcoholics, although any cause of profound thiamine deficiency (e.g. gastric carcinoma, pernicious anemia, hyperemesis gravidarum, malnutrition) can produce the syndrome in a genetically vulnerable individual. The acute phase usually remits rapidly with in-tramuscular thiamine and multivitamins. A residual Korsakoff's syndrome is the most common sequela. Five percent of patients die. Emergency treat-ment comprises restraints when necessary, parenteral thiamine hydrochloride (50 mg.), sedation with chlordiazepoxide (25–50 mg. PO or IV) or diazepam (10–15 mg. PO or IV), and hospitalization. As in the treat-ment of withdrawal syndromes, intravenous fluid and electrolyte replace-ment should not be routinely administered (31, 36).

ALCOHOL-RELATED DELUSIONAL DISORDER
(ALCOHOL PARANOID STATE)

In our experience alcoholic patients with delusional disorder are typically male and chronic heavy drinkers who have had few alcohol-related dif-ficulties until their sixth or seventh decade, when they become increasingly suspicious, sullen, irritable, and finally delusional. Delusional ideas usually involve themes of a spouse's infidelity, a relative's dishonesty, a neighbor's "dirty tricks," or a municipality's illegal action. These patients become neighborhood cranks and are finally hospitalized when local authorities run out of patience from constant complaints or litigation or when family members become exasperated or fearful that the patient may hurt someone. These patients do not appear affectively ill.

Although cortical atrophy and cognitive impairment secondary to chronic heavy alcohol use have not been fully established (39, 40), in our experience patients with alcohol-related delusional disorder exhibit mild to moderate cortical atrophy and cognitive impairment. Occasionally neuroleptics may be required if the delusions do not fully resolve with strict abstinence and multivitamin treatment.

Drug Abusers

The drug abuser who is not suffering from an induced psychosis, delirium, or a coarse brain syndrome secondary to drugs, should not be admitted to a general hospital short-term inpatient unit. These patients are manipulative and often sociopathic. Inevitably they disrupt the care of other patients. In some settings drug abusers will introduce street drugs into the unit.

The chronic abuser is often encountered on medical and surgical services, however, and some knowledge of the principles of detoxification and the treatment for specific street drugs with psychotropic properties is essential. Table 19-3 lists some common drugs of abuse.

BARBITURATE AND SEDATIVE HYPNOTICS: INTOXICATION AND WITHDRAWAL

Sedative hypnotics, all synthetic chemicals, are general CNS depressants which produce sedation in small doses and sleep in larger doses (41, 42). People who habitually use these compounds tend to cluster into two groups, one composed of young, often antisocial males who use these drugs to alter their consciousness; and the other composed of middle-aged, often middle-class individuals, who are initially prescribed a sedative hypnotic for anxiety or a sleep disorder and who then continue to use these drugs as physiological tolerance and eventually addiction develops (43).

The clinical features of sedative hypnotic intoxication are similar to those of simple alcohol intoxication. These patients, however, tend to be systemically healthier than alcoholics. Behavioral management is similar to that for alcohol intoxication, with special attention to the possibility of masked hypoglycemia as the cause of the syndrome. Unlike alcohol, high blood levels of sedative hypnotics are likely to induce respiratory arrest, and patients who are markedly lethargic should be treated in medical intensive care units (41-44).

In mild cases of intoxication behavioral treatment includes a safe, quiet environment in which the patient's behavior, vital signs, and level of consciousness can be regularly observed. Restraints may be necessary for agitated patients. The semicomatose or comatose patient should be intubated following gastric lavage and ventilated if necessary. Activated char-

TABLE 19-3 Common Drugs of Abuse

SEDATIVE HYPNOTICS	OPIATES	SYMPATHOMIMETICS	INHALANTS	HALLUCINOGENS
Chloral hydrate	Opium	Cocaine	Nitrous oxide	Phencyclidine (PCP)
Barbiturates	(10% morphine)	Amphetamines	Glues	Cannabis (marijuana)
a. Long-acting	Heroin	a. Amphetamine	Paints, lacquers	(tetrahydrocannabinol)
(phenobarbital—	(Diacetyl morphine)	(Benzedrine)	(e.g. toluene)	D-lysergic acid
Luminal)	Morphine	b. Dextro-amphetamine	Paint thinner	diethylamide-25 (LSD)
b. Short-acting	Demerol	(Dexedrine)	(e.g. turpentine)	Peyote
(secobarbital—Seconal,	(Meperidine)	c. Methamphetamine	Refrigerants	Mescaline
pentobarbital—Nembutal,	Percodan	(Methedrine)	(e.g. freon)	(trimethoxy-phenylethylamine)
amobarbital—Amytal)	(Oxymorphone)	Amphetamine congeners	Gasoline	Psilocybin (related
Glutethimide (Doriden)	Methadone	a. Methylphenidate	Solvents	to serotonin)
Methyprylon (Noludar)	(Dolophine)	(Ritalin)	(e.g. acetone)	Corymbos (morning
Ethchlorvynol (Placidyl)	Codeine	b. Phenmetrazine	Aerosols	glory seeds) (related
Ethinamate (Valmid)	(Methyl morphine)	(Preludin)	Nitrites	to LSD)
Meprobamate (Miltown,				Myristica (nutmeg)
Equanil)	*Opiate-like*			
Methaqualone	Talwin			
(Quaalude)	(Pentazocine)			
Benzodiazepines	Darvon			
a. Long-acting	(d-propoxyphene)			
(chlordiazepoxide—Librium)				
b. Short-acting				
(clorazepam, oxazepam)				
c. Intermediate-acting				
(diazepam—Valium)				

coal should be introduced into the stomach to absorb any remaining drug, and the urine should be alkalinized with sodium bicarbonate infusion (helpful primarily for phenobarbital intoxication). If meprobamate is the offending agent, a 20 percent intravenous solution of mannitol at a rate of 50 cc. per hour should be administered. Fluid and electrolyte balance should be maintained. Aqueous or lipid hemodialysis may be helpful, as they remove most sedative hypnotic from the blood. Intravenous naloxone, 0.4 mg., and 50 cc. of 50 percent glucose (in nonalcoholics) should be routinely given if the specific coma-causing drug is not known (41-45).

The sedative hypnotic withdrawal syndrome is virtually identical to that of alcohol withdrawal, with the important exceptions that coarse tremor is not always present and that grand mal seizures (also observed in alcohol withdrawal syndromes) may occur early in the withdrawal period. Symptoms begin twelve to forty-eight hours after the last dose but may be delayed up to seven to ten days for long-acting compounds. Severity of symptoms is directly related to the daily dose and the duration of use. For most sedative-hypnotics, the clinician should suspect addiction if daily use at therapeutic doses or above has been longer than thirty days. After ninety days of use at or above the therapeutic dose range addiction is virtually guaranteed. Treatment requires hospitalizing the patient (on a medical service), mildly sedating the patient with a sedative hypnotic and then withdrawing this over a ten- to twelve-day period (43-46).

Withdrawal from barbiturates is best accomplished with pentobarbital, which should be administered initially as a 200 mg. test dose by mouth and again every two hours until the patient exhibits mild ataxia, dysarthria, nystagmus, and lethargy. If 400 mg. or less produces intoxication, no further treatment is needed. If 600 mg. or more is needed to achieve intoxication, the patient should be placed on that daily amount in divided doses given every six hours. Dose reduction should begin after twenty-four hours starting with the morning and midday doses, then rotating the time of dose reduction, retaining the evening dose as long as possible. Thus, for example, a patient requiring 800 mg. of pentobarbital to become intoxicated would receive the following withdrawal schedule (in mg.): Day 1—200, 200, 200, 200; Day 2—160, 160, 200, 200; Day 3—160, 160, 160, 160; Day 4—120, 120, 160, 160; Day 5—120, 120, 120, 120; Day 6—80, 80, 120, 120; Day 7—80, 80, 80, 80; Day 8—80, 80, 80: Day 9—40, 40, 80: Day 10—40, 40; Day 11—40: Day 12—no medication (43, 44, 47).

Nonbarbiturate sedative hypnotic withdrawal is best accomplished by using the offending agent at the dose determined from a benzodiazepine challenge, milligram for milligram. If the patient is addicted to a benzodiazepine, a barbiturate challenge may result in a false negative response. An equivalent challenge can be performed with an initial 50 mg. dose of chlordiazepoxide, administered by mouth and repeated every two hours until intoxication. Intoxication at 100 mg. or less requires no further treatment. If 150 mg. or more is needed to induce intoxication, the patient should be placed on that amount in divided doses given every eight hours for the first twenty-four hours. The dose should be reduced by 25 mg. daily following a schedule similar to that for barbiturates. Thus, a patient requiring 250 mg. of chlordiazepoxide to become intoxicated would receive the following schedule (in mg.): Day 1—75, 75, 100; Day 2—75, 75, 75; Day 3—50, 75, 75; Day 4—50, 50, 75; Day 5—50, 50, 50; Day 6—25, 50, 50; Day 7—25, 25, 50; Day 8—25, 25, 25; Day 9—25, 25; Day 10—25; Day 11—no medication (43, 44).

OPIATE INTOXICATION AND WITHDRAWAL

Opiate addiction in Western countries primarily involves heroin and methadone (see Table 19-3). The latter is often obtained at "methadone clinics." Heroin may be sniffed ("snorting") or injecting subcutaneously ("skin popping") or intravenously ("mainlining"). Methadone is usually taken orally. The number of individuals addicted is not known, although estimates suggest at least 500,000 in the United States. Urban blacks and Hispanics constitute the majority of opiate addicts. Physicians and nurses form the next largest group of opiate users (48–50).

Opiate intoxication is characterized by euphoria or dysphoria followed by apathy, psychomotor retardation, and slurred speech; impaired attention, concentration, and memory; and then somnolence. Pupillary constriction is always initially present, but in comatose anoxic patients pupillary dilation can occur. Other signs of severe intoxication include respiratory distress, apnea with cyanosis, areflexia, hypotension, and tachycardia. Pulmonary edema and grand mal seizures can occur. Needle "tracks" or scarred veins resulting from repeated intravenous injection of drugs is a classic physical feature of addiction (48–50).

The treatment of opiate intoxication involves maintaining adequate oxygenation, preventing aspiration of vomitus, and maintaining cardiac output and blood pressure. Intravenous naloxone (0.4 mg.) is an extremely safe narcotic antagonist, which should be given immediately (diluted in 10 cc. of sterile normal saline) to any patient suspected of medically dangerous opiate intoxication. This dose can be repeated three or four times within the first ten minutes of treatment if no response is seen. Intrajugular or intrafemoral vein administration may be required, as the usual sites of intravenous administration may be scarred and unusable. Pupillary dilatation is often the first sign of a response. Restraints should be applied prior to injection, for if effective, the patient will awake in severe withdrawal and will be agitated, confused, and irritable. If severe, this delirium should be controlled with intravenous benzodiazepines. As most opiates have a longer half-life than naloxone, repeated doses may be necessary, and constant observation is essential during the next twenty-four hours to prevent respiratory arrest (48, 49, 51).

Opiate withdrawal is rarely life-threatening and virtually never as dramatic as its cinematic analogue. As most opiates are short-acting, withdrawal signs, although mild, begin within eight to twelve hours after the last dose. Peak severity occurs between twenty-four and thirty-six hours and may remain at this level for an additional period of twenty-four to thirty-six hours before abating. Residual features such as restlessness, fatigue, and insomnia last for several weeks.

The syndrome begins with restlessness, dysphoria, lethargy, fitful sleep, and then tearing, nasal discharge, sweating, yawning, and deep, sighing respirations. These features can all be self-induced (plucking a nasal hair will produce tearing and nasal discharge) or feigned, and treatment should not begin until the patient experiences piloerection. If severe addiction remains untreated, chills, muscle and joint pain, abdominal cramps, vomiting and diarrhea, tachycardia, hypertension, and fever can occur. Anorexia, insomnia, anxiety, and agitation also may be prominent (48, 49, 52).

Opiate abusers should not be admitted to a general psychiatric unit. These patients are for the most part manipulative, disruptive, untruthful, and unpleasant. Detoxification, however, may be required for patients occasionally admitted to medical or surgical units for drug-related conditions (e.g. hepatitis, thrombophlebitis, subcutaneous abcesses, endocarditis, pulmonary infection or emboli, osteomyelitis). These patients, however, often disrupt medical staff routine; careful counseling and education of nursing personnel is essential if the detoxification period is to proceed without a major uproar.

Detoxification from opiates is accomplished with oral methadone. If an initial test dose of 20 mg. causes intoxication, no further treatment is needed. Rarely does a patient need more than 40 mg. daily, divided into a morning and evening dose. A typical withdrawal schedule reduces the dose by five each day. An example is (in mg.): Day 1—20, 20; Day 2—15, 20; Day 3—15, 15; Day 4—10, 15; Day 5—10, 10; Day 6—5, 10; Day 7—5, 5; Day 8—0, 5; Day 9—no medication. Flurazepam, 30 mg. PO for sleep, should be routinely administered throughout the withdrawal period (48, 49, 52).

Newborns of mothers addicted to opiates will also develop withdrawal within forty-eight hours postpartum if not treated. These infants will be irritable, hyperactive, febrile, tremulous, anorexic, and tachypneic. A high-pitched "catlike" cry is characteristic, and seizures may occur. Friction-induced pressure point skin irritation caused by hyperactivity is also a common clinical sign. Treatment is best accomplished with paregoric, three to ten drops every four hours titrated to mild sedation. The sedative dose should be tapered over a seven-day period (53).

SYMPATHOMIMETICS

The two chief sympathomimetics of abuse are cocaine and the amphetamines. Cocaine is a naturally occurring CNS stimulant extracted from the leaves of the South American coca plant. It has no cross-tolerance with the amphetamines. Cocaine is not physiologically addicting, although psychological dependence often occurs. Because of its extremely high cost, cocaine is primarily used today by the upper middle class and the rich. It can be inhaled as a powder, dissolved in water and injected intravenously, or smoked as an ether extract ("freebasing"). Most street cocaine is adulterated ("cut") with talcum powder or dry milk. Approximately 3 million Americans are repeated users (50, 54).

Cocaine produces peripheral vasoconstriction, increased body temperature and metabolic rate, excessive sweating, mydriasis, increased heart rate and blood pressure, and a sense of expansiveness, unlimited energy, and euphoria. Intoxication is characterized by irritability, suspiciousness, fearfulness, and jerky agitation, stereotypy, tactile hallucinations of insects crawling on or just under the skin ("cocaine bugs"), and visual hallucinations (classically of geometric shapes and patterns). These patients may become violent. Respiratory depression, hyperpyrexia, hypertension, and seizures can occur, and each may lead to sudden death (48, 54, 55).

Amphetamine and dextroamphetamine are synthetic substitutes for ephedrine, which occurs naturally in a desert plant indigenous to China. The oral and intravenous dose of amphetamine and its congeners (methylphenidate and phenmetrazine) have similar but longer-lasting and milder acute effects than cocaine. Unlike cocaine, physical tolerance develops to amphetamine. Chronic amphetamine and cocaine use can result in a delusional, hallucinatory disorder. Stereotypy is common, and emotional unresponsiveness characteristic. These patients move in a jerky, birdlike manner and continually look about them as if scanning for some anticipated danger. They also may engage in prolonged staring at their reflections in mirrors. Withdrawal is characterized by prolonged sleep with increased REM time, fatigue, apathy, and increased appetite (48–50, 56).

In addition to the standard environmental and behavioral strategies generally employed in the treatment of acute drug intoxication (see above), sympathomimetic drug intoxication may require neuroleptic administration. Standard treatments for hyperpyrexia to prevent cardiovascular collapse and seizures, acidification of the urine with ammonium chloride (500 to 1,000 mg. every four hours) to enhance drug excretion, and phentolamine (1 to 5 mg. intravenously) for severe hypertension may also be required. The psychosis secondary to chronic administration is treated symptomatically (48, 56).

INHALANTS

Inhalant use is faddish and in the United States is primarily observed among the young, poor, and Spanish-speaking. Chemicals producing psychoactive vapors are diverse in structure. Recent surveys suggest that 7 million Americans have used these solvents, which include hydrocarbons, freons, ketones, esters, alcohols, and glycols. Inhalant intoxication resembles alcohol intoxication but is of shorter duration. Use of any inhalant may result in aggressive and assaultive behavior requiring restraints and sedation. Diazepam 10 to 30 mg. PO or 10 to 15 mg. IV may be required. Individuals who regularly use organic solvent inhalants are at great risk for brain damage. In one study 40 percent of subjects scored in the severe impairment range on the Halstead–Reitan battery. Chronic use may also affect peripheral nerves and kidney and liver function. Acute intoxication is characterized by delirium, tinnitus, ataxia, tremors and fasciculations, distortions of body image, and visual hallucinations often of colorful images and geometric shapes (57, 58). Nitrites, chemically unrelated to other inhaled substances, specifically produce a transient alteration in consciousness and are used primarily in association with sexual behavior (59).

HALLUCINOGENS

Phencyclidine (PCP)

During the past several years PCP use has increased to epidemic proportions despite inconsistent reports of positive psychotropic experiences (usually an intense euphoria with feelings of unlimited power and energy) and frequent and consistent reports of adverse reactions (intense depression, psychosis, violence). Some hospitals report detectable PCP in the urine of up to 70 percent of psychiatric admissions (60, 61). A white crystalline powder, PCP may be mistaken for cocaine, and "cheap" cocaine highs are commonly reported by patients presenting with PCP intoxication. As many as 2 million to 3 million Americans (most under age twenty-five) have used PCP, which is sold as "angel dust," "hog," "crystal," and "weed," to name but a few sobriquets. PCP users commonly use other street drugs and alcohol and have a history of drug-related arrests. PCP may be snorted, smoked, or injected. There is some evidence that once distributed in body fat as much as 94 percent of a given dose remains in body tissue indefinitely. "Flashbacks" have been attributed to temporary mobilization of the molecule from fat to brain (62, 63).

Because PCP has an affinity for the vestibulocerebellar system, intoxication is always characterized by dizziness, nystagmus, and muscular uncoordination. Tachycardia and hypertension are also common. Behaviorally, a delirium with intense anxiety, suspiciousness, irritability, and violence is characteristic. Psychosis most commonly presents as a typical drug-induced psychotic state or mania (62–64). Treatment is described in Chapter 8 on emergency psychiatry.

Cannabis

Marijuana, derived from the hemp plant, is the most widely used street drug. Nearly 60 percent of high school graduates in the United States have used the drug. Its main active ingredient is tetrahydrocannabinol. Hashish is a form of marijuana with a high concentration of tetrahydrocannabinol. Physiological tolerance to the drug has not been observed, although psychological dependence may occur (50, 65, 66).

Long-term use appears to impair lung function and to suppress the immune system. Heavy cannabis smokers are at greater risk for lung cancer and fungal infections than individuals who smoke equivalent amounts of tobacco. Reproductive and chromosomal aberations have also been reported with chronic use (67).

Acute effects include increased heart rate and blood pressure, impaired concentration and acquisition and storage of information, impaired reaction time and time sense (events appear to proceed more slowly than they actually do), and impaired coordination and judgment. Some individuals, particularly first-time users, experience acute fearfulness, confusion, dysphoria, and occasionally irritability, suspiciousness, delusional ideas, hallucinations, and distortions of body image. Chronic behavioral effects include an "amotivational" syndrome of apathy, loss of drive and ambition, and general mild cognitive impairment (65, 66, 68, 69).

Treatment of the acute syndrome rarely requires sedation, as a quiet, structured environment with friendly and calm staff interactions with the patient is usually sufficient to resolve all symptoms. Anxiolytics are helpful in the more severe cases, and neuroleptics are virtually never required unless the acute psychoses persists for more than a few hours. There is no known effective treatment for the "amotivational" syndrome (48, 49).

LSD, Peyote, Mescaline, Psilocybin, and Corymbos

LSD, a synthetic ergot alkaloid derivative; peyote and mescaline, extracted from a Mexican cactus; psilocybin, extracted from a Mexican mushroom; and corymbos and myristica, the active ingredients in morning glory seeds and nutmeg respectively, are hallucinogenic substances primarily used by middle- and upper-class young adults. Consumption of these drugs, which in relatively low doses can induce psychosis, has decreased during the past ten years. Nevertheless, about 3 percent of people under twenty-five currently use these substances (54).

Acute effects include altered perception of shape, color, and stimulus intensity; synesthesias (the perception in one sensory modality caused by a stimulus in another); and paresthesias, altered consciousness, dizziness, weakness, tremors, and nausea. Intense moods, lability of affect, distorted time sense, oneiroid states, states of religious and philosophic ecstasy, hallucinations (particularly visual), delusional moods and ideas, incoordination, and general cognitive impairment may also occur (48, 67).

Uncomplicated and relatively mild adverse reactions rarely require hospitalization. A calm, structured pleasant environment with moderate light and sound and a calm, supportive staff is usually sufficient. Anxiolytics and, for some psychotic but nonexcited patients, a single intramuscular dose of neuroleptic (e.g. chlorpromazine 25 mg.) may be required. Patients who are extremely agitated and excited or whose symptoms persist past four to six hours generally require hospitalization. In our experience neuroleptics are then needed, and treatment is best achieved with haloperidol. However, as many street drugs have anticholinergic properties, neuroleptics, themselves potent anticholinergic agents, occasionally exacerbate drug-induced psychotic symptoms. Should this occur or if resolution of symptoms is not obtained within three to five days, ECT should be administered, as it is effective and safe in the treatment of most drug-induced states (24, 48, 51).

In some individuals, particularly those experiencing "bad trips" (usually frightening psychotic states) and thus presumably most vulnerable to the neurotropic effects of hallucinogens, a single administration may result in permanent brain dysfunction. Certainly repeated use of hallucinogens can result in cognitive impairment, recurrent psychoses, chronic hallucinosis, and a chronic avolitional state, each of which may persist long after discontinuation of the drug (70, 71). We have seen a number of patients in their late twenties with chronic emotional blunting, formal thought disorder, and complete auditory hallucinations who, in their late teens or early twenties, used hallucinogenic drugs for a one- to two-year period. Despite no further drug use (confirmed by family, friends, and medical observation), these schizophrenic-like symptoms persisted. None of these patients had a premorbid history suggestive of psychiatric disorder or any family history of schizophrenia.

One of us had a patient, a psychiatric technician, who, from all sources, was not previously psychiatrically ill and had never used street drugs of any kind, but who was given LSD (documented) in orange juice by a psychiatric patient who was a drug abuser. The drug abuser was "celebrating" his discharge from the hospital and freely admitted "spiking" the juice. Thirty minutes later, while playing football, the technician began to experience frightening visual perceptual distortions and hallucinations. He was hospitalized and treated with a neuroleptic for three days.

Although his acute symptoms completely abated, he lost all interest in

TABLE 19-4 Poetic Description of Drug States

Barbiturates sedative–hypnotics and alcohol	Labile emotions from friendship to hate; Slurring of language, and stumbling of gait. Vision is blurry, and acts like a clown.
Opiates	Cool to the touch, unresponsive to pain, Hunger diminished, and scars over vein. Pupils pinpointed, and blood pressure low, Urine diminished, and breathing is slow.
Sympathomimetics	Constantly moving, and high as a kite, Pupils dilated, and stays up all night. Acting suspicious, and trying to fight, Blood pressure rising, and no appetite.
Hallucinogens	Fantastic colors and beautiful lights, Great synesthesias, eureka insights. Out of the body, time stops for a while, Pupils dilated, amphetamine style.

SOURCE: Adapted from (Table 15.19, "Drug Rhymes," in Arnold M. Ludwig, *Principles of Clinical Psychiatry* (New York: The Free Press, 1980), p. 315. Copyright © 1980 by the Free Press, a Division of Macmillan, Inc. Used by permission.

pursuing his college education and became emotionally bland (a departure from his premorbid friendly, animated ambitious behavior). A year later he was encountered on a busy street corner "standing around," vacantly watching the crowds pass by. Although without any recurrent acute symptoms during the year, he had not entered school, had stopped seeing his friends, and spent his time doing nothing, supported on disability insurance. He had no family history of psychiatric disorder.

A poetic summation of the characteristics of drug states is presented in Table 19–4.

References

1. Jellinek, E. M. *The Disease Concept of Alcoholism.* New Haven: College & University Press, 1960.

2. Cohalan, D.; Cisin, I. H.; Crossley, H. M. *American Drinking Practices: A National Survey of Behavior and Attitudes,* monograph no. 6. New Brunswick, N.J.: Rutgers University Center of Alcohol Studies, 1969.

3. Goodwin, D. W.; Guze, S. B. *Psychiatric Diagnosis.* 2d ed. New York and Oxford: Oxford University Press, 1979, Ch. 7, pp. 118–44.

4. DeLint, J.; Schmidt, W. The Epidemiology of Alcoholism. In Israel, Y.; Mardones, J. (eds.), *Biological Basis of Alcoholism.* Toronto: Wiley–Interscience, 1971, pp. 423–42.

5. Maddox, G. L.; Williams, J. R. Drinking behavior of negro collegians. *Quart. J. Stud. Alcohol 29:* 117–29, 1968.

6. Robins, L. N.; Murphy, G. E.; Breckenridge, M. B. Drinking behavior of young negro men. *Quart. J. Stud. Alcohol 29:* 657–84, 1968.

7. Pemberton, D. A. A comparison of the outcome of treatment in female and male alcoholics. *Br. J. Psychiat. 113:* 367–73, 1967.

8. Goodwin, D. W. Alcoholism and heredity: A review of the hypothesis. *Arch. Gen. Psychiat. 36:* 57–61, 1979.

9. Goodwin, D. W. Hereditary factors in alcoholism. *Hosp. Pract. 13:* 121–30, 1978.

10. Cadoret, R. J.; Gath, A. Inheritance of alcoholism in adoptees. *Br. J. Psychiat. 132:* 252–58, 1978.

11. Goodwin, D. W.; Schulsinger, F.; Knop, J.; *et al.* Alcoholism and depression in adopted-out daughters of alcoholics. *Arch. Gen. Psychiat. 34:* 751–55, 1977.

12. Goodwin, D. W.; Crane, J. B.; Guze, S. B. Alcoholic "blackouts": A review and clinical study of 100 alcoholics. *Am. J. Psychiat. 126:* 191–98, 1969.

13. Goodwin, D. W. *Alcoholism: The Facts.* New York and London: Oxford University Press, 1981.

14. Shaw, S.; Lue, S. L.; Lieber, C. S. Biochemical tests for the detection of alcoholism: Comparison of plasma alpha-amino-n-butyric acid with other available tests. *Alcoholism: Clin. Exper. Res. 2:* 3–7, 1978.

15. Lieber, C. S. Pathogenesis and early diagnosis of alcoholic liver injury. *New Eng. J. Med. 298:* 888–93, 1978.

16. Ries, R.; Bokan, J.; Schuckit, M. A. Modern diagnosis of schizophrenia in hospitalized psychiatric patients. *Am. J. Psychiat. 137:* 1419–21, 1980.

17. Guze, S. B. *Criminality and Psychiatric Disorders.* New York: Oxford University Press, 1976.

18. Goodwin, D. W. Alcohol in suicides and homicides. *Quart. J. Stud. Alcohol 34:* 144–56, 1973.

19. Schuckit, M.; Pitts, F. N., Jr.; Reich, T.; *et al.* Alcoholism. *Arch. Environ. Health 18:* 301–6, 1964.

20. Goodwin, D. W. Substance induced and substance use disorders: Alcohol. In Greist, J. H.; Jefferson, J. W.; Spitzer, R. L. (eds.), *Treatment of Mental Disorders.* New York and Oxford: Oxford University Press, 1982, pp. 44–61.

21. Winokur, F.; Clayton, P. J.; Reich, T. *Manic Depressive Illness.* St. Louis, Mo.: C. V. Mosby, 1969.

22. Merry, J.; Reynolds, C. M.; Bailey, J.; *et al.* Prophylactic treatment of alcoholism by lithium carbonate. *Lancet 2:* 481–82, 1976.

23. Kline, N. S.; Wren, J. C.; Cooper, T. B.; *et al.* Evaluation of lithium therapy in chronic and periodic alcoholism. *Am. J. Med. Sci. 268:* 15–22, 1974.

24. Taylor, M. A. Indications for Electroconvulsive Treatment. In Abrams, R.; Essman, W. B. (eds.), *Biological Foundations and Clinical Applications.* New York: SP Medical and Scientific Books, 1982, pp. 7–39.

25. Miller, A. I.; D'Agostino, A.; Minsky, R. Effects of combined chlordiazepoxide and alcohol in man. *Quart. Stud. Alcohol 1:* 9–13, 1963.

26. Lieber, C. S. The metabolism of alcohol. *Sci. Amer. 234:* 25–31, 1974.

27. Victor, M.; Adams, R. D. The Effect of Alcohol on the Nervous System. In Merritt, H. H.; Hare, C. C. (eds.), *Metabolic and Toxic Diseases of the Nervous System.* Baltimore: Williams & Wilkins, 1953, pp. 526–73.

28. Tavel, M. E.; Davidson, W.; Batteron, T. D. A critical analysis of the mortality associated with delirium tremens. *Am. J. Med. Sci. 242:* 18–29, 1961.

29. Victor, M. The Pathophysiology of Alcoholic Epilepsy. In Wikler, A. (ed.), *Addictive States,* vol. 46. Baltimore: Williams & Wilkins, Association for Research in Nervous and Mental Disease, 1968, pp. 431–54.

30. Marinacci, A. A. Electroencephalography in Alcoholism. In Thompson, G. N. (ed.), *Alcoholism.* Springfield, Ill.: C. C. Thomas, 1956, pp. 484–536.

31. Victor, M.; Adams, R. D.; Collins, G. H. *The Wernicke–Korsakoff Syndrome.* Philadelphia: F. A. Davis, 1971.

32. Mendelson, J. H. Biological concomitants of alcoholism. *New Eng. J. Med. 283:* 24–32, 1970.

33. Ogata, M.; Mendelson, J.; Mello, N. Electrolytes and osmolality in alcoholics during experimental intoxication. *Psychosom. Med. 30:* 463–88, 1968.

34. Freinkel, N.; Arky, R. A. Effects of alcohol on carbohydrate metabolism in man. *Psychosom. Med. 28:* 551–63, 1966.

35. Kaim, S.; Klett, C. J.; Rothfeld, B. Treatment of the acute alcohol withdrawal state: A comparison of four drugs. *Am. J. Psychiat. 125:* 1640–46, 1969.

36. Shader, R. I. *Manual of Psychiatric Therapeutics: Practical Psychopharmacology and Psychiatry.* Boston: Little, Brown, 1975, pp. 211–35.

37. Victor, M.; Hope, J. M. The phenomenon of auditory hallucinations in chronic alcoholism: A critical evaluation of the status of alcoholic hallucinosis. *J. Nerv. Ment. Dis. 126:* 451–81, 1958.

38. Schuckit, M. A.; Winokur, G. Alcoholic hallucinosis and schizophrenia: A negative study. *Br. J. Psychiat. 119:* 549–50, 1971.

39. Carlen, P. L.; Wortzman, G.; Holgate, R. C.; et al. Reversible cerebral atrophy in recently abstinent chronic alcoholics measured by computed tomography scans. *Science 200:* 1076–78, 1978.

40. Epstein, P. S.; Pisoni, V. D.; Fawcett, J. A. Alcoholism and cerebral atrophy. *Alcoholism: Clin. Exp. Res. 1:* 61–65, 1977.

41. Harvey, S. C. Hypnotics and Sedatives: Miscellaneous Agents. In Goodman, L. S.; Gilman, A. (eds.), *The Pharmacological Basis of Therapeutics.* New York: Macmillan, pp. 124–36, 1975.

42. Harvey, S. C. Hypnotics and Sedatives: The Barbiturates. In Goodman, L. S.; Gilman, A. (eds.), *The Pharmacological Basis of Therapeutics.* New York: Macmillan, pp. 102–23, 1975.

43. Shader, R. I.; Caine, E. D.; Meyer, R. E. Treatment of Dependence on Barbiturates and Sedative Hypnotics. In Shader, R. I. (ed.), *Manual of Psychiatric*

Therapeutics: Practical Psychopharmacology and Psychiatry. Boston: Little, Brown, 1975, pp. 195–202.

44. Hofmann, F. G. *A Handbook on Drug and Alcohol Abuse: The Biomedical Aspects.* New York: Oxford University Press, 1975, pp. 116–28.

45. Davis, J. M.; Benvenuto, J. A. Acute Reactions from Drug Abuse Problems. In Resnick, H. L. P.; Ruben, H. L. (eds.), *Emergency Psychiatric Care.* Bowie, Md.: Charles Press, 1975, pp. 81–101.

46. Liskow, B. Substance Induced and Substance Use Disorders: Barbiturates and Similarly Acting Sedative Hypnotics. In Greist, J. H.; Jefferson, J. W.; Spitzer, R. L. (eds.), *Treatment of Mental Disorders.* New York: Oxford University Press, 1982, pp. 62–77.

47. Wikler, A. Diagnosis and treatment of drug dependence of the barbiturate type. *Am. J. Psychiat. 125:* 758–65, 1968.

48. Berger, P. A.; Tinklenberg, J. R. Medical Management of the Drug Abuser. In Freeman, A. M.; Sack, R. L.; Berger, P. A. (eds.), *Psychiatry for the Primary Care Physician.* Baltimore: Williams & Wilkins, 1979, pp. 359–80.

49. Berger, P. A.; Tinklenberg, J. R. Treatment of Abusers of Alcohol and Other Addictive Drugs. In Barchas, J. D.; Berger, P. A.; Ciaranello, R. D. (eds.), *Psychopharmacology from Theory to Practice.* New York: Oxford University Press, 1977, pp. 355–85.

50. National Commission on Marijuana and Drug Abuse. *Drug Use in America: Problem in Perspective.* 2d report, 1973.

51. Greenblatt, D. J.; Shader, R. I. Psychotropic Drug Overdosage. In Shader, R. I. (ed.), *Manual of Psychiatric Therapeutics: Practical Psychiatry and Psychopharmacology.* Boston: Little, Brown, 1975, pp. 237–67.

52. Blachly, P. H. Management of the opiate abstinence syndrome. *Am. J. Psychiat. 122:* 742–44, 1966.

53. Mahander, R. A. The Management of the Narcotic Withdrawal Syndrome in the Neonate. In Bourne, P. G. (ed.), *A Treatment Manual for Acute Drug Abuse Emergencies.* Washington, D.C.: U.S. Government Printing Office, DHEW, 1974, pp. 27–28.

54. Berger, P. A.; Dunn, M. J. Substance Induced and Substance Use Disorders. In Greist, J. H.; Jefferson, J. W.; Spitzer, R. L. (eds.), *Treatment of Mental Disorders.* New York: Oxford University Press, 1982, pp. 78–142.

55. Peterson, R. C.; Stillman, R. C. *Cocaine 1977.* Washington, D.C.: U.S. Government Printing Office, *NIDA Research,* monograph no. 13, DHEW, 1977.

56. Ellinwood, E. H. Amphetamines/Anorectics. In Dupont, R. I.; Goldstein, A.; O'Donnell, J. (eds.), *Handbook on Drug Abuse.* Washington, D.C.: U.S. Government Printing Office, NIDA, DHEW, 1979, pp. 221–31.

57. Cohen, S. Inhalants. In Dupont, R. I.; Goldstein, A.; O'Donnell, J. (eds.), *Handbook on Drug Abuse.* Washington, D.C.: U.S. Government Printing Office, NIDA, DHEW, 1979, pp. 213–20.

58. Sharp, C. W.; Brehm, M. L. *Review of Inhalants: Euphoria to Dysfunction.*

Washington, D.C.: U.S. Government Printing Office, *NIDA Research,* monograph no. 15, DHEW, 1977.

59. Sigell, L. T.; Kapp, F. T.; Fusaro, G. A.; *et al.* Popping and snorting volatile nitrites: A current fad for getting high. *Am. J. Psychiat. 135:* 1216–18, 1978.

60. Jain, N. C.; Budd, R. D.; Budd, B. S. Growing abuse of phencyclidine: California "angel dust." *New Eng. J. Med. 297:* 673, 1977.

61. Showalter, C. V.; Thornton, W. E. The increasing abuse of phencyclidine. *Ill. Med. J. 151:* 387–89, 1977.

62. Pittel, S. M.; Oppedahl, M. C. The Enigma of PCP. In Dupont, R. I.; Goldstein, A.; O'Donnell, J. (eds.), *Handbook on Drug Abuse.* Washington, D.C.: U.S. Government Printing Office, NIDA, DHEW, 1979, pp. 249–54.

63. Peterson, R. C.; Stillman, R. D. *Phencyclidine (PCP) Abuse: An Appraisal.* Washington, D.C.: U.S. Government Printing Office, *NIDA Research,* monograph no. 21, DHEW, 1978.

64. Cohen, S. Angel dust. *Am. J. Psychiat. 238:* 515–16, 1977.

65. Harris, L. S. Cannabis: A Review of Progress. In Lipton, M. A.; DiMascio, A.; Killam, K. F. (eds.), *Psychopharmacology: A Generation of Progress.* New York: Raven Press, 1978, pp. 1565–74.

66. Meyer, R. E. Behavioral pharmacology of marijuana. In Lipton, M. A.; DiMascio, A.; Killam, K. F. (eds.), *Psychopharmacology: A Generation of Progress.* New York: Raven Press, 1978, pp. 1639–52.

67. Nicholi, A. M., Jr. The nontherapeutic use of psychoactive drugs. *New Eng. J. Med. 16:* 925–33, 1983.

68. *Marijuana and Health.* 2d Annual Report to Congress from the Secretary of Health, Education, and Welfare, 1972.

69. Scher, J. The marijuana habit. *JAMA 214:* 1120, 1970.

70. Grant, I.; Mohns, L.; Miller, M.; *et al.* A neuropsychological study of polydrug users. *Arch. Gen. Psychiat. 33:* 973–78, 1976.

71. Grant, I.; Judd, L. L. Neuropsychological and EEG disturbances in polydrug users. *Am. J. Psychiat. 133:* 1039–42, 1976.

72. Ludwig, A. M. Principles of Clinical Psychiatry. New York: The Free Press, 1980, p. 315.

CHAPTER 20

The Elderly Patient

Introduction

Compared to other age groups, the elderly are increasing more rapidly in numbers, have the highest prevalence of psychiatric illness, and are the most "underserved" psychiatrically. Aging involves anatomic and physiologic decline, which occurs to widely varying degrees among elderly individuals. For that reason, the aged are more likely than the young to have disease in multiple organ systems and are more vulnerable to iatrogenic (particularly drug-induced) illnesses. Among the commonest syndromes of the elderly are affective disorders (especially depression) and coarse brain diseases (particularly dementia and delirium). Despite the influence of the above factors, the prognosis for recovery for some of the chief psychiatric syndromes (e.g. mania, endogenous depression, some of the dementias, and deliria) and those of other branches of medicine is excellent, as the following case example illustrates.

An eighty-six-year-old retired widower was brought to the hospital by his son-in-law, because for several weeks he was continually crying and stating that he was a burden, that he was too old and had lived long enough, and that "if I had the guts, I'd jump off a roof." He had lost his appetite, and his clothing was becoming baggy. Although for years he had been awakening several times nightly to urinate, now when he first awoke he could not return to sleep. He also had an increased frequency of urination. He reported that his memory and his vision had not been as good as they used to be and that his left eye looked bloody (in the mirror) since he'd bumped his head into a cabinet several days previously.

Since he had had brain surgery at age sixty for reasons uncertain to him and his family, he had had weakness of the right hand and grand mal seizures, which were excellently controlled when he took his phenytoin properly. During the past six months he had been taking his phenytoin regularly and had had no seizures. At ages sixty-five and seventy-five he had been hospitalized and successfully treated with medication for severe depression.

The physical examination revealed a gaunt, bespectacled, cooperative man with an omega sign who cried continually, begged for relief of symptoms, and had suicidal ideation. He had a left subconjunctival hematoma, bilateral lens opacities, increased intraocular tension, and impaired vision for reading despite glasses. There was a nontender skin nodule on the left side of his nose. Cerumen partially occluded both ear canals, and systolic and diastolic murmurs were heard in the second intercostal space just to the right of the sternum. The prostate gland was enlarged. There was weakness of right hand grip. The minimental state score was 21/30, indicative of diffuse cognitive impairment. The EEG revealed left temporal slowing, and the EKG suggested an old healed myocardial infarction. The chest x-ray revealed right upper lobe calcification due to previous healed granulomatous disease.

The diagnoses were endogenous depression secondary to decreased frequency of epileptic seizures, subconjunctival hematoma secondary to trauma, cataracts and glaucoma, presbyopia, actinic keratosis of the skin over the nose, epilepsy and right hand flexion weakness secondary to brain surgery, asymptomatic aortic stenosis and regurgitation, old healed pulmonary tuberculosis and myocardial infarction, and benign prostatic hypertrophy.

On the second hospital day he had several grand mal seizures, and serum phenytoin levels were drawn and later found to be low. By the third hospital day his mood had returned to normal, and his appetite and sleep improved. Apparently the resolution of his depression was due to the spontaneous seizures. Therapeutic blood levels of phenytoin could be maintained at his prehospital dose, and he had no more seizures. His subconjunctival hematoma resolved spontaneously. Intraocular pressure was reduced by timolor maleate eye drops, and his reading vision was improved by prescription for stronger glasses. He successfully underwent a transurethral prostatic resection, and his urinary tract symptoms almost completely disappeared. Soon afterward he was discharged home and was most grateful for the care he had received.

The principles of diagnosis and treatment of the elderly are identical to those of the young, but the physician must be more cautious in his medical therapeutics lest he cause or intensify illness. The rest of this chapter is devoted to elaborating upon those generalizations.

The Psychiatrically "Underserved" Elderly

In 1979 there were 23 million (10 percent of the population) Americans over sixty-five. By 2030 they will constitute 20 percent of our population (1). This will greatly increase the need for psychiatric services, for the probability of developing mental illness increases steeply after middle age (2). Between 1904 and 1950 the number of people fifty-five or older increased fourfold, but their first admissions to psychiatric facilities increased ninefold (2).

The elderly are a psychiatrically underserved group. Of 30,000 admissions to one teaching hospital, 17 percent were over seventy, but only 9.7 percent of referrals for psychiatric consultations were in this group (3). This lack of referral was not because the patients were psychiatrically well. In another study 80 percent of the cognitive disorders of elderly patients were not identified by general practitioners (4). Other studies (5) show that physicians of all specialties underdiagnose cognitive dysfunctions. Ouslander (6) writes: "On medical and surgical services, little time and effort is placed on meaningful mental status examinations."

Lack of physician awareness about cognitive dysfunction in the elderly is only one factor. All studies of geriatric populations demonstrate that the elderly underutilize psychiatric facilities (7–12). Another problem is physician bias against treating old people (1). The intern "hero" of one popular novel (13) puts it this way: "For before the House of God, I had loved old people. Now they were no longer old people, they were gomers, and I did not, I could not, love them, any more . . . .Gomer is an acronym: Get Out of My Emergency Room—it's what you want to say when one's sent in from the nursing home at 3 a.m." Contributing to this are the correct perception that geriatric patients are more likely to have disease in multiple systems (14) and the usually incorrect notion that the prognosis for recovery of the aging for given psychiatric (15, 16) and systemic illnesses (17, 18) is poorer than that for younger people. One of our students stated that she wanted to enter a specialty "in which you cured people," and ruled out "geriatrics" as a result. When told that lots of illnesses in the elderly were curable, she responded by saying "being old is a terminal illness."

In a questionnaire mailed to psychiatrists case studies were presented in which all the details were the same except for the patient's age. When the case study described an elderly patient, the psychiatrists were more likely to regard the prognosis as poor and to treat the patient differently (19).

Undertreatment occurs in private office practice as well. A national survey of psychiatrists in private practice revealed that only 4 percent of the patients were over sixty (9). Freud recommended that patients over fifty not be psychoanalyzed because he thought the "egos" of the elderly are too "rigid" (20) to benefit from psychotherapy. That the elderly are less able to afford out-of-pocket fees also limits the treatments available to them.

The 1980 Rand Report (21) noted a need for 1,130 geriatric psychiatrists, a number far different from the seventeen board-certified psychiatrists identified as specialists in geropsychiatry. While there is a need for research and teaching in geropsychiatry, it would be a mistake to identify the field as being so specialized that treatment of the elderly should be excluded from the mainstream of psychiatric practice. Despite the expanding base of information about aging and the particular concerns that must be addressed in treating the elderly, the principles of diagnosis and treatment for the psychiatric syndromes of the aged are the same as for the young.

The Biology and Pathophysiology of Aging

The exact nature of aging is unknown. There are two perspectives on the subject:

1. There is a genotype "programmed into the cells" so that specific disease is not required to cause cell death, which will occur after a fixed and predetermined number of cell replications. Evidence for this comes from the work of Hayflick and Moorhead (22), who demonstrated that human fibroblast cells, both in vivo and in vitro, underwent a fixed number of replications, regardless of environmental events.

2. Aging is the product of events such as DNA damage, mutation, formation of free radicals, formation of cross-linkages between molecules, wear and tear, accumulation of toxic metabolites, and impaired supply of nutrients (23). Some combination of these factors probably determines the aging of the individual.

Because of public health and other medical interventions life expectancy has greatly increased. In the late eighteenth century old age began in the thirties and forties. Children who lived to age five survived to thirty-eight or thirty-nine (24). However, there is no evidence that the aging process itself, and hence the life span, has been altered. Adams and Victor (25) write: "Since biblical times, when human beings were allotted three score and ten years, human life has not lengthened greatly."

Aging (senescence) involves decline in physiologic function as the years progress. From individual to individual and from organ to organ in each individual, the rate of decline varies considerably. For almost every test of systemic health or brain functioning, the variability is significantly greater among groups of old people than among groups of young people (26–28). Thus many individuals can function outstandingly to advanced ages. Slater and Roth (2) list Leonardo, Titian, Dürer, Michelangelo, Voltaire, Goethe, Verdi, Renoir, and Picasso as examples of "artistic genius that continued to flower in old age." Just recently, a sixty-five-year-old man swam the English Channel (29).

TABLE 20-1 Deterioration with Age

PHYSICAL CHARACTERISTIC	PERCENTAGE DETERIORATION FROM AGE 30 TO AGE 75
Number of taste buds	64
Power of hand grip	45
Vital capacity	44
Number of kidney glomeruli	44
Number of fibers in nerves	37
Glomerular filtration rate	31
Maximum rate of work	30
Resting cardiac output	30
Blood flow to brain	20
Total body water content	18
Basal metabolic rate	16
Body weight in men	12
Brain weight	10

SOURCE: [Modified from] Table 1, "Physiologic and Anatomic Deterioration with Age," in "The Physiology of Aging" by N. Shock. *Scientific American* (January 1962), p. 101. Copyright © 1962 by Scientific American, Inc. All rights reserved.

For the group of elderly as a whole, however, there is a distinct anatomic and physiologic decline. Table 20-1 lists these changes (30). In addition to the table list there are shortened stature, stooped posture,* depigmentation and loss of hair, wrinkling of skin, decrease in muscle mass and strength, slowing of movements and halting of gait, redistribution of fat, loss of teeth, altered facial architecture, loss of high-frequency hearing, decrease of visual acuity, and decalcification of bones (31–33). There is a decrease in total number of cells in the body (34). Systolic blood pressure increases (35). Neuropathological changes include decrease in number of dendrites, neurofibrillary degeneration, granulovascular degeneration, lipofuscin accumulation, lewy bodies, hirano bodies, senile plaques, amyloid deposits, shrinkage of dendritic arbor, decrease of extracellular space, corpora amylacea, and myelin remodeling of the glia (25).

There is a decrease in the total sleep time (36) and in the amount of rapid eye movement sleep, and stage four sleep almost disappears (37). There is EEG slowing in the alpha, delta, and beta frequencies. Cerebral blood flow is harder to maintain in the presence of drops in blood pressure, so that fainting and consequent injury are more likely (38). There are a dramatic decrease in estrogen levels and subtle changes in the levels of other hormones. There is decreased responsivity of the immune system (35). Pain and fever are less effective warning signals of disease. Thus silent myocardial infarctions and infections without fever occur and may be missed (14).

---

*Shortened stature and stooped posture may be avoided in old age if a person makes a lifetime habit of eating foods with a high calcium content.

There is probably a reduction of biogenic amine neurotransmitters in the brain and spinal cord, including a decreased supply of choline, choline acetyl transferase, and dopamine (15, 39–42). The amount of monoamine oxidase increases in the brain, which probably contributes to the diminution of dopamine and other neurotransmitters (43). There is an increase in the level of cerebrospinal fluid lactate (44). Plasma norepinephrine levels increase both at rest and in response to stress (45).

During stressful learning tasks the elderly have larger increases in free fatty acids, which do not peak until forty-five minutes after completion of the task. By contrast, younger individuals have only a slight increase in free fatty acid levels in the early stages of learning (26). According to Wilkie *et al.*, difficulty in learning among the aged is associated with heightened autonomic nervous system activity secondary to increased neuroendocrine sensitivity in target organs (26). This could contribute to the severity of the "catastrophic response" of some patients confronted with cognitive deficits. Propanolol, which reduces autonomic nervous system end organ activity, improved learning in one sample of old people (46). (It should be noted, however, that propanolol can also produce delirium.) Creativity involving truly inventive solutions to problems, in contrast to applying previously used strategies, declines with age (47). However, memory impairment is not always present (5).

The elderly are vulnerable to first occurrence and recurrence of most diseases that affect younger adults and have a higher frequency of some conditions, many of which are serious or fatal. The latter include cerebral arteriosclerosis and infarction, arteriosclerotic heart disease, certain cancers, Parkinson's disease, and primary degenerative dementia. They are more likely to have disease in multiple systems (14). Because of this, there can be an additive effect, so that in 26 percent of the autopsies of one sample of elderly decedents, in no organ system was there found a disease of sufficient severity that could itself account for the patient's death in a younger person (47). The authors of that study therefore attributed these deaths to "aging itself" (48).

Nevertheless, despite these many signs of decline the diseases that are curable in younger people are usually curable in the elderly. One example in the field of internal medicine is that, excluding other causes of death, survival rates for cancers are as high for the elderly as for the young (17). This also applies to psychiatric illnesses (e.g. in mania, major depression, and many deliria) that are curable in the young. In fact, first episodes of mania in the elderly were found to be less severe than for younger counterparts, and the recurrence rate is lower (15). However, because of the abovementioned physiologic differences between old and young a number of precautions must be taken, and vigilance must be greater. This is most important in the area of psychopharmacology.

Psychopharmacology

Among the most important issues in the care of elderly is the use of medication. The elderly are more likely to receive drugs, including psychotropic
drugs, to receive multiple drugs, to develop drug toxicity, and to have unfavorable drug interactions. In a study of 242 elderly people in one community, only 2.5 percent reported having no illness at all, and only 7.4 percent were not under the care of a physician (49). These individuals were
using a total of 301 types of medications, 60 percent by prescription, with 83
percent of them taking two to six drugs and 14 percent seven to fifteen drugs.
In this same study misuse of medications due to physician misunderstanding
of drug interactions was found in 14 percent (49). Prescriptions for one sample of aged were 35–40 percent for anxiolytics, neuroleptics, sedatives, or
combinations of these categories (50). The use of psychotropic drugs is increasing among the elderly (51). In a sample of patients in skilled nursing
homes, 47 percent were receiving tranquilizers, 35 percent sedative–hypnotics, and 8.5 percent antidepressants; 25 percent were taking more than
one tranquilizing medication (50). The depressed elderly are heavy users of
all medications, especially psychotropics: 48 percent of one survey of
depressed elderly in the community took psychotropic medications (52). Approximately 50 percent of the elderly who use psychotropic drugs feel that
they cannot perform daily activities unless they use a drug (53). One-third of
medically ill patients in a general hospital receive at least one psychotropic
drug (54, 55). Some geriatric tonics contain alcohol, which can cause sedation (56).

This high frequency of use of medication is particularly important
because the elderly are less able to metabolize and eliminate medicines,
leading to an increased risk of side effects for a given dose. And for some
medications (e.g. diazepam and nitrazepam) there is greater toxicity (e.g.
depression of the central nervous system) at any plasma level as well as for
any dose (57). Such effects are in large part due to a combination of
diminished hepatic blood flow (resulting from decreased cardiac output),
decreased hepatic metabolism, reduced plasma albumen causing larger frac-
tions of unmetabolized drug, increased proportion of body fat causing
greater drug retention, and reduced renal clearance of drugs (57, 58).
However, unless the patient is taking anticholinergic drugs or has a disease
affecting intestinal absorption, the absorption of medications from the gut
occurs as readily in the elderly as in the young (58–60).

Among the most serious side effects is diminished cognitive function,
most prominent in the nondominant hemisphere, and often manifested by
delirium or dementia. The worst offenders include anxiolytics, sedatives,
hypnotics (26), anticholinergics, and antihypertensives, although the list of
drugs capable of producing behavioral changes is enormous. For certain an-

tihypertensives such as reserpine and alphamethyldopa, there is a serious risk of depression.

One study (61) reported impaired cognition in 35 percent of patients over sixty who were taking antidepressants. Another study (62) reported that the abnormal behavior of 16 percent of 236 patients receiving psychotropic drugs before admission to a geropsychiatric hospital unit was caused by side effects of the drugs. Straker (63) writes: "Clinicians in the geriatric field have all shared the experience of seeing a confused, demented older patient rapidly clear to a normal sensorium when all drug intake was stopped." The following is such an example:

An eighty-four-year-old man had never experienced any psychiatric difficulty until he went to his family doctor for back pain, which had resulted from a small spontaneous compression fracture of a lumbar vertebra. The patient was instructed to rest and given prescriptions for meprobamate, ibuprofen, and acetaminophen with codeine for the pain. During the following two weeks, the patient developed the belief that the Russians had invaded his radio and were controlling its musical programs, and frequently called for his (deceased) daughter to enter his room. He stopped eating, was agitated and pacing, became totally sleepless, cried, spoke of suicide, and was disoriented to time and place. A diagnosis of drug-induced delirium was made, all medications were discontinued, and his mental status gradually improved to normal within the next three weeks.

Because of the altered physiology of aging, when abnormal behavior does occur as a side effect, it is more likely to last longer once the drug is discontinued or the dose reduced. For example, digoxin-induced delirium often lasts for several days after digoxin is discontinued (64). In some cases (e.g. the improper monitoring of insulin) the drug-induced psychopathology can be permanent, or even a harbinger of the patient's death. Behavioral toxicity is but one type of serious drug toxicity to which the elderly are more prone. Postural hypotension is more likely and is particularly common with the use of low-potency neuroleptics, tricyclic antidepressants, and MAOIs. Concomitantly prescribed diuretics, nitrates, and low-salt diets can all enhance this effect (65). Postural hypotension often leads to falls, which sometimes produce hip fractures or subdural hematomas.

Tricyclic antidepressants can precipitate congestive heart failure (65, 66). Tricyclic antidepressants, neuroleptics, and lithium can produce cardiac arrhythmias. For the elderly, lithium-induced EKG changes are more common than for the young (67). Tardive dyskinesia is more likely to occur when neuroleptics are first prescribed for elderly persons (68), and is far more common in the elderly, because many elderly have had years of exposure to neuroleptics. Urinary and fecal incontinence, more common in the elderly to begin with, particularly in the demented elderly (the majority of incontinent patients have cognitive impairment and 45 percent are demented) (69), can be caused or aggravated by laxatives, which are often routinely prescribed without good indication (69).

Drug interactions are an important consideration. Tricyclic antidepressants and neuroleptics can negate the antihypertensive effect of guanethidine. Indomethacin increases lithium retention, which can cause severe lithium toxicity (70). Theophylline enhances the renal excretion of lithium, and unless these two agents are properly titrated the lithium can be rendered ineffective (71). Antacids containing aluminum, magnesium, and calcium can decrease the absorption of benzodiazepines and neuroleptics (72). In one nursing home survey (72), antacids combined with phenothazines accounted for 15 percent of all drug combinations. Milk of magnesia decreases the absorption and efficacy of all psychotropic drugs (73).

Psychopathology

The most common major psychiatric disorders of old age are depression (of all types) and coarse brain syndromes. Of the coarse disorders, dementia and delirium are both the most common and the most severe. The community prevalence (95 percent of the elderly live outside of institutions) of all types of depression (major depression, dysthymic disorder, mourning reaction, organic affective disorder) is between 11 and 44 percent, depending upon the source (74). Again depending on source, the rates of depression among the hospitalized elderly are between 12 and 68 percent (74). The prevalence of depression in the elderly is even higher in people with systemic illness (74). These figures are sufficiently high that one author (15) wrote, "Every physician suspecting early dementia in a patient would do well to reflect for a moment on the simple statistical fact that the patient is twice as likely to be depressed as demented" (75).

As is the case for all psychiatric syndromes, criteria for the diagnosis of depression are the same for the elderly as for the young. It should be noted, however, that cognitive dysfunction secondary to depression ("pseudodementia") is more common among the elderly (76), that there is a statistical trend toward higher rates of cortisol secretion and dexamethasone nonsuppression among older melancholic patients (77, 78), and that unrealistic concerns about physical health are more frequent among the elderly depressed (79–81). In one sample 64 percent of depressed aged patients had "physically unjustified bodily complaints, most frequently involving the GI tract, head and cardiovascular system" (81).

Endogenous depression is a common manifestation of coarse brain disease. Usually, if the underlying coarse disease is cured, the depression will remit. On occasion, when the underlying coarse process remits, the depression "takes on a life of its own" and must be treated like any endogenous depression (15). When the coarse disease is incurable, the depression can still be treated successfully (15). The treatment of melancholia has already been discussed in Chapter 11 and will be touched upon later in this chapter.

The combination of being old and depressed (especially with major depression) is highly associated with suicide. The odds are yet higher when the patient has a systemic illness. In one study 85 percent of those over sixty who committed suicide had had an active systemic illness, and in 70 percent of those cases the illness contributed to the suicide (82). A suicide attempt by an older person is much more likely to be fatal than an attempt by a younger person (83). For women, suicide rate (82) and prevalence of depression (34, 85) peak and reach a plateau in middle age, and the plateau persists during the senium (82). For men the suicide rates continue to rise with age, although the steepness of the rise in suicide rates in males varies greatly from country to country (86). In fact, in Finland the suicide rate drops in very old age (86).

The majority of severe depressions in the elderly are relapses, although new cases of depression or mania may occur over the age of seventy-five (87). The ratio of depressed to manic episodes increases with age, with the "unipolar" elderly being much more numerous than the "bipolar" elderly (87). Attacks of mania or hypomania constitute about 5–10 percent of affective disorders in old age (2). In approximately half of the cases of mania this is a recurrence of illness that had already been manifest earlier. In the other half the first attack occurred in the senium (2). Lehmann (15) reported a case where the onset was at seventy-two. The prognosis for mania in the elderly is very good if the patient is not neurologically impaired or a drug abuser (88). In the latter two categories, patients tend to develop chronic mania (88).

Coarse brain diseases, particularly dementia and delirium, are also extremely common in the elderly. Rates of organic mental syndromes are twice as high in those seventy-five or over as in those between sixty-five and seventy-five (83). For dementia specifically, the population prevalence is under 3 percent between the ages of sixty-five and sixty-nine, and greater than 20 percent over the age of eighty (83). Forty percent of elderly residents and two-thirds of elderly admissions at long-stay psychiatric facilities have a primary diagnosis of dementia (83). And for every individual with severely disabling dementia in an institution, there are two living in the community (83). The prevalence rates for delirium are not known (89).

Dementia no longer need be associated with progressive deterioration with no hope of recovery. In one sample of one hundred patients with recent onset of dementia, 15–20 percent may be caused by remediable conditions (83, 90, 91). Of this 15–20 percent, one-third had depressive "pseudodementia," one-fourth had normal-pressure hydrocephalus, one-fifth had intracranial mass lesions, and one-half of the rest had drug-related disorders (90, 91). The same drugs that cause delirium (see Chapter 10) can cause dementia (62). Of those patients who do not recover from dementia, 55 percent have primary degenerative dementia, 24 percent have multi-infarct dementia, and the rest have a variety of other disorders (92). Physicians often miss the diagnosis of dementia when the patient is compliant (93, 94). Our research (94) suggests that routine cognitive screening is much more likely to detect cognitive abnormalities in the elderly than in the young.

Besides the common causes listed above, there are other afflictions of the elderly that cause dementia. Compared to an age-matched population, Parkinson's disease (common in the aged) is more likely to be associated with dementia (95). The frequency of dementia in Parkinson's disease is between 22 and 40 percent (95, 96). Creutzfeld–Jakob's disease, a rare disorder (2 to 7 per 100,000 is the prevalence) usually begins between fifty and sixty, and the patient usually does not survive to sixty-five. However, the condition can have a later onset; one patient developed the condition at seventy (97). Huntington's chorea, the prevalence of which is also 2 to 7 cases per 100,000, usually begins at about age forty, but a case has been recorded with onset at seventy (98).

Besides medication, the commonest precipitants of delirium in the medically ill elderly are fever, dehydration, decreased cardiac output, electrolyte imbalance, and hypoxia (99). In cases where the patient already has comprised cerebral functioning, the very processes of admission to the hospital (100), extensive laboratory testing (101), or placement in a single hospital room (102) can precipitate delirium or intensify dementia. Delirium can be superimposed upon dementia, and this is more likely in the elderly.

Besides affective disorder and coarse brain disease, other conditions are also seen. Alcoholism often persists into the senium, and 10 percent of alcoholics reportedly have a late onset (103). Late-onset alcoholism appears to be rare unless associated with other psychiatric illness. Significant numbers of young opiate addicts persist with their addictions into old age. One study identified forty-four opiate abusers age fifty and older. Half were employed, had no family to support, and maintained a small habit (104).

Not much is known about anxiety disorders in the elderly. Such disorders certainly can persist into old age, but it is not known whether there is a general tendency for these conditions to intensify, to stay the same in severity, or to decrease in old age. The onset of a severe anxiety disorder, or of any psychiatric illness for that matter, in an old person warrants a careful search for coarse brain disease or systemic illness. When cognitive functioning, motor coordination, hearing or vision has become impaired, and the elderly person is aware of this, anxiety associated with avoidance of risky tasks such as driving a car may represent good judgment and should not be viewed as phobic. In some sociopaths the frequency of antisocial behavior is reported to diminish.

Exhibitionism, genital play with children, and sexual assault of young people account for more than 12 percent of the offenses for which old people are prosecuted (2). Homosexual and heterosexual assaults against adults are less common (2). Cerebral degeneration is responsible for some of these misdemeanors, but in the majority of cases cognitive dysfunction is absent (2). Although violence committed by the elderly is less frequent than by the young, it does occur. In one sample the commonest diagnoses among hospitalized violent geriatric patients were, in order of frequency, late paraphrenia, coarse brain disease of unspecified type, bipolar illness (manic), senile dementia, and alcoholic dementia (105).

Several authors (2, 106) have described a syndrome called late paraphrenia, characterized by onset in the senium of hallucinations or delusions with relatively good cognitive function and no evidence for coarse brain disease. It is more common in women than in men, and accounts for 8–9 percent of all female first admissions in Great Britain over the age of sixty-five. Formal thought disorder occurs in 30 percent of cases. Life expectancy is the same as for the general population of elderly (2).

Primary Prevention

Primary prevention efforts during youth and adulthood are relevant to geriatric dementia and delirium. Attention to diet; avoidance of smoking, heavy drinking, and drug abuse; regular exercise; and proper treatment of hypertension could contribute to avoiding such conditions as buccolingual, respiratory, and other cancers; arteriosclerotic dementias; cirrhosis of the liver; and alcoholic dementias.

Childhood and old age are the two age groups where periodic examinations, even when the patient is apparently well, are unarguably in order. Elderly patients and their families are sometimes prone to attributing treatable disabilities to irreversible effects of age or withholding information about symptoms for fear that an examination will reveal something ominous (1). Relatively simple interventions arising from such checkups, such as the removal of cerumen from an ear canal, can have a significant effect on the patient's behavior.

Care of the Hospitalized Elderly Patient

EVALUATION

Given the elderly patient's greater vulnerability to illness in all systems, the thoroughness of the history and physical examination has particular significance. If the patient's cognitive functioning or cooperativeness is such that the history is incomplete, a history from a relative, a friend, or a landlady may be invaluable. A telephone call to another physician who has cared for the patient may help. Old medical records should be reviewed. The fact that the patient may have recently been examined by a physician in another specialty should not deter the psychiatrist from performing his own physical examination and referring the patient for consultation if a finding is not readily explainable.

GENERAL MANAGEMENT ON THE PSYCHIATRIC UNIT

Psychogeriatric Units

Some hospitals have psychogeriatric units. Use of such units, as compared to assignment of patients to general psychiatric wards, has not been studied sufficiently to determine their efficacy. One of our colleagues (107) noted that at one large Veteran's Administration hospital with a large number of elderly and chronically ill patients, frail elderly patients were the most prone to being injured by other patients. As a result a separate unit was established for frail geriatric patients. The impression was that this significantly reduced the number of such injuries. If a psychogeriatric unit is established, it must be with an eye to the continued availability of well-trained nurses and physicians who are enthusiastic about the care of such patients. This requires ongoing in-service teaching of psychogeriatrics, and physician interest in teaching and research in psychogeriatrics. Problems with establishing such units may include staff cynicism and bias about work with old patients.

Room Assignments

Patients should not automatically be assigned to private rooms, even when they are affordable. For patients who prefer sharing a room with others or who have significant cognitive impairment, semiprivate arrangements may be preferable.

Laboratory Testing

Regardless of the patient's age, the scheduling of laboratory tests requires some planning. The object is to be thorough and safe, to minimize delay, to avoid unnecessary phlebotomies and trips to laboratories, and to reduce waiting times in unfamiliar locations. All procedures should be discussed with the patient to the extent that he can comprehend. When a test is scheduled in the hospital laboratory, a patient with significant cognitive dysfunction should be accompanied by a staff member.

General Care

Although there should be some times each day when the patient can sit and rest, every effort should be made to reduce isolation and boredom. If the patient wears glasses or a hearing aid, he should also use these in the hospital. (These should be placed in the same location every night.) If he can read and concentrate sufficiently, he should have access to favorite newspapers, magazines, or books. If reading is impossible, staff should offer to read newspaper or magazine articles. Television and radio should be available. When the patient is watching television, his chair should be located to give him a good view of the screen. In preference to his spending long periods of time alone in his room, he could be seated in a chair near the nurses' station or another orderly high-traffic area.

In general visiting by family and close friends who are aware of the patient's condition and are not perceived by him as a nuisance should be encouraged. Visits by chaplains and hospital volunteers may be helpful. Hospital staff should regularly engage the patient in conversation, encouraging discussion of subjects about which the patient is interested. This may range from asking the patient what he would be doing if he were not ill to listening while he talks about the past or about death and dying.

A daily program of activities, geared to the patient's level of functioning, should be established by the nursing staff and by occupational and recreational therapists. An in-hospital "field trip," such as to the cafeteria or kitchen, may provide a welcome change of scenery for long-term patients. Giving the patient a regular task that he can manage with some success (even if it is folding towels or watering plants) is often helpful, especially when coupled with praise for these accomplishments.

Allowances must be made for cognitive and other disabilities. Compared to the younger patient, extra nursing time will usually need to be allotted. Often elderly patients need assistance in eating, washing, dressing, and bathing. When the patient has to be fed by another person, it may be useful to have him hold a piece of bread in one hand to give him a sense of helping with the meal.

Staff should usually sit close to the patient. If he has a hearing problem, staff should sit face to face and speak slowly and loudly. The staff should be prepared to explain instructions or answer the same questions multiple times.

A paper bag for waste should be taped to the patient's bed. Dentures should never be placed in a tissue or napkin; they could be lost or, if small, choked upon. If restraints are ever needed, body jackets are preferable. Chest and waist straps are easier to put in place but are often physically irritating.

Although these allowances will often need to be made for disabilities, the patient should always be accorded the highest degree of respect. Calling the patient by his first name (unless he asks you to do so), using phrases like "good boy," or talking in a condescending manner is inexcusable.

Medical Treatments

As a rule treatments indicated for a younger person are also indicated for an elderly one. However, in most cases the starting doses of psychoactive (and almost all other) medications should be one-third (15) to two-thirds the usual adult starting dose; dosage increments will usually be lower than for younger patients. On occasion, however, very high doses may eventually be needed. For example, a sixty-five-year-old 135-pound man, with mania and chronic obstructive lung disease, had to receive 2,700 mg. of lithium daily to achieve therapeutic blood levels, as he was simultaneously receiving theophylline for his pulmonary condition (71). Combinations of psychotropic drugs should be avoided wherever possible. Drugs that impair alertness should be avoided if possible and, if prescribed, given with caution. Laxatives and antacids should not be prescribed routinely; there must be good indication.

Major Depression

The treatment of choice for major depression in the elderly is ECT. For this condition it is more effective and safer (108) than tricyclic antidepressants or lithium. It will usually alleviate pseudodementia associated with major depression in the elderly. It is the treatment of choice for suicidal major depression in an ICU or CCU and should be administered to the patient in the ICU or CCU itself (64). It can also be safely given to patients with pacemakers (109, 110). Nevertheless, certain precautions must be taken in giving ECT to an elderly patient. One should usually stop treatments whenever full remission of an acute episode has occurred, rather than necessarily completing a "routine course" of six treatments. Monitoring of cognitive functioning with brief screening tests may identify newly developed cognitive dysfunction that may be a predictor of a prolonged post-ECT delirium. The latter syndrome is more common in the elderly. Maintenance ECT can be given following remission of an episode of major depression, just as in younger adults.

If the patient has major depression and refuses ECT, antidepressants or lithium could be used, but with caution. The newer antidepressants (such as trazodine, nomifensine, and mianserin) are reported to have less cardiotoxicity and fewer anticholinergic side effects than the tricyclics. Antidepressants and lithium are contraindicated in patients with active heart disease. If lithium is prescribed, serum levels should be checked regularly.

Mania

The treatment of choice for mania is lithium carbonate, regardless of the patient's age. Following remission of a manic episode, prophylactic lithium should be given for three to six months. Continued use of lithium after that depends upon the frequency of prior manic and depressive episodes. If such episodes occurred every several years or more frequently, continued use of lithium would be indicated.

If the patient's mania manifests as catatonic stupor, ECT is the treatment of choice. If the patient develops severe excitement, ECT or a neuroleptic such as haloperidol must be used initially. ECT is the treatment of choice of an acute manic patient in an ICU/CCU and should be administered on the unit (64). ECT is preferable to lithium when a manic patient must be on a low-salt diet, must take diuretics, or must receive a medication (such as theophylline or indomethacin) that creates major problems when used in combination with lithium.

Schizophrenia

For decades schizophrenia has been overdiagnosed, and neuroleptics have consequently been overprescribed. One consequence has been that there is a large cohort of elderly who carry the diagnosis of schizophrenia and the long-term effects of treatment with neuroleptics. One such effect is tardive dyskinesia. Whether long-term neuroleptic use produces additional brain dysfunction is uncertain, but it is quite likely. Additional cortical dysfunction could, in turn, increase the likelihood of a diagnosis of schizophrenia in a patient for whom it was never the correct diagnosis.

For this reason the diagnosis of schizophrenia in an elderly patient needs to be reviewed. Regardless of diagnosis, if the patient has been taking neuroleptics for years and his situation has stabilized, an attempt should be made to withdraw the neuroleptics gradually within several weeks. When patients have for at least several months been receiving anticholinergic antiparkinson agents for extrapyramidal side effects of neuroleptics, they can be discontinued abruptly with only a small risk of relapse of extrapyramidal symptoms.

Reactive Depressions

The treatments of choice for dysthymia, MAOIs or cognitive psychotherapy, are the same for the elderly as for the young. While starting dosages of MAOIs must be lower for the elderly, it should be noted that the elderly have lower brain catecholamine levels, and because of this it has even been suggested (111) that they could benefit from MAOIs more than the young. Many patients with reactive depression can be treated outside the hospital.

Anxiety Disorders

Late onset of panic attacks or generalized anxiety require, as stated before, a careful search for systemic illness or coarse brain disease. In cases where the diagnosis of panic disorder, agoraphobia, or obsessive–compulsive disorder is clear, treatment (MAOIs, imipramine, or propanolol) is the same as for younger people. For animal or situational phobias (other than agoraphobia) behavior modification is the treatment of choice. For panic disorder and situational phobias the patient can usually be treated outside of the hospital.

Late Paraphrenia

Late paraphrenia, a term more prevalent in the British literature, usually refers to a first-episode delusional psychosis developing after age sixty to sixty-five, characterized by a broad affect; an intense mood of anxiety, suspiciousness, irritability, euphoria, or sadness; systematized delusional ideas; and signs of cognitive dysfunction. This condition more frequently affects women than men and appears to be a functional rather than a structural morbid process, unrelated to senile or atherosclerotic dementia. It is extremely responsive to convulsive treatment. Because of complicating nutritional imbalance and systemic illness in people in this age group, their particular adverse sensitivity to psychotropic drugs, and their high death rate during chronic hospitalization, ECT, the most effective and safest therapeutic strategy (112), can be lifesaving.

Coarse Brain Diseases

As stated before, 20 percent of cases of dementia and many cases of delirium are curable (83, 90, 91). These include cases of major depression, drug toxicity, vitamin deficiency, Wernicke–Korsakoff syndrome (15–20 percent of cases fully recover) (83, 90, 91), normal pressure hydrocephalus, bacterial and viral infections, fluid and electrolyte imbalance, endocrine disorders, head injuries due to falls, some brain tumors (1), and transient ischemic attacks due to carotid artery occulsion. Laboratory diagnostic tests for most of these conditions are reported in the section on delirium in Chapter 18. The primary treatments of these conditions are listed in Table 20–2.

It should be apparent from Table 20–2 that some of the dementias, once diagnosed, will require that the psychiatrist obtain medical or surgical con-

TABLE 20-2 Treatments of Curable Causes of Dementia

CONDITION	TREATMENT
1. Major depression with pseudodementia	1. ECT (second choice: antidepressants or lithium)
2. Drug toxicity	2. Remove offending drug, give antidote if one exists
3. Vitamin deficiency	3. Replacement of deficient vitamin
a. "Megaloblastic madness" due to B_{12} or folic acid deficiency	a. Vitamin B_{12} or folic acid
b. Pellagra	b. Niacin
c. Beriberi or Wernicke–Korsakoff syndrome	c. Thiamine hydrochloride
4. Normal pressure hydrocephalus	4. Surgical shunting
5. Bacterial infections	5. Antibiotics following obtaining of cultures
6. Endocrine disorders	6.
a. Hypothyroidism	a. Levothyroxine (T_4)
b. Hyperthyroidism	b. Depending on cause, may include surgery, methimazole, propylthiouracil, I^{131} or other treatments
c. Hypoglycemia	c. Glucose; treat underlying cause
d. Diabetic ketoacidosis	d. Insulin, fluid and electrolyte replacement
e. Addison's disease	e. Cortisol, fluid and electrolyte management if needed, treat underlying cause
f. Cushing's disease	f. Treat underlying cause
g. Hypoparathyroidism	g. Calcium, vitamin D
7. Electrolyte imbalance	7. Treat underlying cause; replace deficient electrolytes or hydrate as needed
8. Epidural or subdural hematoma	8. Surgical evacuation
9. Brain tumor	9. Neurosurgical removal (if operable) or irradiation
10. Transient ischemic attacks due to carotid occlusion	10. Carotid endarterectomy or aspirin

sultation and possible transfer to a medical or surgical ward. When there is no antidote (e.g. physostigmine for anticholinergic toxicity) for drug toxicity, as is often the case, the physician may need to wait for as long as several days or weeks for the condition to clear fully. However, when the diagnosis of drug toxicity is correct and the offending drug is removed or the dosage markedly reduced, the physician should expect progressive improvement (be it gradual or rapid) in the patient's condition.

As stated before, by far the most common incurable cause of dementia is primary degenerative dementia (Alzheimer's–senile brain disease). Despite its incurability there is evidence (113) that the use of Hydergine (dihydroergotoxine mesylate), an ergot derivative, can improve cognitive functioning to some degree in some patients. One recent report (114) states that intravenous physostigmine can do the same on a transient basis, but at this time that finding cannot be applied to clinical practice. There is no solid evidence that lecithin, choline, metrazole, hyperbaric oxygen, vasopressin, or procaine is effective in reducing cognitive dysfunction or improving general health of patients with primary degenerative dementia (113).

The general ward management of the demented patient is the same as that for the delirious patient, discussed in Chapter 18.

References

1. Butler, R. Overview of Aging. In Usdin, G. (ed.), *Aging: The Process and the People*. New York: Brunner/Mazel, 1978, pp. 1–19.

2. Slater, E.; Roth, M. *Mayer-Gross' Clinical Psychiatry*. New York: Oxford University Press, 1971, p. 537.

3. Shevitz, S. A.; Silberfarb, P. M.; Lipowski, Z. J. Psychiatric consultations in a general hospital: A report on 1000 referrals. *Dis. Nerv. Syst. 37:* 295–300, 1976.

4. Williamson, J.; Stokoe, I. H.; Gray, S.; *et al.* Old people at home: Their unreported needs. *Lancet 1:* 1117–20, 1964.

5. Folstein, M.; Rabins, P. Psychiatric evaluation of the elderly patient. *Primary Care 6:* 609–20, 1979.

6. Ouslander, J. G. Illness and Psychopathology in the Elderly. In Jarvik, L. (ed.), *Psychiatric Clinics of North America: Aging*, 1982, pp. 145–59.

7. Stever, J. Psychotherapy with the Elderly. In Jarvik, L. (ed.), *Psychiatric Clinics of North America: Aging*, 1979, pp. 199–213.

8. Blank, M. L. Raising the age barrier to psychotherapy. *Geriatrics 29:* 141, 1974.

9. Marmor, J. *Psychiatrists and Their Patients: A National Survey of Private Office Practice*. Washington, D.C.: American Psychiatric Association, 1975.

10. Dye, C. J. Psychologists' role in the provision of mental health care for the elderly. *Profess. Psychol. 9:* 38, 1978.

11. Dorken, H.; Webb, J. T. Licensed Psychologists in Health Care: A Survey of Their Practices. In Kiesler, C. A.; Cummings, N. A.; vandenBos, G. R. (eds.), *Psychology and National Health Insurance: A Source Book*. Washington, D.C.: American Psychological Association, 1979, pp. 129–60.

12. Straker, M. The Psychiatric Emergency. In Pasnau, R. (ed.), *Consultation-Liaison Psychiatry*. New York: Grune & Stratton, 1975, pp. 177–94.

13. Shem, S. *The House of God*. New York: Dell, 1978, p. 38.

14. Reichel, W. (ed.), *The Geriatric Patient*. New York: Hospital Practice Publishing Co., 1978.

15. Lehmann, H. E. Affective Disorders in the Aged. In Jarvik, L. (ed.), *Psychiatric Clinics of North America: Aging*. Philadelphia: W. B. Saunders, 1982, pp. 27–44.

16. Feigenbaum, E. Ambulatory Treatment in the Elderly. In Busse, E.; Pfeiffer, E. (eds.), *Mental Illness in Later Life*. Washington, D.C.: American Psychiatric Association, 1973, pp. 153–66.

17. Serpick, A. Cancer in the Elderly. In Reichel, W. (ed.), *The Geriatric Patient*. New York: Hospital Practice Publishing Co., 1978, pp. 105–17.

18. Schuster, M. Disorders of the Aging GI system. In Reichel, W. (ed.), *The Geriatric Patient*. New York: Hospital Practice Publishing Co., 1978, pp. 73–86.

19. Ford, C. V.; Shordone, R. J. Attitudes of psychiatrists towards elderly patients. *Am. J. Psychiat.* 137: 571–75, 1980.

20. Freud, S. On Psychotherapy. In Jones, E. (ed.), *Collected Papers*. London: Hogarth, 1924, pp. 249–63.

21. Kane, R. L.; Solomon, D. H.; Beck, J. C.; *et al. Geriatrics in the United States: Manpower Projections and Training Considerations*. Santa Monica, Calif.: Rand Corporation, 1980.

22. Hayflick, L.; Moorhead, P. The serial cultivation of human diploid cells. *Exp. Cell Res.* 25: 585–621, 1961.

23. Shock, N. Biological Theories of Aging. In Birren, J.; Schaie, K.; Warner, K. (eds.), *Handbook of the Psychology of Aging*. New York: Van Nostrand Reinhold, 1977, pp. 103–15.

24. Estes, J. W. The practice of medicine in Eighteenth Century Massachusetts. *New Eng. J. Med. 305:* 1040–47, 1981.

25. Adams, R.; Victor, M. *Principles of Neurology*. New York: McGraw–Hill, 1977, pp. 396–407.

26. Wilkie, F. L.; Eisdorfer, C.; Staub, J. Stress and Psychopathology in the aged. In Jarvik, L. (ed.), *Psychiatric Clinics of North America: Aging*. Philadelphia: W. B. Saunders, 1982, pp. 131–43.

27. Savage, R. D.; Gaber, L. B.; Bolten, N.; *et al. Personality Adjustment in the Aged*. New York: Academic Press, 1979.

28. Siegler, I. C. The Psychology of Adult Development and Aging. In Busse, E. W.; Blazer, D. G. (eds.), *Handbook of Geriatric Psychiatry*. New York: Van Nostrand Reinhold, 1980, pp. 169–22.

29. Sun–Times Wire Service. 65-year-old man swims English Channel. *Chicago Sun Times*, August 29, 1982, p. 40.

30. Shock, N. The physiology of aging. *Sci. Am.* 208: 104, 1963.

31. Rossman, I. Bodily Changes with Aging. In Busse, E. W.; Blazer, D. G. (eds.), *Handbook of Geriatric Psychiatry*. New York: Van Nostrand Reinhold, 1980, pp. 125–46.

32. Marsh, G. R. Perceptual Changes with Aging. In Busse, E. W.; Blazer, D. G. (eds.), *Handbook of Geriatric Psychiatry*. New York: Van Nostrand Reinhold, 1980, pp. 147–68.

33. Paulson, G. W. The Neurologic Evaluation in Dementia. In Wells, C. E. (ed.), *Contemporary Neurology Series: Dementia.* 2d ed. Philadelphia: F. A. Davis, 1977, pp. 169–88.

34. Shock, N. Intrinsic Factors in Aging. In Hansen, P. F. (ed.), *Age with a Future.* Proceedings of Sixth International Congress, Copenhagen and Philadelphia, Munksgaard and F. A. Davis, 1964.

35. Bortz, W. M. Disease and aging. *JAMA 248:* 1203–8, 1982.

36. Feinberg, I. Effects of Age on Human Sleep Patterns. In Kales, A. (ed.), *Sleep: Physiology and Pathology.* Philadelphia: Lippincott, 1968.

37. Pickering, C. M. Sleep circadian rhythm and cardiovascular disease. *Cardiovasc. Rev. Rep. 1:* 37, 1980.

38. Wollner, L.; McCarthy, S. T.; Soper, N. D. W.; *et al.* Failure of cerebral autoregulation as a cause of brain dysfunction in the elderly. *Br. Med. J. 1:* 1117–18, 1979.

39. White, P.; Hiley, C. R.; Goodhart, M. J.; *et al.* Neocortical cholinergic neurons in elderly people. *Lancet 1:* 668–70, 1977.

40. Adolfson, R.; Gottries, C. G.; Roos, B. E.; *et al.* Postmortem distribution of dopamine and homovanillic acid in human brain, variations related to age, and a review of the literature. *J. Neurotrans. 38:* 271–76, 1976.

41. Carlson, A.; Winblad, B. Influence of age and fuse interval between death and autopsy on dopamine and 3-methoxy tyramine levels in human basal ganglia. *J. Neurotrans. 38:* 271–76, 1976.

42. McGeer, E.; McGeer, P. L. Neurotransmitter Metabolism in the Aging Brain. In Lerry, R. D.; Gershon, S. (eds.), *Aging,* vol. 3. New York: Raven Press, 1976, pp. 389–403.

43. Robinson, D. S. Changes in monoamine oxidase and monoamines with human development and aging. *Fed. Proc. 34:* 103–7, 1975.

44. Yesavage, J.; Belger, P. A. Correlation of cerebrospinal fluid lactate with age. *Am. J. Psychiat. 137:* 976–77, 1980.

45. Barnes, R.; Rasking, M.; Halter, J.; *et al.* The effect of mental stress on plasma catecholamine levels in young and old men. Pt. 2. *Gerontologist 20:* 60, 1980.

46. Eisdorfer, C.; Nowlin, J.; Wilkie, F. Improvement of learning in the aged by modification of automatic nervous system activity. *Science 170:* 1327–29, 1970.

47. Horn, J.; Cattell, R. Age differences in fluid and crystallized intelligence. *Acta Psychol. 26:* 107–219, 1967.

48. Kohn, R. R. Causes of death in very old people. *JAMA 247:* 2793–97, 1982.

49. Chien, C. P.; Townsend, E. J.; Ross-Townsend, A. Substance Use and Abuse Among the Community Elderly: The Medical Aspect. In Peterson, D. M. (ed.), *Drug Use Among the Aged.* New York: Spectrum, 1979, pp. 357–72.

50. Busse, E. W.; Blazer, D. Disorders Related to Biological Functioning. In Busse, E. W.; Blazer, D. G. (eds.), *Handbook of Geriatric Psychiatry.* New York: Van Nostrand Reinhold, 1980, pp. 390–414.

51. Salzman, C. Polypharmacy and Drug–Drug Interactions in the Elderly. In

Nandy, K. (ed.), *Geriatric Psychopharmacology*. Amsterdam: Elsevier North Holland, 1979, pp. 117–26.

52. Gurland, B.; Dean, L.; Cross, P.; *et al*. The Epidemiology of Depression and Dementia in the Elderly: The Use of Multiple Indicators of These Conditions. In Cole, J.; Barrett, J. (eds.), *Psychopathology in the Aged*. New York: Raven Press, 1980, pp. 37–60.

53. Guttman, D. A Study of Drug-taking Behavior of Older Americans. In Beber, C. R.; Lamy, P. P. (eds.), *Medication Management and Education in the Elderly*. Washington, D.C.: Excerpta Medica, 1978, pp. 18–19.

54. Salzman, C.; Van Der Kolk, B. A. Psychotropic drugs and polypharmacy in elderly patients in a general hospital. *J. Am. Geriat. Soc. 28:* 18–22, 1980.

55. Salzman, C.; Van Der Kolk, B. A. Psychotropic drugs and polypharmacy in a general hospital. *J. Geriat. Psychiat. 12:* 167–76, 1979.

56. Salzman, C. Update in geriatric psychopharmacology. *Geriatrics 34:* 87–90, 1979.

57. Greenblatt, D. J.; Sellers, E. M.; Shader, R. I. Drug disposition in old age. *New Eng. J. Med. 306:* 1081–87, 1982.

58. Salzman, C. Key Concepts in Geriatric Psychopharmacology. In Jarvik, L. (ed.), *Psychiatric Clinics of North America: Aging*. Philadelphia: W. B. Saunders, 1982, pp. 181–90.

59. Larny, P. P. *Prescribing for the Elderly*. Littleton, N.H.: P. S. G. Publishing, 1980.

60. Trounce, J. R. Drug metabolism in the elderly. *Br. J. Clin. Pharmacol. 2:* 289, 1975.

61. Davies, R. K.; Tucker, G. I.; Harrow, M.; *et al*. Confusional episodes and antidepressant medication. *Am. J. Psychiat. 128:* 95, 1971.

62. Learoyd, B. M. Psychotropic drugs in the aging patient. *Med. J. Aust. 1:* 1131–33, 1972.

63. Straker, M. Adjustment Disorders and Personality Disorders in the Aged. In Jarvik, L. (ed.), *Psychiatric Clinics of North America: Aging*. Philadelphia: W. B. Saunders, 1982, pp. 121–129.

64. Neshkes, R. E.; Jarvik, L. Clinical Psychiatry and Cardiovascular Disease in the Aged. In Jarvik, L. (ed.), *Psychiatric Clinics of North America: Aging*. Philadelphia: W. B. Saunders, 1982, pp. 171–99.

65. Rubenstein, E.; Felderman, D. D. (eds.). Scientific American Medicine, vol. 4, no. 2. New York: *Scientific American*, 1982.

66. Glassman, A. H.; Bigger, J. T. Cardiovascular effects of therapeutic doses of tricyclic antidepressants. *Arch. Gen. Psychiat. 38:* 815–20, 1981.

67. Roose, S. P.; Bone, S.; Hardorfer, C.; *et al*. Lithium treatment in older patients. *Am. J. Psychiat. 136:* 843–44, 1979.

68. Chouinard, G.; Annable, L.; Ross-Chouinard, A.; *et al*. Factors related to tardive dyskinesia. *Am. J. Psychiat. 136:* 79–82, 1979.

69. Ouslander, J. G.; Kane, R. L.; Abrams, I. B. Urinary incontinence in elderly nursing home patients. *JAMA 248:* 1194–98, 1982.

70. Frolich, J. C.; Leftwich, R.; Ragheb, M.; et al. Indomethocin increases plasma lithium. Br. Med. J. 1: 1115–16, 1979.

71. Sierles, F. S.; Ossowski, M. G. Concurrent use of theophylline and lithium in a patient with chronic obstructive lung disease and bipolar disorder. Am. J. Psychiat. 139: 117–18, 1982.

72. Shader, R. I.; Georgotus, A.; Greenblatt, D. J.; et al. Impaired desmethyldiazepam from chlorazepate by magnesium aluminum hydroxide. Clin. Pharmacol. Ther. 24: 308–15, 1978.

73. Blaschke, T. F.; Cohen, S. N.; Latro, D. S.; et al. Drug–Drug Interactions and Aging. In Jarvik, L.; Greenblatt, D. F.; Harmon, D. (eds.), Clinical Pharmacology and the Aged Patient. New York: Raven Press, 1981, pp. 11–26.

74. Blazer, D. G. Depression in Late Life. St. Louis: C. V. Mosby, 1982.

75. David, W. K.; Klaus, B. Epidemiology of Mental Disorders Among the Aged in the Community. In Birren, J. E.; Sloane, P. B. (eds.), Handbook of Mental Health and Aging. Englewood Cliffs, N. J.: Prentice-Hall, 1980, pp. 34–56.

76. Folstein, M.; Folstein, S.; McHugh, P. The "minimental state" examination. J. Psychiat. Res. 12: 189–98, 1975.

77. Asnis, G. M.; Nathan, R. S.; Halbreich, W.; et al. Cortisol secretion in relation to age in major depression. Psychosom. Med. 41: 586, 1979.

78. Brown, W. A.; Shuey, I. Response to dexamethasone and subtypes of depression. Arch. Gen. Psychiat. 37: 747–51, 1980.

79. Gurland, B. J. The comparative frequency of depression in various adult age groups. J. Gerontol. 31: 283–92, 1976.

80. Pfeiffer, E.; Busse, E. W. Affective Disorders: Paranoid, Neurotic, and Situational Reactions. In Busse, E. W.; Pfeiffer, E. (eds.), Mental Illness in Later Life. Washington, D.C.: American Psychiatric Association, 1973, pp. 107–44.

81. Salzman, C.; Van Der Kolk, B.; Shader, R. I. Psychopharmacology and the Geriatric Patient. In Shader, R. I. (ed.), Manual of Psychiatric Therapeutics. Boston: Little, Brown, 1975, pp. 171–84.

82. Dorpat, T. L.; Anderson, W. F.; Ripley, H. S. The Relationship of Physical Illness to Suicide. In Resnik, H. (ed.), Suicidal Behaviors. Boston: Little, Brown, 1968, pp. 209–19.

83. Gurland, B. J.; Cross, P. S. Epidemiology of Psychopathology in Old Age. In Jarvik, L. (ed.), Psychiatric Clinics of North America: Aging. Philadelphia: W. B. Saunders, 1982, pp. 11–26.

84. Ban, T. A. The treatment of depressed geriatric patients. Am. J. Psychother. 32: 93–104, 1978.

85. Weissman, M. M.; Myers, J. K. Affective disorders in a U.S. urban community. Arch. Gen. Psychiat. 35: 1304–11, 1978.

86. World Health Association. World Health Statistical Report 21: 6, 1968.

87. Post, F. The Functional Psychoses. In Isaacs, A.; Post, F. (eds.), Studies in Geriatric Psychiatry. New York: Wiley, 1978, pp. 77–94.

88. Himmelhoch, J. M.; Neil, J. F.; May, S. J.; et al. Age, dementia, dyskinesias and lithium response. Am. J. Psychiat. 137: 941–45, 1980.

89. Kay, D. W. K. Epidemiologic Aspects of Organic Brain Disease in the Aged. In Gaity, C. M. (ed.), *Aging and the Brain*. New York: Plenum, 1972, pp. 15–27.

90. Liston, E. H. Delirium in the Aged. In Jarvik, L. (ed.), *Psychiatric Clinics of North America: Aging*. Philadelphia: W. B. Saunders, 1982, pp. 49–66.

91. Wells, C. E. Chronic brain disease: An overview. *Am. J. Psychiat. 24:* 259–63, 1978.

92. Terry, R. Senile Dementia, and Alzheimer's Disease. In Katymen, R.; Terry, D. (eds.), *Alzheimer's Disease, Senile Dementia, and Related Disorders*, vol. 7, *Aging*. New York: Raven Press, 1978, pp. 11–14.

93. Engel, G. L.; Romano, J. Delirium: A syndrome of chronic cerebral insufficiency. *J. Chronic Dis. 9:* 260–77, 1959.

94. Sierles, F. S.; Taylor, M. A.; Herschberg, S. M.; *et al.* Cognitive deficits in medical inpatients. Manuscript in preparation, 1984.

95. Celesia, G. C.; Wanameker, W. M. Psychiatric disturbances in Parkinson's disease. *Dis. Nerv. Sys. 33:* 577, 1972.

96. Sroka, H.; Elizan, T. S.; Yahr, M. D.; *et al.* Organic mental syndrome and confusional states in Parkinson's disease: Relationship to computerized tomographic signs of cerebral atrophy. *Arch. Neurol. 38:* 399–42, 1981.

97. May, W. W.; Itabasi, H. H.; DeJong, R. N. Creutzfeld–Jakob disease: 2. Clinical, pathologic and genetic study of a family. *Arch. Neurol. 19:* 137–49, 1968.

98. Myreanthopoulos, N. C. Huntington's chorea: Review article. *J. Med. Genet. 3:* 248–314, 1966.

99. Ouslander, J. G. Illness and Psychopathology in the Elderly. In Jarvik, L. (ed.), *Psychiatric Clinics of North America: Aging*. Philadelphia: W. B. Saunders, 1982, pp. 145–58.

100. Roslaniec, A.; Fitzpatrick, J. J. Changes in mental status in older adults with four days of hospitalization. *Res. Nurs. Health 2:* 177–87, 1979.

101. Etienne, P. E.; Dastoor, D.; Goldapple, E.; *et al.* Adverse effects of medical and psychiatric workup in six demented geriatric patients. *Am. J. Psychiat. 138:* 520–21, 1981.

102. Warshaw, G. A.; Moore, J. T.; Friedman, W.; *et al.* Functional disability in the hospitalized elderly. *JAMA 248:* 847–50, 1982.

103. Gaitz, C.; Baer, P. Characteristics of elderly patients with alcoholism. *Arch. Gen. Psychiat. 24:* 372–78, 1971.

104. Capel, W. C.; Stewart, G. T. The management of drug abuse in aging populations. *J. Drug Issues 1:* 114–21, 1971.

105. Petrie, W. M.; Lawson, E. C.; Hollender, M. H. Violence in geriatric patients. *JAMA 248:* 443–44, 1982.

106. Roth, M. The natural history of mental disorder in old age. *J. Ment. Sci. 101:* 281–301, 1955.

107. Almy, G. Personal communication, 1982.

108. Gaspar, D.; Samarsinghi, L. A. ECT in psychogeriatric practice: A study of risk factors, indicators and outcome. *Comp. Psychiat. 23:* 170–75, 1982.

109. Abiuso, P.; Dukleman, R.; Proper, M. Electroconvulsive therapy in patients with pacemakers. *JAMA* 240: 2459–60, 1975.

110. Jauher, P.; Weller, M.; Hirsch, S. R. Electroconvulsive therapy for a patient with a cardiac pacemaker. *Br. J. Psychiat. 1:* 90–91, 1979.

111. Ashford, J. W.; Ford, C. V. Use of MAO inhibitors in elderly patients. *Am. J. Psychiat. 136:* 1466–67, 1979.

112. Taylor, M. A. Indications for electroconvulsive treatment. In Abrams, R.; Essman, W. B. (eds.), *Electroconvulsive Therapy in Theory and Practice.* New York: SP Medical and Scientific Books, 1982, pp. 7–39.

113. Reisberg, B.; Ferris, S. H.; Gershon, S. An overview of pharmacologic treatment of cognitive decline in the aged. *Am. J. Psychiat. 138:* 593–600, 1981.

114. Davis, K. L.; Mohs, R. C. Enhancement of memory processes in Alzheimer's disease with multiple-dose intravenous physostigmine. *Am. J. Psychiat. 139:* 1421–24, 1982.

CHAPTER 21

Anorexia Nervosa

Anorexia nervosa is an uncommon but serious condition in which the patient, typically a teenage girl, develops a gross misperception or overvalued idea that she is significantly overweight and that she must diet or use other means (e.g. self-induced vomiting, exercise programs, use of diuretics or laxatives) to lose large amounts of weight. She consequently experiences massive weight loss, associated physiologic changes (most but not all of which are the product of starvation), and has a 9 percent chance of dying during the illness from starvation or other causes (1). Despite the weight loss, which renders her cachectic, she does not perceive herself as gaunt, continues to be fearful of gaining weight, and (until there are profound effects of starvation) remains physically active, even overactive. Despite the use of the term anorexia, the patient usually maintains a good appetite and may be preoccupied with food, a collector of recipes, a reader of cookbooks, and an enthusiastic cook for others (1). She may at times gorge herself with food (bulimia) and avoid weight gain by immediately inducing vomiting. It has been proposed that there is a specific subtype of bulimic anorexic patient, or that bulimia is a separate disorder, but these propositions remain unproved.

Diagnostic Criteria

We use the *DSM-III* criteria for anorexia nervosa, which are as follows:

1. Intense fear of becoming obese, which does not diminish as weight loss progresses.

2. Disturbance of body image, e.g. claiming to "feel fat" even when emaciated.
3. Weight loss of at least 25 percent of original body weight or, if under eighteen years of age, weight loss from original body weight plus projected weight gain expected from growth charts may be combined to make up the 25 percent.
4. Refusal to maintain body weight over a minimal normal weight for age and height.
5. No known physical illness that would account for the weight loss.

Epidemiology

Although an uncommon disorder, anorexia nervosa is thought to be increasing in incidence, which is between 0.37 and 1.6 per 100,000 population per year (2). Regardless of the population surveyed, 94–96 percent of anorexia nervosa patients are women (3–5), for reasons yet to be explained. It is usually described as more common among people of middle and upper socioeconomic status (6) and less common among blacks (7), but these conclusions are not based upon adequate controlled sampling (7). Eighty-five percent of the patients develop the illness between the ages of thirteen and twenty, and onset is rare below the age of ten or over thirty (6).

There is an increased frequency of major affective disorders and of alcoholism in the families of patients with anorexia nervosa as compared with the general population (8–10). To consider the possibility that affective disorder, alcoholism, and anorexia nervosa could represent manifestations of the same genotype, there is a need for studies using specialized analytic techniques (11), to determine whether affective disorder, alcoholism, and anorexia nervosa show genetic overlap or cluster independently in families.

Parent–child concordance for anorexia nervosa is uncommon (1). Compared with the general population, however, more mothers (16 percent) and fathers (23 percent) of anorexia nervosa patients had "weight phobia" or significantly reduced adolescent weight (9), suggesting the genetic transmission of a recessive disorder. The concordance for anorexia nervosa among monozygotic twins is 52 percent and for dizygotic twins 11 percent (1). There are a number of case reports of two or more members of a sibship with anorexia nervosa (1).

Additional Clinical Manifestations

Amenorrhea is extremely common among anorectics, and for some patients the amenorrhea precedes significant weight loss (7, 12). Usually, but not always, menses return when weight is restored (6, 13–15). Interest in sex is considerably decreased or absent; often it was diminished or absent prior to onset of the illness. (Decreased interest in sex is also noted in normals voluntarily starving themselves) (16). Pregnancy is a rare explanation of some of the symptoms, although conception has been reported (14) during periods of prolonged amenorrhea.

Constipation is very frequent, usually the product of diminished food intake, and disappears soon after the patient begins eating normally (1). Diarrhea is frequent in patients who abuse laxatives.

In addition to gauntness findings sometimes include narrowing of the shoulders and hips, bradycardia (with the lowest recorded pulse rate being 28) (17), reduced basal temperature, dry skin, and loss of scalp hair with retention of pubic and axillary hair. Often lanugo hairs (blond, short, "downy" hairs) are seen on cheeks, neck, forearms, and thighs. If the patient has vomited repeatedly, dental problems are common because of gastric acidity. These problems include dissolution of enamel and dental caries (18). Parotid gland enlargement may occur, usually in patients with repeated bouts of emesis and hypochloremic alkalosis (19–23). Irritation of the skin or scarring is occasionally seen on the dorsum of the hand close to the metacarpophalangeal joint, where a finger inserted in the pharynx to induce vomiting has rubbed against upper incisor teeth (24).

Occasionally edema (1), acrocyanosis (a circulatory problem in which the hands or feet are persistently cold, blue, and sweaty) (6), Raynaud's phenomenon (a circulatory problem in which the fingers or toes become pale and painful when exposed to cold temperatures) (6), or orange pigmentation of palms and soles (probably due to dietary faddism with overingestion of carotene-containing foods) (6, 25) may be observed. Moderate anemia (26–28) with associated pallor or petechiae because of reduced numbers of platelets (1, 28, 29) are occasionally seen. Some patients with anorexia nervosa are prone to developing infections (1, 6); in some, this is in part a product of the leukopenia that occasionally occurs (30). In rare cases beriberi (31, 32), pellagra (33), vitamin K deficiency (34), or Korsakoff's encephalopathy may occur.

Vomiting and laxative abuse may lead to electrolyte abnormalities (see below) and consequent weakness, cardiac arrhythmias, tetany, or convulsions (1). An unusual complication is duodenal compression by the superior mesenteric artery, which may occur in patients with weight loss from any cause and should be suspected in patients with postprandial abdominal pain or intractable vomiting (35). The probable mechanism is the dissolution of the fat pad lying between the duodenum and the superior mesenteric artery, which crosses it, as well as the bogginess and lack of coordinated contraction of the duodenum during starvation.

Additional behavioral problems include insomnia, diminished concentration, depressed mood, suicidal ideation, suicide attempts, and a resistance to agreeing that one is seriously ill and in danger of dying. In advanced cases delirium may occur. The depressions that have been reported have not been well characterized, but it has been noted that upon follow-up after initial recovery endogenous depression is sometimes observed months or years later (8). The patient's capacity to experience hunger is intact, but the ingestion of minute amounts of food produces satiation far more readily than it would for normal controls (36). It is also important to note that in some series (37, 38) misperceptions about body shape and size also occur among nonanorectic age-matched controls, but the latter individuals do not engage in anorectic eating patterns.

Laboratory Testing

Many laboratory abnormalities have been noted in patients with anorexia nervosa, none of which occur in all patients or are pathognomonic, and most of which are the product of starvation and disappear when weight becomes normal. These include hypokalemia (a serious complication of vomiting or diuretic abuse), hyponatremia (39), hypochloremic alkalosis (39), hypercholesterolemia (6, 40), hypercarotenemia (6) (sometimes due to ingestion of high quantities of carotene-containing foods associated with faddish diets), anemia, thrombocytopenia, leukopenia, hypofibrinogenemia (7), increased blood urea nitrogen (1, 41), diminished glomerular filtration rate (42), decreased basal metabolic rate (6), decreased erythrocyte sedimentation rate (7), electroencephalographic (1, 6, 43) and electrocardiographic abnormalities (29, 44–46), reversible atrophy on computerized tomographic brain scan (47), and delayed gastric emptying (48, 49).

The following endocrine abnormalities are very common:

Dexamethasone nonsuppression (7, 50)
Increased A.M. plasma cortisol (51–53)
Flattened diurnal variation of plasma cortisol (54, 55)
Increased 24-hour excretion of urinary free cortisol (56, 57)
Mild hypoglycemia (58, 59)
Flat curve or hyperglycemic response to glucose load on the glucose
   tolerance test (1)
Plasma luteinizing hormone (LH) secretion pattern resembling that of
   prepubescent children (1, 60)
Impaired LH response to luteinizing hormone releasing hormone (52, 61)
Low T_3 (62, 63)
Low/low normal thyroxine (T_4) levels (64, 65)

Slightly increased reverse T_3 levels (62)
Increased growth hormone (52, 66)
Reduced growth hormone response to apomorphine (66, 67)
Low nocturnal prolactin levels and absence of sleep-induced rise in
    prolactin (68, 69)
Diminished urinary MHPG (50)
Decreased urinary estrogens and gonadotropins (70, 71)
Diminished testosterone levels in male patients (72, 73)
Increased testosterone levels in female patients (74)
Decreased urinary 17-ketosteroids (75, 76)
Abnormal responses of argenine vasopressing in plasma and
    cerebrospinal fluid in response to an intravenous sodium load (77)

Typically normal findings include normal levels of thyrotropin (TSH) (52, 78), thyrotropin response to thyrotropin-releasing hormone (52, 78), cortisol binding globulin capacity (56, 79), resting prolactin level (80, 81), prolactin response to chlorpromazine (80, 82), and prompt release of growth hormone following administration of thyrotropin releasing hormone (83, 84).

Prognosis

As noted above, there is a serious risk of death (1). In one series 82 percent of the deaths were the product of starvation and its complications, and 18 percent the result of suicide (1). The complications of starvation included bronchopneumonia or other infections, renal failure, cardiac failure, electrolyte abnormalities resulting from vomiting and the use of purgatives, and complications of invasive medical treatments (1). The latter included gastric dilatation from too rapid feeding, aspiration of tube feedings, and electrolyte imbalance from intravenous fluids (1). The first two of these complications can be avoided by intravenous hyperalimentation.

Regarding overall prognosis of the condition, Garfinkel and Garner (1) write: "Overall the evaluations which are of long duration and which include primarily pediatric samples show that over 40% of patients are fully remitted and 30% are considerably improved at follow-up. However, at least 20% are unimproved or seriously impaired, and 9% have died as a result of the illness." The prognosis is worse if the age of onset is over twenty (85, 86), if the patient has failed to respond to previous treatment (27, 87), if the patient demonstrates bulimia (87), or if the patient had significant behavior problems prior to the onset of anorexia nervosa (88, 89).

Treatment

Although there is an improvement in the condition of most patients with anorexia nervosa, to our knowledge there are only two controlled studies (90, 91), each with very small sample size, demonstrating the efficacy of any of the many forms of treatment of anorexia nervosa. The two studies are those of Gross *et al.* (90), which showed significant weight gain with use of lithium in patients meeting Feighner criteria (92) for anorexia nervosa, and of Pope *et al.* (91), who showed diminished frequency of binge eating with use of imipramine in patients meeting *DSM-III* criteria for bulimia.

The other types of treatment for anorexia nervosa have been the subject of case reports (of varying series size) linking that mode of treatment with recovery (1, 93). These treatments have included psychotherapy (94), psychotherapy with hyperalimentation in severe cases (95), behavior modification (96), behavior modification with chlorpromazine (97), amitryptyline (97–100), phenelzine (101) in anorectics with reactive depressions, carbamazepine (102) in (one of six) patients with bulimia, lithium carbonate (1, 103), leukotomy (104), and electroconvulsive therapy (105). That five of these treatments are also used in the treatment of affective disorders, coupled with the familial association of affective disorders, the dexamethasone suppression test abnormalities, and the high frequency of suicide, has provided evidence for some authors (8–10) to suggest a link (as yet ill defined) between anorexia nervosa and major affective disorders.

The initial evaluation should include a thorough physical examination and laboratory tests. These should include complete blood count, urinalysis, chest x-ray, electrocardiogram, serum electrolytes, cholesterol, blood urea nitrogen, uric acid, alkaline phosphatase, creatine phosphokinase, cortisol, serum vitamin levels, electroencephalogram, computerized tomographic brain scan, and dexamethasone suppression test. Electrolyte levels should be monitored weekly, or more frequently if an abnormality was detected initially or if vomiting or diarrhea occur.

Although it is possible to treat a patient with a mild case as an outpatient, employing lithium carbonate or imipramine, we recommend admission of those patients who have weight loss exceeding 25 percent of body weight or significant medical sequelae of starvation, who are significantly depressed or suicidal, or whose family lives have become chaotic as a result of the illness. Many of these can eventually be persuaded to be treated voluntarily in the hospital. Involuntary hospitalization is occasionally necessary, and legally justifiable, when the patient refuses admission, and starvation or depression are so advanced that there is an imminent risk of death (1).

This does not mean that patients are eager to be admitted, for the opposite is the case. Few such patients perceive themselves as gaunt and seriously ill (1). Many accept admission in order to placate their relatives, who, after the illness has progressed, have become frankly intolerant of it or distraught about it. Also, some of the medical complications of starvation, such as hair loss, edema, impaired concentration, amenorrhea, insomnia, and suicidal ideation may be sources of discomfort for the patient and contribute to her consenting to admission (1). The physician should tell the patient that these are medical problems produced by starvation and that in the absence of weight gain they are likely to intensify and render her vulnerable to dying. Unless medical complications are severe, admission to a psychiatry service is usually preferable to admission on a medical unit because of a greater acceptance by psychiatric staff of abnormal behavior and because of their greater familiarity with the use of behavioral management programs.

Prior to admission the patient and her family should receive an extensive description of the program (including the possibility that involuntary tube feeding might have to be employed) and should be told that if this program is not fully agreeable, admission will not be feasible (24). They should sign consent to participate in the behavioral management program to be described below. This program (24) includes the following:

The patient begins on the unit's step system (see Chapter 9) with absolutely no privileges. This means no visitors, no phone calls, no television or radio, no reading, no school activities, no recreational or occupational therapy activities, and no off-ward activities. For every kilogram increase in weight, privileges precisely specified in advance (e.g. one telephone call per day and television for one hour daily for the first kilogram of weight gained) are added according to a schedule tailored to the individual patient. The final privilege is discharge, which will occur only after the patient has reached a specified weight (typically 90 percent of the average weight for her age and height) and maintained it for two weeks (1). She is also told that she will not be allowed to exceed this weight or to gain weight too quickly. This is actually reassuring, since the patient is usually terrified of experiencing unlimited weight gain (1).

To verify accurately that weight gain is occurring and that the patient is not feigning it by carrying heavy objects in her clothes, she should be weighed in pajamas, at the same time each day, on the same scale, with weight recordings taken only by a small number of designated staff members who are very familiar with her. She is expected to eat three balanced meals daily, beginning with an intake of 1,500–2,000 calories per day and progressing gradually to 3,000–3,500 calories daily over two to three weeks. If the increase in food intake is too rapid, gastric dilatation may occur (1, 6, 106). The dietitian presents her with some choices on the menu, but once she has made her selection and the tray is presented, she is encouraged to finish all the food on her plate. Some physicians recommend that if the patient leaves food, it should be pureed in a blender and force-fed by nasogastric tube. It is rare for patients to require force-feeding twice. Force-feeding can be justified on the grounds that advanced starvation from anorexia nervosa is a potentially fatal condition and that the patient and her family were informed prior to admission that involuntary feeding might be necessary. Also, if this or any other aspect of the treatment regimen is unacceptable to the patient and her family and she is not immediately at risk for dying, she may be allowed to leave the hospital against medical advice.

The patient should be observed carefully as she eats, because many anorectic patients may secretly dispose of their food if they are not watched or give the appearance of eating busily while they are actually just laboriously cutting their food. For one hour following the meal the patient should continue to be on one-to-one observation to prevent self-induced vomiting. If the patient does induce vomiting, this observation should extend to an hour and a half or two hours postprandially.

If the patient was hyperactive prior to admission, if she is hyperactive on admission, or if her starvation is extensively debilitating, she should be placed initially on bed rest with the exception of dining room or bathroom privileges. If she is normoactive or hypoactive, then she should initially be expected to spend all her time outside her room with the exception of sleep times. As she reaches a specified weight, this can be modified as a privilege. Since the hyperactivity of anorexia nervosa (in contrast to the hyperactivity of mania) is willed, there is no need to prescribe medication to diminish it.

If major systemic abnormalities (e.g. electrolyte imbalance, cardiac arrhythmia, signs of heart failure) are noted, these must be treated, and consultation with an internist is usually in order. During daily rounds the patient should be examined for the development of tachycardia, edema, gallop rhythm, or basilar rales, all signs of the cardiac malfunction or failure that occasionally occurs in anorexia nervosa patients (1, 45, 46).

Although the focus of the admission must be the reversal of the effects of starvation by weight gain, conversations with the patient should (as for any patient) cover nondietary aspects of the patient's life. She is entitled to the same degree of interpersonal sensitivity as any other patient. Her family should be apprised of developments and should be assisted in reinforcing normal eating habits upon the patient's discharge.

Concurrent with the behavior modification program the patient should receive a trial of lithium carbonate if she has not manifested bulimia, self-induced vomiting, or diarrhea, or a trial of imipramine if she has manifested bulimia, self-induced vomiting, or diarrhea. If vomiting continues and is considerable, imipramine can be administered intramuscularly. If the patient has lost considerable weight, which is usually the case, dosages of lithium or imipramine must be reduced below the standard adult doses that would ordinarily be used for the treatment of mania or endogenous depression.

If, on admission or at any other time, the patient demonstrates melancholia, the above-mentioned behavior management program should be postponed, and the patient should be treated primarily for melancholia with ECT, lithium, or imipramine. If the patient manifests a dysthymic/reactive type of depression, phenelzine should be prescribed instead of lithium or imipramine in conjunction with the behavioral management program. It should be repeated that although some of the symptoms and signs (e.g. weight loss, insomnia) and laboratory findings (e.g. dexamethasone nonsuppression) of melancholia can occur in anorectics, the two syndromes are usually fairly easy to distinguish. For example, the weight loss in anorexia nervosa is usually accompanied by a good appetite, and in endogenous depression usually by diminished appetite (anorexia). If all attempts at treatment of anorexia nervosa fail, nasogastric tube feeding or hyperalimentation (94) should be initiated.

Following discharge the patient should be seen regularly, ideally on the hospital unit itself, where she can be weighed on the same scale by the same people in the setting where she began her recovery. She should be told that a return to her preadmission anorectic behaviors will require readmission. She should be maintained for six months on whatever somatic therapies had been employed in the hospital. Because many anorexia patients conform to the behavioral regimen simply to get discharged, to avoid physical symptoms of starvation, or to please their families and never relinquish their overvalued ideas about their weight, recurrences are common and a considerable source of frustration for physicians involved in their care.

References

1. Garfinkel, P. E.; Garner, D. M. Anorexia Nervosa: A Multidimensional Perspective. New York: Brunner/Mazel, 1982.

2. Kendell, R. E.; Hall, D. J.; Harley, A.; et al. The epidemiology of anorexia nervosa. Psychol. Med. 3: 200-203, 1973.

3. Halmi, K. A. Anorexia nervosa: Demographic and clinical features in 94 cases. Psychosom. Med. 36: 18-25, 1974.

4. Decourt, J. Sur l'anorexie mentale de l'adolescence dans le sex masculin. Rev. Neuropsychiatr. Infant 12: 499, 1964.

5. Dally, P. J. Anorexia Nervosa. New York: Grune & Stratton, 1959.

6. Halmi, K. A. Anorexia Nervosa. In Freeman, A. M.; Kaplan, H. I.; Sadock, B. J. (eds.), Comprehensive Textbook of Psychiatry. 3d ed. Baltimore: Williams & Wilkins, 1980, pp. 1882-91.

7. Goodwin, D. M.; Guze, S. B. Psychiatric Diagnosis. New York: Oxford University Press, 1979.

8. Cantwell, D. P.; Sturzenburger, S.; Burroughs, J.; et al. Anorexia nervosa: An affective disorder? Arch. Gen. Psychiat. 34: 1087-93, 1977.

9. Winokur, A.; March, V.; Mendels, J. Primary affective disorder in relatives of patients with anorexia nervosa. *Am. J. Psychiat. 137*(6): 695–98, 1980.

10. Hudson, J. I.; Pope, H. G., Jr.; Jonas, J. M.; *et al.* Family history study of anorexia nervosa and bulimia. *Br. J. Psychiat. 142:* 133–38, 1983.

11. Reich, T. R.; Cloninger, C. R.; Guze, S. B. The multifactorial model of disease transmission: 1. Description of the model and its use in psychiatry. *Br. J. Psychiat. 127:* 1–10, 1975.

12. Fries, H. Studies on Secondary Amenorrhea, Anorectic Behavior, and Body Image Perception: Importance for the Early Recognition of Anorexia Nervosa. In Vigersky, R. (ed.), *Anorexia Nervosa.* New York: Raven Press, 1977, pp. 163–76.

13. Beck, J. C.; Brochner–Mortensen, J. Observations on the prognosis in anorexia nervosa. *Acta Med. Scand. 149:* 409–30, 1954.

14. Theander, S. Anorexia nervosa: A psychiatric investigation of 94 female patients. *Acta Psychiat. Scand.* (suppl.) *214:* 1–194, 1970.

15. Kay, D. W. K.; Leigh, D. Natural history, treatment and prognosis of anorexia nervosa, based on study of 38 patients. *J. Ment. Sci. 100:* 411–31, 1954.

16. Keys, A.; Brozek, J.; Henschel, A.; *et al. The Biology of Human Starvation,* vol. 1. Minneapolis: University of Minnesota Press, 1950.

17. Brotman, A. W.; Stein, T. A. A case report of cardiovascular abnormalities in anorexia nervosa. *Am. J. Psychiat. 140*(9): 1227–28, 1983.

18. Hurst, P. S.; Lacey, J. H.; Crisp, A. H. Teeth, vomiting and diet: A study of the dental characteristics of seventeen anorexia nervosa patients. *Postgrad. Med. J. 53:* 298–305, 1977.

19. Simon, D.; Lauderbach, P.; Lebovici, M.; *et al.* Parotidomegalie au cours des dysorexies mentales: 10 observations. *Nouv. Presse Med. 8:* 2399–2402, 1979.

20. Dawson, J.; Jones, C. Vomiting-induced hypokalemia, alkalosis, and parotid swelling. *Practitioner 218:* 267–68, 1977.

21. Lavender, A. Vomiting and parotid enlargement. *Lancet 1:* 426, 1969.

22. Levin, P. A.; Falko, J. M.; Dixon, K.; *et al.* Benign parotid enlargement in bulimia. *Ann. Int. Med. 93:* 827–29, 1980.

23. Watt, J. Benign parotid swellings: A review. *Proc. Roy. Soc. Med. 70:* 483–86, 1977.

24. Almy, G. Personal communication, 1983.

25. Lucas, A. R. On the meaning of laboratory values in anorexia nervosa. *Mayo Clin. Proc. 52:* 748–50, 1977.

26. Berkman, J. M. Anorexia nervosa, anterior pituitary insufficiency, Simmonds' cachexia and Sheehan's disease, including some observations in water metabolism associated with starvation. *Postgrad. Med. J. 3:* 237–46, 1948.

27. Morgan, H. G.; Russell, G. F. M. Value of family background and clinical features as predictors of long-term outcome in anorexia nervosa: Four-year follow-up study of 41 patients. *Psychol. Med. 5:* 355–71, 1975.

28. Warren, M. P.; Vande Wiele, R. L. Clinical and metabolic features of anorexia nervosa. *Am. J. Obstet. Gynecol. 117:* 435–49, 1973.

29. Silverman, J. A. Anorexia nervosa: Clinical and Metabolic Observations in a Successful Treatment Plan. In Vigersky, R. (ed.), *Anorexia Nervosa*. New York: Raven Press, 1977, pp. 331-39.

30. Gotch, F. M.; Spry, C. J. F.; Mowat, A. G.; *et al.* Reversible granulocyte killing defect in anorexia nervosa. *Clin. Exp. Immunol. 21:* 244-49, 1975.

31. Palmer, H. A. Beriberi complicating anorexia nervosa. *Lancet 1:* 269, 1939

32. Smitt, J. W. Case of anorexia nervosa complicated by beriberi. *Acta Psychiat. Neurol. 21:* 887-900, 1946.

33. Clow, F. E. Anorexia nervosa. *New Eng. J. Med. 207:* 613-17, 1932.

34. Aggeler, P. M.; Lucia, S. P.; Fishbon, H. M. Purpura due to vitamin K deficiency in anorexia nervosa. *Am. J. Digest. Dis. 9:* 227-29, 1942.

35. Burrington, J. D.; Wayne, E. R. Obstruction of the duodenum by the superior mesenteric artery: Does it exist in children? *J. Pediatr. Surg. 9:* 733-41, 1974.

36. Garfinkel, P. E. Perception of hunger and satiety in anorexia nervosa. *Psychol. Med. 4:* 309-15, 1974.

37. Garner, D. M.; Garfinkel, P. E.; Stancer, H. C.; *et al.* Body image disturbances in anorexia nervosa and obesity. *Psychosom. Med. 38:* 227-336, 1976.

38. Button, E. J.; Fransella, F.; Slade, P. D. A reappraisal of body perception disturbance in anorexia nervosa. *Psychol. Med. 7:* 231-43, 1977.

39. Elkington, J. R.; Huth, E. J. Body fluid abnormalities in anorexia nervosa and undernutrition. *Metabolism 8:* 376-403, 1959.

40. Klinefelter, H. F. Hypercholesterolemia in anorexia nervosa. *J. Clin. Endocrinol. Metab. 25:* 1520, 1965.

41. Lampert, F.; Lau, B. Bone marrow hypoplasia in anorexia nervosa. *Eur. J. Pediatr. 124:* 65-71, 1976.

42. Klahr, S.; Alleyne, G. A. O. Effects of protein-calorie malnutrition on the kidney. *Kidney Int. 3:* 129-41, 1973.

43. Lundberg, O.; Walinder, J. Anorexia nervosa and signs of brain damage. *Int. J. Neuropsychiat. 3:* 165-73, 1967.

44. Thurston, J.; Marks, P. Electrocardiographic abnormalities in patients with anorexia nervosa. *Br. Heart J. 36:* 719-23, 1974.

45. Gottdiener, J. S.; Gross, H. A.; Henry, W. L.; *et al.* Effects of self-induced starvation on cardiac size and function in anorexia nervosa. *Circulation 58:* 425-33, 1978.

46. Drossman, D. A.; Ontjes, D. A.; Heizer, W. D. Clinical conference: Anorexia nervosa. *Gastroenterology 77:* 1115-31, 1979.

47. Heiny, E. R.; Martinez, J.; Haenggeli, A. Reversibility of cerebral atrophy in anorexia nervosa and Cushing's syndrome. *J. Comput. Assist. Tomog. 1(4):* 415-18, 1977.

48. Dubois, A.; Gross, H. A.; Ebert, M. H.; *et al.* Altered gastric emptying and secretion in primary anorexia nervosa. *Gastroenterology 77:* 319-23, 1979.

49. Saleh, J. W.; Lebwohl, P. Metaclopramide-induced gastric emptying in patients with anorexia nervosa. *Am. J. Gastroenterol. 74:* 127-32, 1980.

50. Gerner, R. H.; Gwirtsman, H. E. Abnormalities of dexamethasone suppression test and urinary MHPG levels in anorexia nervosa. *Am. J. Psychiat. 138:* 650–53, 1981.

51. Alvarez, L. C.; Dimas, C. O.; Castro, A.; *et al.* Growth hormone in malnutrition. *J. Clin. Endocrinol. Metab. 43:* 400–409, 1972.

52. Brown, G. M.; Garfinkel, P. E.; Jeuniewic, N.; *et al.* Endocrine Profiles in Anorexia Nervosa. In Vigersky, R. (ed.), *Anorexia Nervosa.* New York: Raven Press, 1977, pp. 123–35.

53. Casper, R. C.; Chatterton, R. T.; Davis, J. M. Alteration in serum cortisol and its binding characteristics in anorexia nervosa. *J. Clin. Endocrinol. Metab. 49:* 406–11, 1979.

54. Boyar, R. M.; Katz, J. Twenty-four-hour Gonadotropin Secretion Patterns in Anorexia Nervosa. In Vigersky, R. (ed.), *Anorexia Nervosa.* New York: Raven Press, 1977, pp. 177–87.

55. Garfinkel, P. E.; Brown, G. M.; Stancer, H. C.; *et al.* Hypothalamic-pituitary function in anorexia nervosa. *Arch. Gen. Psychiat. 32:* 739–44, 1975.

56. Boyar, R. M.; Hellman, L. D.; Roffwarg, H.; *et al.* Cortisol secretion and metabolism in anorexia nervosa. *New Eng. J. Med. 296:* 190–93, 1977. '

57. Walsh, B. T.; Katz, J. L.; Levin, J.; *et al.* Adrenal activity in anorexia nervosa. *Psychosom. Med. 40:* 499–506, 1978.

58. Mecklenberg, R. S.; Loriaux, D. L.; Thompson, R. H.; *et al.* Hypothalamic dysfunction in patients with anorexia nervosa. *Medicine 53:* 147–59, 1974.

59. Vigersky, R. A.; Loriaux, D. L.; Andersen, A. E.; *et al.* Delayed pituitary hormone response to LRF and TRF in patients with anorexia nervosa and with secondary amenorrhea associated with simple weight loss. *J. Clin. Endocrinol. Metab. 43:* 893–900, 1973.

60. Katz, J. L.; Boyar, R. M.; Roffwarg, H.; *et al.* Weight and circadian luteinizing hormone secretory pattern in anorexia nervosa. *Psychosom. Med. 40:* 549–67, 1978.

61. Akande, E. O.; Carr, P. J.; Dutton, A.; *et al.* Effect of synthetic gonadotropin-releasing hormone in secondary amenorrhea. *Lancet 2:* 112–16, 1972.

62. Burman, K. D.; Vigersky, R. A.; Loriaux, D. L.; *et al.* Investigations Concerning Thyroxine Deiodinative Pathways in Patients with Anorexia Nervosa. In Vigersky, R. (ed.), *Anorexia Nervosa.* New York: Raven Press, 1977.

63. Groxson, M. S.; Ibbertson, H. K. Low serum triiodothyronine (T_3) and hypothyroidism in anorexia nervosa. *J. Clin. Endocrinol. Metab. 44:* 167–74, 1977.

64. Miyai, K.; Yamamoto, T.; Azukizawa, M.; *et al.* Serum thyroid hormones and thyrotropin in anorexia nervosa. *J. Clin. Endocrinol. Metab. 40:* 334–38, 1975.

65. Wakeling, A.; DeSouza, V. A.; Oore, M. B. R.; *et al.* Amenorrhea, body weight and serum hormone concentrations, with particular reference to prolactin and thyroid hormones in anorexia nervosa. *Psychol. Med. 9:* 265–72, 1979.

66. Casper, R. C.; Davis, J. M.; Pandey, C. N. The Effect of the Nutritional Status and Weight Changes on Hypothalamic Function Tests in Anorexia Nervosa. In

Vigersky, R. (ed.), *Anorexia Nervosa*. New York: Raven Press, 1977, pp. 137-47.

67. Sherman, B. M.; Halmi, K. A. Effect of Nutritional Rehabilitation on Hypothalamic-Pituitary Function in Anorexia Nervosa. In Vigersky, R. (ed.), *Anorexia Nervosa*. New York: Raven Press, 1977, pp. 211-23.

68. Brown, G. M.; Kirwan, P.; Garfinkel, P.; *et al.* Overnight patterning of prolactin and melatonin in anorexia nervosa. (abstr.) Venice: 2d International Symposium on Clinical Psycho–Neuro–Endocrinology in Reproduction, June, 1979.

69. Kalucy, R. C.; Crisp, A. H.; Chard, T.; *et al.* Nocturnal hormonal profiles in massive obesity, anorexia nervosa, and normal females. *J. Psychosom. Res. 20:* 595-604, 1976.

70. Russell, G. F. R.; Loraine, J. A.; Bell, E. T.; *et al.* Gonadotropin and estrogen excretion in patients with anorexia nervosa. *J. Psychosom. Res. 9:* 79-85, 1965.

71. Russell, G. F. R.; Beardwood, C. J. The Feeding Disorders, with Particular Reference to Anorexia Nervosa and Its Associated Gonadotrophin Changes. In Michael, R. P. (ed.), *Endocrinology and Human Behaviour*. London: Oxford University Press, 1968, pp. 310-29.

72. Beumont, P. J. V. Anorexia nervosa: A review. *S. Afr. Med. J. 44:* 911-15, 1970.

73. Davidson, D. M. Anorexia nervosa in a serviceman: Case report. *Milit. Med., 617-19,* September, 1976.

74. Baranowska, B.; Zgliczynski, S. Enhanced testosterone in female patients with anorexia nervosa: Its normalization after weight gain. *Acta Endocrinol. Copen. 90:* 328-35, 1979.

75. Danowski, T. S.; Livstone, E.; Gonzales, A. R.; *et al.* Fractional and partial hypopituitarism in anorexia nervosa. *Hormones 3:* 105-18, 1972.

76. Emanuel, R. W. Endocrine activity in anorexia nervosa. *J. Clin. Endocrinol. Metab. 16:* 801-16, 1956.

77. Gold, P. W.; Kaye, W.; Robertson, G. L.; *et al.* Abnormalities in plasma and cerebrospinal fluid vasopressin in patients with anorexia nervosa. *New Eng. J. Med. 308*(19): 1117-23, 1983.

78. Beumont, P. J. V.; George, G. C. W.; Pimstone, B. L.; *et al.* Body weight and the pituitary response to hypothalamic-releasing hormones in patients with anorexia nervosa. *J. Clin. Endocrinol. Metab. 43:* 487-96, 1976.

79. Casper, R. C.; Chatterton, R. T.; Davis, J. M. Alteration in serum cortisol and its binding characteristics in anorexia nervosa. *J. Clin. Endocrinol. Metab. 49:* 406-11, 1979.

80. Beumont, P. J. V.; Friesen, H. G.; Gelder, M. G.; *et al.* Plasma prolactin and luteinizing levels in anorexia nervosa. *Psychol. Med. 4:* 219-21, 1974.

81. Isaacs, A. J.; Leslie, R. D. G.; Gomez, J.; *et al.* The effect of weight gain on gonadotrophins and prolactin in anorexia nervosa. *Acta Endocrinol. 94:* 145-50, 1980.

82. Hafner, R. J.; Crisp, A. J. McNeilly, A. S. Prolactin and gonadotrophin activity in females treated for anorexia nervosa. *Postgrad. Med. 52:* 76-79, 1976.

83. Gold, M. S.; Pottash, A. L. C.; Sweeney, D. R.; *et al.* Further evidence of hypothalamic–pituitary dysfunction in anorexia nervosa. *Am. J. Psychiat. 137:* 101–2, 1980.

84. Malda, K.; Kato, Y.; Yamaguchi, N.; *et al.* Growth hormone release following thyrotrophin-releasing hormone injection into patients with anorexia nervosa. *Acta Endocrinol. 81:* 8, 1976.

85. Ryle, J. A. Discussion on anorexia nervosa. *Proc. Roy. Soc. Med. 32:* 735–46, 1939.

86. Theander, S. Anorexia nervosa: A psychiatric investigation of 44 female cases. *Acta Psychiat. Scand. Suppl. 214:* 1–194, 1970.

87. Hsu, L. K. G.; Crisp, A. J.; Harding, B. Outcome of anorexia nervosa. *Lancet 1:* 61–65, 1979.

88. Garfinkel, P. E.; Moldofsky, H.; Garner, D. M. The Outcome of Anorexia Nervosa: Significance of Clinical Features, Body Image, and Behavior Modification. In Vigersky, R. (ed.), *Anorexia Nervosa.* New York: Raven Press, 1977, pp. 315–29.

89. Halmi, K.; Brodland, G.; Loney, J. Prognosis in anorexia nervosa. *Ann. Int. Med. 78:* 907–9, 1973.

90. Gross, H. A.; Ebert, M. H.; Faden, V. B.; *et al.* A double-blind controlled trial of lithium carbonate in primary anorexia nervosa. *J. Clin. Psychopharm. 1(6):* 376–81, 1981.

91. Pope, H. G.; Hudson, J. I.; Jonas, J. M.; *et al.* Bulimia treated with imipramine: A placebo-controlled, double-blind study. *Am. J. Psychiat. 140(5):* 554–58, 1983.

92. Feighner, J. P.; Robins, E.; Guze, S. B.; *et al.* Diagnostic criteria for use in psychiatric research. *Arch. Gen. Psychiat. 26:* 56–63, 1972.

93. Russell, G. F. M. The Management of Anorexia Nervosa. In *Symposium on Anorexia Nervosa and Obesity.* Royal College of Physicians in Edinburgh, 1973, p. 43.

94. Bruch, H. *Eating Disorders: Obesity, Anorexia Nervosa, and the Person Within.* New York: Basic Books, 1973.

95. Maloney, M. J.; Farrell, M. K. Treatment of severe weight loss in anorexia nervosa with hyperalimentation and psychotherapy. *Am. J. Psychiat. 137(3):* 310–14, 1980.

96. Cincirpini, P. M.; Kornblith, S. J.; Turner, S. M.; *et al.* A behavioral program for the management of anorexia nervosa and bulimia. *J. Nerv. Ment. Dis. 171(3):* 186–89, 1983.

97. Dally, P. J.; Sargant, W. A new treatment of anorexia nervosa. *Br. Med. J. 1:* 1770–73, 1960.

98. Needleman, H. L.; Waber, D. Amitryptiline therapy in patients with anorexia nervosa (letter). *Lancet 2:* 580, 1976.

99. Moore, D. C. Amitryptiline therapy in anorexia nervosa. *Am. J. Psychiat. 34:* 1303–4, 1977.

100. Kendler, K. S. Amitryptiline induced obesity in anorexia nervosa: A case report. *Am. J. Psychiat. 135:* 1107–8, 1978.

101. Walsh, B. T.; Stewart, J. W.; Wright, L.; *et al.* Treatment of bulimia with monoamine oxidase inhibitors. *Am. J. Psychiat. 139*(12): 1629–30, 1982.

102. Kaplan, A. J.; Garfinkel, P. E.; Darby, P. L.; *et al.* Carbamazepine in the treatment of bulimia. *Am. J. Psychiat. 140*(9): 1225–26, 1983.

103. Barcai, A. Lithium in adult anorexia nervosa. *Acta Psychiat. Scand. 55:* 97–101, 1977.

104. Crisp, A. H.; Kalucy, R. S. The effect of leukotomy in untractable adolescent weight phobia. *Postgrad. Med. J. 49:* 883, 1973.

105. Bernstein, I. C. Anorexia nervosa treated successfully with electroshock therapy. *Am. J. Psychiat. 120:* 1023, 1964.

106. Jennings, K. P.; Klidjian, A. M. Acute gastric dilatation in anorexia nervosa. *Br. Med. J. 2:* 477–78, 1974.

CHAPTER 22

Anxiety Disorder, Obsessional Disorder

Two disorders infrequently encountered in a psychiatric inpatient unit (although they are quite common in a busy medically oriented psychiatric practice) are included here for thoroughness's sake and because on rare occasions hospitalization will be indicated for intensive somatic therapy.

Anxiety Disorder

This disorder, which has a population prevalence of 5 percent (1) and is more common in women than in men (2), usually has its onset in the third decade of life and is characterized by subjective, unjustified, and occasionally overwhelming sensations of tension, depersonalization, fear, and panic, variably accompanied by such manifestations of autonomic nervous system hyperactivity as tachycardia, tachypnea, dry mouth, hyperperistalsis, sweating, pallor, and mydriasis. When the first attack chances to occur suddenly while the patient is away from home, he may subsequently develop a profound disinclination ever again to travel alone for fear that another such attack might render him helpless and without succor. For unknown reasons, such agoraphobics (also described as having phobic anxiety–depersonalization syndrome) are frequently women ("housebound housewives") who become utterly dependent on their family or friends for even the shortest trips away from home.

In other instances anxiety symptoms gradually insinuate themselves into a previously normal existence until their accumulated weight over the years results in a socially and occupationally crippling disability.

In one or another patient individual clinical features may predominate, giving a characteristic stamp and title to the syndrome. Thus, hyperventilation syndrome (tachypnea, light-headedness, facial pallor), neurocirculatory asthenia (palpitations, chest pain, fatigue, exercise intolerance), panic disorder (sensation of impending doom, depersonalization, muscular weakness), and agoraphobia are probably all manifestations of the same underlying disorder, may be observed at various times in the same patient, and may respond to the same treatment.

Anxiety disorders are familial and may also be associated with an increased risk for affective disorder in first-degree relatives (3). Two physiological markers, mitral valve prolapse (4) and lactate intolerance (5), have been identified in some patients with anxiety disorders, but their etiological significance remains to be defined. They may be responsible, however, for the frequent complaint of exercise intolerance in many patients so afflicted. A lactate tolerance test has been proposed as a diagnostic laboratory procedure in patients with anxiety disorders (6). In this procedure a 500 molar solution of sodium lactate is given intravenously at a rate of 20 ml./minute, producing a typical anxiety attack in patients so predisposed. Although sensitivity, specificity, and diagnostic confidence of the test remain to be defined, the procedure is increasingly used clinically to identify patients with atypical syndromes and to demonstrate to them the biological nature of their disorder.

Most patients with anxiety disorders should receive outpatient treatment, usually with tricyclic antidepressants or MAOIs, alone or in combination with behavioral therapies (e.g. systematic desensitization). According to one method the primary anxiety or panic disorder is treated by the medication, and the acquired (conditioned) phobic behavior is then treated by behavioral means (7). The beta-adrenergic blocking agent propranolol has also been used in doses of 30–120 mg./day and provides equivalent anxiolysis to diazepam but without its addictive potential (8). An occasional patient, however, may be so crippled by his symptoms that a brief removal to the protective environment of a hospital is justified, the more so if an intensive course of high-dose MAOI is contemplated. (More frequent, however, is the patient who requires admission to be detoxified from the high-dose, chronic benzodiazepine treatment he is receiving, often combined with excessive amounts of self-administered alcohol.)

A variety of psychosurgical procedures (e.g. limbic leucotomy, subcaudate tractotomy) are claimed as effective in the treatment of chronic anxiety disorders, with reported results of about 50–60 percent much improved or recovered in uncontrolled trials (9, 10). Although a definitive statement on the value of psychosurgery in anxiety states awaits the results of randomized, controlled studies, there are nevertheless some patients who fail a multitude of other biological therapies expertly administered, yet experience marked improvement after psychosurgery. We therefore recommend careful consideration of this form of treatment in patients who remain unresponsive to the standard approaches and whose anxiety symptoms seriously impair their daily functioning. The best results are obtained in patients who have supportive families, who do not abuse drugs or alcohol, and who have not exhibited any social or personality deterioration.

Obsessional Disorder

Obsessional disorder has a population prevalence of less than 1 percent (11) and is equally distributed between the sexes. There is a tendency to familial clustering (12), but its extent is undefined as yet. Obsessional disorder is in many ways more severe than anxiety disorder and is characterized primarily by the subjective experience of tortured self-doubt. Obsessional thoughts of contamination with dirt and germs typically lead to compulsive washing and cleaning rituals, which may be totally out of the patient's control (they are not, however, experienced by him as resulting from any external agency). "Checking" behaviors are common, as the patient repeatedly has to reassure himself that he has not left the gas on, left the door unlocked, inadvertently insulted someone in a letter, or accidentally run over a pedestrian on the highway without realizing it. There is a driven quality to the patient's behavior, and extreme anxiety is produced by any attempt to prevent or interfere with the compulsive rituals. The condition, although fluctuating in intensity, is generally chronic, and frequently worsens with time and the accumulation of new rituals, which add to, rather than replace, existing ones. It is apparent to the patient that his obsessional fear (for example, of asphyxiating on his own saliva while asleep) is absurd—even ludicrous—but this in no way obviates his compelling need to awaken himself by alarm every fifteen minutes throughout the night in order to prevent such an outcome.

Obsessional disorders are notoriously resistant to treatment, and neuroleptics, anxiolytics, standard antidepressants, and ECT are all generally ineffective. Recently a chlorinated form of the tricyclic antidepressant imipramine (chlorimipramine) has been reported successful in treating obsessional patients, but large-scale controlled trials of this compound have not yet been reported, and the drug has not yet been introduced for use in the United States.

As for anxiety disorder, it is occasionally justified to administer a brief course of bilateral ECT for temporary relief in a patient whose severe, intractable, obsessional disorder has brought him to a standstill or to the verge of suicide (13). The comments on psychosurgery made above apply equally to patients with obsessional disorders.

References

1. Cohen, M.; White, P. Life situations, emotions, and neurocirculatory asthenia (anxiety neurosis, effort syndrome). *Ass. Res. Nerv. Dis. Proc. 29:* 832–69, 1950.

2. Woodruff, R. A.; Goodwin, D. W.; Guze, S. B. *Psychiatric Diagnosis.* New York: Oxford University Press, 1974, p. 47.

3. Wheeler, E. O.; White, P. D.; Reed, E. W.; *et al.* Familial incidence of neurocirculatory asthenia (anxiety neurosis, effort syndrome). *J. Clin. Invest. 27:* 562, 1948.

4. Kantor, J. S.; Zitrin, C. M.; Zeldis, S. M. Mitral valve prolapse syndrome in agoraphobic patients. *Am. J. Psychiat. 137:* 467–69, 1980.

5. Pitts, F. N.; McClure, J. N., Jr. Lactate metabolism in anxiety neurosis. *New Erg. J. Med. 277:* 1329–36, 1967.

6. Liebowitz, M. R.; Klein, D. F. Differential diagnosis and treatment of panic attacks and phobic states. *Ann. Rev. Med. 32:* 583–99, 1981.

7. Shader, R. I.; Goodman, M.; Gever, J. Panic disorders: Current perspectives. *J. Clin. Psychopharm. 2* (suppl. to no. 6): 25–105, 1982.

8. Wheatley, D. Comparative effects of propranolol and chlordiazepoxide in anxiety states. *Br. J. Psychiat. 115:* 1411–12, 1969.

9. Guptepe, E. O.; Young, L. B.; Bridges, P. K. A further review of the results of stereotactic subcaudate tractotomy. *Br. J. Psychiat. 126:* 270–80, 1975.

10. Mitchell–Heggs, N.; Kelly, D.; Richardson, A. Stereotactic limbic lencotomy: A follow-up at 16 months. *Br. J. Psychiat. 128:* 226–40, 1976.

11. Weissman, M.; Meyers, J.; Harding, P. Psychiatric disorders in a U.S. urban community: 1975–1976. *Am. J. Psychiat. 135:* 459–67, 1978.

12. Brown, F. W. Heredity in the psychoneuroses. *Proc. Roy. Soc. Med. 35:* 785–90, 1942.

13. Goldney, R. D.; Simpson, I. G. Female genital self-mutilation, dysorexia and the hysterical personality: The Caenis syndrome. *Can. Psychiat. Assoc. J. 20:* 435–41, 1975.

CHAPTER 23

Somatization Disorder (Briquet's Syndrome)

A working knowledge of somatization disorder (Briquet's syndrome, hysteria), coupled with a willingness to obtain a medical systems review, will sometimes solve a diagnostic puzzle in a patient who has experienced unnecessary, invasive, and expensive diagnostic studies; needless medical treatments (including surgery); and considerable physician and patient frustration and resentment. The patient with classic somatization disorder is a woman with a long history of medically unexplained complaints and multiple hospitalizations. She reports that her physicians rarely offer a diagnosis and dismiss her complaints with such statements as, "It's all in your head." She answers questions dramatically and is suggestible, answering "yes" to questions about myriad medical symptoms. In the absence of superimposed disorders, the initial physical examination and laboratory tests reveal no clear abnormalities.

The *DSM-III* (1) criteria for somatization disorder, modified from the Perley and Guze (2) and Feighner *et al.* (3) criteria for the syndrome, are as follows:

1. A history of physical symptoms of several years' duration beginning before the age of thirty
2. Complaints of at least fourteen symptoms for women and twelve for men, from thirty-seven symptoms listed below

To count a symptom as present, the individual must report that the symptom caused him or her to take medicine (other than aspirin), alter his or her life pattern, or see a physician. The symptoms, in the judgment of the clinician, are not adequately explained by physical disorder or physical injury and are not side effects of medication, drugs, or alcohol. The clinician need not be convinced that the symptom was actually present, e.g. that the individual actually vomited throughout her entire pregnancy; report of the symptom by the individual is sufficient. The symptoms are:

Sickly. Believes that he or she has been sickly for a good part of his or her life

Conversion or pseudoneurological symptoms. Difficulty swallowing, loss of voice, deafness, double vision, blurred vision, blindness, fainting or loss of consciousness, memory loss, seizures or convulsions, trouble walking, paralysis or muscle weakness, urinary retention or difficulty urinating

Gastrointestinal symptoms. Abdominal pain, nausea, vomiting spells (other than during pregnancy), bloating (gassy), intolerance (e.g. gets sick) of a variety of foods, diarrhea

Female reproductive symptoms. Judged by the individual as occurring more frequently or severely than in most women: painful menstruation, menstrual irregularity, excessive bleeding, severe vomiting throughout pregnancy or causing hospitalization during pregnancy

Psychosexual symptoms. For the major part of the individual's life after opportunities for sexual activity: sexual indifference, lack of pleasure during intercourse, pain during intercourse

Pain. Pain in back, joints, extremities, genital area (other than during intercourse); pain on urination; other pain (other than headaches)

Cardiopulmonary symptoms. Shortness of breath, palpitations, chest pain, dizziness

Most of the symptoms of somatization disorder do not mimic neurologic disease. However, conversion disorders, which by definition do mimic symptoms of neurologic disease, are more common in patients with somatization disorder (4). The appendix to this chapter consists of a second interview of a twenty-five-year-old woman with Briquet's syndrome. This interview is presented because some readers will not be familiar with typical responses of patients with Briquet's syndrome.

The prevalence of Briquet's syndrome is unclear. In one urban community, .04 percent of those interviewed satisfied diagnostic criteria for it (5). It occurs in 1–2 percent of women and is relatively rare in men (6); however, it may be somewhat more common among homosexual men or among men seeking or receiving disability compensation (7, 8). Briquet's syndrome runs in families, occurring in 20 percent of first degree relatives of patients with the disorder (9, 10). For reasons not yet clear (one hypothesis is that Briquet's syndrome and sociopathy share similar genotypes), there is an increased prevalence of sociopathy and alcoholism among male relatives of patients with Briquet's syndrome, as well as an increased prevalence of Briquet's syndrome among female relatives of patients with sociopathy or alcoholism (9, 10). Also, individuals with somatization disorder are more likely than others to marry sociopaths, alcoholics, or drug abusers (11, 12).

As mentioned before, people with somatization disorder (as well as those with sociopathy) have an increased prevalence of conversion disorders (4), and increased rates of hospitalization (4) and unnecessary surgical procedures (13). Briquet's syndrome is common among female felons, 41 percent of whom meet the Feighner *et al.* (3) criteria for Briquet's syndrome (14, 15). Of these female criminals, the majority have a concurrent diagnosis of sociopathy (14).

Another correlation is that patients with somatization disorder have an increased frequency of suicidal thoughts and suicidal attempts. Completed suicide is rare in Briquet's syndrome, however, only one such case having been reported (15). At the current state of our knowledge, Briquet's syndrome cannot be cured, but individual symptoms usually subside spontaneously.

If a diagnosis of Briquet's syndrome is made in an emergency room or consultation service, the patient will rarely need to be admitted to the psychiatric ward. Occasionally, however, the diagnosis is overlooked, and the patient may be admitted because of a depressed mood or a suicide attempt.

The medical systems review needed for the diagnosis may extend the initial diagnostic interview by as much as a half-hour or require a follow-up interview. When the diagnosis is established, this should be presented and explained to the patient. Some patients are grateful for what is probably the first cohesive explanation of their recurrent symptoms they have ever received. However, the degree of genuine acceptance of this diagnosis is highly variable.

Despite the temptation for us to recommend seemingly reasonable "prescriptions" (16, 17) for the management of patients with somatization disorder, there is no known effective treatment. The patient with Briquet's syndrome, like the sociopath, should be told that there is nothing that medical science can do to alter the overall course of the condition. If the patient has been referred by another physician, the consulting psychiatrist should personally inform the referring physician of the diagnosis and provide a detailed explanation about somatization disorder if the referring physician does not have a working knowledge of this syndrome.

Appendix: A Diagnostic Interview with a Patient with Somatization Disorder

DOCTOR: Perhaps we could begin by your telling me about the symptoms for which you came here.

PATIENT: I had painful blackouts and I had the swelling in the head and a funny feeling like I wanted to scream or something, and I would just pass out and then when I wake up I don't have any feelings and I can't use my legs to walk.

DOCTOR: Your legs get paralyzed?

PATIENT: Uh-huh.

DOCTOR: And they don't have any feeling in them either?

PATIENT: A little feeling but I just can't move them. I had it before and it's about the same.

DOCTOR: Could you describe the blackouts a bit more?

PATIENT: Sometimes I can remember blacking out and sometimes I can't.

DOCTOR: What happens when you black out?

PATIENT: I'd just fall backwards. My head swims and I'd get a funny feeling inside and I'd just pass out, falling backwards.

DOCTOR: Any other symptoms that go along with that?

PATIENT: With the blackouts?

DOCTOR: Yes.

PATIENT: The headaches.

DOCTOR: Describe those for me.

PATIENT: They're here, on the right side, real bad headaches, and it seemed like nothing would help me. I'd wake up with them and go to sleep with them. The only thing they're giving me now is Fiorinal, and trying to help me, but it's not helping me, only calms me down a little bit. But I still have the headaches.

DOCTOR: Any other symptoms that go along with these symptoms?

PATIENT: Blurred vision.

DOCTOR: Can you describe that a little bit?

PATIENT: Okay. If I'm reading, the words like go together, and if I'm walking or something, it's like some hairy stuff is coming over my eyes and I can't see. And lately I've been seeing spots, you know.

DOCTOR: Does that happen at the same time as the headaches or at different times?

PATIENT: No, with the headaches, and at nighttime, driving. Well, I haven't been driving but riding in the car with somebody. Now the lights bother me coming from the other way.

DOCTOR: Did the visual problem or the blurring of vision ever get to the point where you are actually temporarily blind?

PATIENT: Yes, I went blind for three days.

DOCTOR: What happened when you were blind?

PATIENT: Nothing; I just lost it and I went to an eye specialist in Jacksonville and he said that I had to overcome it and just wait and wait for a couple days and it would go away. That's when I was paralyzed then too and couldn't walk for twenty-one days. All that was included with the blindness.

Doctor: Now, has any of this been satisfactorily explained to you by a doctor?

Patient: No. They just said, "It's just your nerves."

Doctor: It's got to be your nerves, since it's affecting your nervous system. But did they label any disease or condition that was causing this?

Patient: No.

Doctor: Now let me ask you a series of questions like I said I would, going through system by system of your body. Would you describe yourself as having been sickly all of your life?

Patient: I never had any headaches before I went into service—1971—only when I got out of the service.

Doctor: Would you describe yourself as having been a sickly child?

Patient: Yes.

Doctor: In what way were you a sickly child?

Patient: Stomach pains a lot, and they thought I had an ulcer, and the doctor said it was the burning from the acid, and he put me on like a bland diet.

Doctor: Did they say you definitely had an ulcer, or possibly?

Patient: Possibly.

Doctor: Did they ever prove it with a barium x-ray?

Patient: The only thing they did that for was for an attorney that I spoke to.

Doctor: Did you have trouble with your hearing?

Patient: A little. I told the doctor about it. Yeah, I can see your mouth moving, maybe I'm just blinking an eye, but I can't hear what you're saying.

Doctor: You actually become temporarily deaf. Did you tell the doctor about it?

Patient: Yes.

Doctor: What did he tell you?

Patient: Nothing. You're deaf. It's okay. Nothing.

Doctor: It seems like you've been going to doctors with medical symptoms and they can't find the cause.

Patient: You see, most of the doctors I was going to were my family.

Doctor: You mean, doctors in the family?

Patient: My uncle.

Doctor: Would he treat you like a real patient?

Patient: Sometimes.

Doctor: Besides these symptoms you've mentioned, have you ever had trouble swallowing?

Patient: Yes.

Doctor: Under what circumstances?

Patient: Spitting up sometimes, you know.

Doctor: Would you have trouble swallowing when you would be eating or drinking?

Patient: Yes, even my own saliva I can't get it down. I get up at night coughing and choking.

Doctor: Along the same lines, have you ever had a lump in your throat?

Patient: No, only when I was pregnant.

Doctor: And what happened then?

Patient: That's when I found out I was pregnant. I had a lump in my throat and I thought there was something in it. I just kept eating bread, just kept eating bread. I thought I had something caught in it that wouldn't go down.

DOCTOR: I guess it turned out there was nothing in your throat, but something in your belly. Did you tell any doctors about the trouble swallowing?

PATIENT: Um-hum, when I was pregnant. They just mashed my throat and checked it and told me to swallow.

DOCTOR: Did they tell you what was wrong?

PATIENT: Nothing.

DOCTOR: To change subjects again, were there times when you had trouble breathing?

PATIENT: Yes. Nighttime, like I say, even now. My husband had to get up during the night and jump up and get me water. I'd sit up and kind of breathe. Dr. Wise gave me a bag. He said maybe I was having—oh, wow—shoot!

DOCTOR: Did they say you were hyperventilating?

PATIENT: Yeah.

DOCTOR: Was that the only explanation that was offered to you?

PATIENT: Yeah.

DOCTOR: What about chest pains?

PATIENT: Yes, I told the doctor about it the other day and she said it was probably a muscle spasm or something.

DOCTOR: Did she know for sure?

PATIENT: No.

DOCTOR: How long have you been having chest pains?

PATIENT: For just a little while ago.

DOCTOR: Back pains?

PATIENT: No back pains, but the breathing. If I'm around somebody smoking I can't catch my breath. My husband won't let them smoke in the house.

DOCTOR: Coughing?

PATIENT: No. Just a little, very little.

DOCTOR: What about your appetite?

PATIENT: Bad.

DOCTOR: You had a bad appetite?

PATIENT: Yes, I went down to 98 pounds.

DOCTOR: From what?

PATIENT: From just not eating.

DOCTOR: You went down to 98 pounds from how many pounds?

PATIENT: From 135.

DOCTOR: To 98?

PATIENT: Um-hum.

DOCTOR: Do you know why you lost your appetite and lost that much weight?

PATIENT: No, I just lost it. My mom was cooking this and that. Everything I like to eat, but no good.

DOCTOR: Did you tell a doctor about it?

PATIENT: Yes, then I started back eating. The more I was eating, the more weight I was losing. And the doctor said it was my nerves.

DOCTOR: No other explanation?

PATIENT: No, that was it.

DOCTOR: What about being nauseated?

PATIENT: Yes.

DOCTOR: What circumstances?

PATIENT: I eat a lot of salt for that. The doctor told me to take a little pinch of salt and lick it to soothe my stomach.

DOCTOR: Did the doctor tell you why?

PATIENT: That's all he told me to do.

DOCTOR: What about vomiting?

PATIENT: No.

DOCTOR: Do you mean you don't vomit or that you haven't vomited recently?

PATIENT: I do vomit.

DOCTOR: What were the circumstances? When you would vomit?

PATIENT: I wake up in the middle of the night and I'm nauseated.

DOCTOR: Even when you're not pregnant?

PATIENT: I had bowel obstructions and I had constipation real bad. I had to take enemas just about every day.

DOCTOR: Even now?

PATIENT: Yes.

DOCTOR: Was that explained to you?

PATIENT: No. My father had the same problem.

DOCTOR: What about diarrhea?

PATIENT: No.

DOCTOR: Just constipation?

PATIENT: Constipation. An enema every day. If I don't take an enema, I go two or three weeks without going to the rest room.

DOCTOR: Other than that your dad had it, do you know what caused the constipation?

PATIENT: No.

DOCTOR: Does your weight shift around and change a great deal?

PATIENT: Yes, um-hum, suddenly very heavy and very light. That's what I'm doing now.

DOCTOR: Has that been explained to you?

PATIENT: No. Nothing. It's going up and down.

DOCTOR: That's a mystery, isn't it? The doctors don't know anything?

PATIENT: That's why I've tried to take all these pills and tried to kill myself so many times, because I'm tired of people not telling me what's wrong. You get tired of living a life like that.

DOCTOR: Do you have feelings of life not worth living?

PATIENT: I'm getting fed up.

DOCTOR: Do you have thoughts of suicide?

PATIENT: Yes.

DOCTOR: You took pills to kill yourself?

PATIENT: Ten times.

DOCTOR: Were you depressed during those times?

PATIENT: Yes. My husband got on my nerves. Not just him, just going to the hospital all the time, not knowing anything and talking to my parents, but they're not talking to me.

DOCTOR: During those times or any other times, have you had crying spells or cry very easily?

PATIENT: Crying. My husband and I, now we just got married and I've already threatened to kill him. It's real bad.

DOCTOR: Feelings of being hopeless?

PATIENT: Yes, I asked Dr. Brown about my grandfather, just died January first. I'm still seeing him and I'm still crying every night. How long is this supposed to last? I don't know if this has a lot to do with it or what because I was close to my grandfather. My grandfather raised me.

DOCTOR: Do you have visions or hallucinations of him, or any other hallucinations?

PATIENT: I can see him plain, just like he is here, right here.

DOCTOR: During the day?

PATIENT: Day, night, any time. I want to talk with him.

DOCTOR: Hallucinations of him?

PATIENT: Yes.

DOCTOR: Is it just that you think of him or do you actually, literally, see him?

PATIENT: I see him. He clears his throat. He used to clear his throat a lot. I can hear it. I was the only one close to my grandfather because my grandfather and grandmother raised me. I don't know whether my mother's other kids—none of them feel the same way. None of them took it like I took it. And I asked my mother, Why is it supposed to be like that? I'm the only one who's supposed to suffer and nobody else. None of my brothers or sisters.

DOCTOR: Do you also suffer with nervous attacks or nervous spells?

PATIENT: Yes.

DOCTOR: What symptoms do you get when you have a nervous spell?

PATIENT: Shaky.

DOCTOR: Anything else?

PATIENT: I just have to get up and walk or go and I just have to get up and go.

DOCTOR: When you get nervous attacks or get worried, what is it that you worry about?

PATIENT: I don't know. And everyone I talk to, somebody to understand me, says, "Oh, it's nothing." It has to be something.

DOCTOR: I think there is, and I'm going to talk to you about it in a little while.

PATIENT: Okay.

DOCTOR: Are there any things you are particularly afraid of that the average person wouldn't be afraid of?

PATIENT: I have a fear of losing my grandmother.

DOCTOR: Any fear of animals or fear of heights or fear of being closed in?

PATIENT: I can't stay in a room that's closed.

DOCTOR: What happens if you have to stay in a room that's closed?

PATIENT: Then I get these spells.

DOCTOR: Does it scare you? What do you do?

PATIENT: I get out.

DOCTOR: Any room, or only a small room?

PATIENT: I have to go outside.

DOCTOR: Are you more fearful of being in rooms than the average person?

PATIENT: Um-hum, yes.

DOCTOR: Are you sure of it?

PATIENT: Um-hum.

DOCTOR: To change subjects on you again, are there any foods that absolutely don't agree with you, that make you extremely sick?

PATIENT: No. The only thing I can't is drink orange juice. It just breaks me out. That's all.

DOCTOR: You get a rash from orange juice. What about oranges?

PATIENT: Oranges or orange juice, or peaches. But peach juice I can drink. Maybe it's just the furry hair on the peaches, you know.

DOCTOR: What would happen if you ate the peaches?

PATIENT: I'd break out with a rash.

DOCTOR: Okay. Do you ever get very bloated in the belly?

PATIENT: In the night time. My husband asked me what's wrong with my stomach.

DOCTOR: What do you experience when you are bloated?

PATIENT: It's just like I'm pregnant.

DOCTOR: Is it always right after you've eaten, or nighttime or any time?

PATIENT: Mostly nighttime when I'm lying down or something, and when I want to get up and go to the restroom, my stomach is out.

DOCTOR: Has it ever been explained to you.

PATIENT: No.

DOCTOR: You saw a doctor?

PATIENT: The doctor said it was nerves.

DOCTOR: It seems the reason for everything.

PATIENT: I had a private psychiatrist. She said, I understand you and understand your problems. And she talked with my mother and father, and they came and took me home and they gave me anything I want.

DOCTOR: At what age did you have the private psychiatrist?

PATIENT: In 1975. That's before I left home.

DOCTOR: To get back to specific medical symptoms, do you get burning when you urinate?

PATIENT: No.

DOCTOR: Has your urine ever been trapped inside of you like it couldn't come out?

PATIENT: Um-hum.

DOCTOR: Did you tell the doctor about that?

PATIENT: Um-hum. Yes, nothing. Nerves, nothing else. Everything is my nerves.

DOCTOR: Okay. Your menstrual periods—are they regular?

PATIENT: I had a hysterectomy in 1975 or '76.

DOCTOR: Before 1975 did you have any problems with your menstruation?

PATIENT: I went a whole year without stopping. There were tumors in my womb.

DOCTOR: Before that year when you menstruated daily, were your periods regular?

PATIENT: No, they were irregular.

DOCTOR: Always irregular?

PATIENT: Ever since I first started, they were irregular.

DOCTOR: At what age?

PATIENT: Fourteen, fifteen. Okay, I went to dental school in Atlanta and I got real sick with cramps, and the doctor put me on birth control pills to regulate my periods.

DOCTOR: Did it work?

PATIENT: It worked. I had them for only two days on the pills.

DOCTOR: After that, did you continue to have menstrual cramps?

PATIENT: Yes, always.

DOCTOR: Even after you were put on the birth control pills when you were fourteen or fifteen?

PATIENT: I still had the pain, but it was less. Before they put me on the pills, my mother had to put heat on my stomach or I would pull my clothes back and I'd put my stomach on the cold floor.

DOCTOR: At any time before the year before your hysterectomy, when you weren't pregnant, did you ever miss a period for a very long time?

PATIENT: Yes, I missed it just for one month, for one or two months, because he said the ovary wasn't throwing out enough so it couldn't produce, so that's why. When it did come, it just ran like you turned on the water. For five or six days. And clogs came out.

DOCTOR: Was that even before that year when you were bleeding heavily because of tumors?

PATIENT: Um-hum.

DOCTOR: Have there ever been times when you would go for months and you didn't care at all about sex?

PATIENT: Yes. I'm doing that now.

DOCTOR: You mean you could just take it or leave it?

PATIENT: I'm doing that now, since May of last year, 1981.

DOCTOR: You've gone for a year and two months and you haven't cared about sex?

PATIENT: Yes.

DOCTOR: Do you go along with him with having sex?

PATIENT: Every once in a while.

DOCTOR: Is it ever painful?

PATIENT: Um-hum.

DOCTOR: Is it often very painful?

PATIENT: Every time we do something.

DOCTOR: Was it always like that?

PATIENT: No.

DOCTOR: When did it change?

PATIENT: When I had the oophorectomy.

DOCTOR: Why did you have an oophorectomy?

PATIENT: Because my ovary was infected. They took it out. The other ovary is still there.

DOCTOR: And since then, sex has been painful?

PATIENT: Yes. I told the doctor about it. He said maybe I had some adhesions, or something. At times there is no pleasure or no feeling.

DOCTOR: Has your husband been reasonably tolerant of you in terms of your medical symptoms?

PATIENT: I'm jumping on him so much and he just sits there and says it's okay. It's all right. You know, he's trying as hard as he can, but boy, I'm giving it to him. I know it, and I feel it.

DOCTOR: How many times have you been pregnant?

PATIENT: Twice.

DOCTOR: During either of the two pregnancies, did you vomit a lot?

PATIENT: Yes.

DOCTOR: How often did you vomit during that first pregnancy?

PATIENT: The first one, every time you turned around.

DOCTOR: For the whole pregnancy?

PATIENT: Yes.

DOCTOR: All nine months?

PATIENT: They put me in the hospital. I got toxemia. I was weighing 105 and I went up to 180 pounds.

DOCTOR: Most folks with toxemia get it during the third trimester of their pregnancy. Did you vomit through the whole nine months, every day?

PATIENT: Yes.

DOCTOR: Were you hospitalized for the vomiting?

PATIENT: The vomiting and the toxemia, in the fifth month, and again in the seventh month because I went into false labor.

DOCTOR: Do you ever get any seizures, where you fall to the ground and shake?

PATIENT: I had it. I told the doctor about it and he said it came from my taking too many pills, from the overdose, and my mother pushed a spoon in my mouth.

DOCTOR: You mean immediately after the overdose you began to shake with the seizure?

PATIENT: Uh-huh.

DOCTOR: Did you ever have a seizure at any other time?

PATIENT: When I hit my head on the floor a couple of weeks ago.

DOCTOR: Describe that seizure. What did you do?

PATIENT: Shaking, going up and down.

DOCTOR: Do you remember that yourself?

PATIENT: My husband told me about it.

DOCTOR: Were you given an explanation about that?

PATIENT: They said I was having a seizure. When I woke up, the doctor said, "Did you know you just had a seizure?" My husband said it didn't look like a seizure, but that's what the doctor said.

DOCTOR: Did they explain why you were having a seizure?

PATIENT: No. Nothing. I know I hit my head on the floor because I woke up with a headache and because I remember going down, but my husband didn't catch me, and I hit the floor.

References

1. American Psychiatric Association Task Force on Nomenclature and Statistics. *Diagnostic and Statistical Manual of Mental Disorders.* 3d ed. *DSM-III.* Washington, D.C.: American Psychiatric Association, 1980.

2. Perley, M. S.; Guze, S. B. Hysteria: The stability and usefulness of clinical criteria. *New Eng. J. Med. 266:* 421–26, 1962.

3. Feighner, J. P.; Robins, E.; Guze, S. B.; *et al.* Diagnostic criteria for use in psychiatric research. *Arch. Gen. Psychiat. 26:* 56–63, 1972.

4. Goodwin, D. W.; Guze, S. B. *Psychiatric Diagnosis.* 2d ed. New York: Oxford University Press, 1979.

5. Weissman, M. M.; Myers, J. K.; Harding, P. S. Psychiatric disorders in a U.S. urban community. *Am. J. Psychiat. 135:* 459–62, 1978.

6. Woodruff, R. A., Jr.; Clayton, P. J.; Guze, S. B. Hysteria: Studies of diagnosis, outcome and prevalence. *JAMA 215:* 425–28, 1971.

7. Sierles, F. S. Correlates of malingering. *Behav. Sci. and the Law* 2(1): 113–18, 1984.

8. Sierles, F. S.; Chen, J. J.; McFarland, R. E.; *et al.* Posttraumatic stress disorder and concurrent psychiatric illness: A preliminary report. *Am. J. Psychiat.* 140(9): 1077–79, 1983.

9. Arkonac, O.; Guze, S. B. A family study of hysteria. *New Eng. J. Med. 268:* 239–42, 1963.

10. Woerner, P. I.; Guze, S. B. A family and marital study of hysteria. *Br. J. Psychiat. 114:* 161–68, 1968.

11. Cloninger, C. R.; Guze, S. B. Female criminals: Their personal, familial and social backgrounds. *Arch. Gen. Psychiat. 23:* 554–58, 1970.

12. Cloninger, C. R.; Guze, S. B. Psychiatric illness and female criminality: The role of sociopathy and hysteria in antisocial women. *Am. J. Psychiat. 126:* 303–10, 1970.

13. Cohen, M. E.; Robins, E.; Purtell, J. J.; *et al.* Excessive surgery in hysteria. *JAMA 151:* 977–86, 1953.

14. Guze, S. B. *Criminality and Psychiatric Disorders.* New York: Oxford University Press, 1976.

15. Morrison, J. R. Suicide in a case of Briquet's syndrome. *J. Clin. Psychiat.* 42(3): 123, 1981.

16. Murphy, G. E. The clinical management of hysteria. *JAMA* 247(18): 2559–64, 1982.

17. Ford, C. V. *The Somatizing Disorders: Illness as a Way of Life.* New York: Elsevier, 1983.

CHAPTER 24

Conversion Disorder, Psychogenic Pain Disorder, and Hypochondriasis

Among the most controversial diagnoses in psychiatry are conversion disorder, psychogenic pain disorder, and hypochondriasis. For these "somatoform disorders" (1), the clinical presentations resemble those of systemic illnesses or coarse brain diseases. For example, a patient labeled as having conversion disorder manifests paralysis, one diagnosed as having psychogenic pain disorder complains of headache, and one with hypochondriasis fears that her dizziness is a sign of brain cancer. The controversy centers about their validity as distinct disorders (2–5), as against their being manifestations of other syndromes. Also, the *DSM-III* standards for conversion disorder and psychogenic pain disorder are unique because they "imply specific mechanisms to account for the disturbance," those mechanisms being "primary gain" ("keeping an internal conflict or need out of awareness") and "secondary gain" ("avoiding a particular activity that is noxious . . . or getting support from the environment that otherwise might not be forthcoming") (1).

Conversion Disorders

The classic concept of conversion disorder is that of a pseudoneurologic condition, whose signs and symptoms incompletely resemble those of neuro-

422

logic disorders. These include "paralysis, aphasia, seizures, coordination disturbances, akinesia, dyskinesia, blindness, tunnel vision, anosmia, anesthesia, and paresthesia" (1). The classic concept also includes the requirement that unless the pseudoneurologic condition (e.g. anesthesia due to conversion disorder) is "superimposed" upon a clear-cut neurologic disorder (e.g. multiple sclerosis), the signs that are present (e.g. hemianesthesia to the midline only) do not fit what is currently known about nervous system structure and function (e.g. that dermatomes cross the midline). An extension of this is that unless the conversion disorder is "superimposed," laboratory studies reveal no classic abnormalities such as spiking on the electroencephalogram or infarction on computerized tomographic scanning.

The *DSM-III* does not limit conversion disorder to pseudoneurologic symptoms; it includes symptoms associated with the automatic or endocrine system, such as vomiting or pseudocyesis. It also states that these signs and symptoms may be the symbolic representation of unconscious phenomena, for example, "vomiting as a conversion symptom can represent revulsion and disgust. Pseudocyesis (false pregnancy) can represent both a wish for. and a fear of, pregnancy." Although pain has been called the most common manifestation of conversion disorder, the *DSM-III* places "psychogenic pain disorder" in a separate category. The *DSM-III* criteria for conversion disorder are as follows:

A. The predominant disturbance is a loss of or alteration in physical functioning suggesting a physical disorder.
B. Psychological factors are judged to be etiologically involved in the symptom, as evidenced by one of the following:
   1. There is a temporal relationship between an environmental stimulus that is apparently related to a psychological conflict or need and the initiation or exacerbation of the symptom.
   2. The symptom enables the individual to avoid some activity that is noxious to him or her.
   3. The symptom enables the individual to get support from the environment that otherwise might not be forthcoming.
C. It has been determined that the symptom is *not* under voluntary control.
D. The symptom cannot, after appropriate investigation, be explained by a known physical disorder or pathophysiological mechanism.
E. The symptom is not limited to pain or to a disturbance in sexual functioning.
F. It is not due to somatization disorder or schizophrenia.

Research of conversion disorder raises doubts about its validity as a distinct disorder. As Slater (3) has written: "Looking back over the long history of hysteria we see that the null hypothesis has never been disproved.

No evidence has yet been offered that the patients diagnosed as suffering from hysteria are in medically significant terms anything more than a random selection."

Slater and Glithero (4) performed a follow-up study on eighty-five hospitalized patients with a diagnosis of conversion disorder. Twelve had died, a mortality rate in excess of what could be expected after an interval of about ten years following diagnosis. Of the seventy-three living patients, nineteen had a diagnosis of conversion disorder coupled with another medical diagnosis. Follow-up of twenty-two additional cases indicated that medical illness was present but undetected when the conversion disorder diagnosis was made. Of the remaining thirty-two patients with no evidence of systemic illness or coarse brain disease, two had schizophrenia, nine had affective disorders, and only twenty-one had "no demonstrable organic pathology."

In another follow-up study Gatfield and Guze (6) found that of twenty-four patients diagnosed as having conversion disorders, six had somatization disorder, six had neurologic disease, one had "rubbery legs" when his hemoglobin was 8 grams, one was a malingerer, two were unexplained (one of them being a "compensation case"), and only one could be identified as an "isolated conversion reaction."

Molitch and Rechlin (7) found that the combination of galactorrhea and amenorrhea, which typifies pseudocyesis, is associated with hyperprolactinemia in 50–70 percent of cases and with prolactinomas 35–60 percent of the time. Whitlock (8) found that 62.5 percent of patients with symptoms of conversion disorder had significant coexisting or preceding coarse brain disorder, in contrast to only 5.5 percent of controls. Stefansson *et al.* (9) diagnosed "organic illness" for 56 percent of sixty-four patients seen on a consultation service who were diagnosed as having a conversion disorder. Stefansson *et al.* also noted that of seventy-two patients in a large county case register with an antemortem diagnosis of conversion disorder, twenty (28 percent) died within a year of the date of the conversion diagnosis (9). That was significantly more than the authors expected.

In another sample McKegney (10) found that 47 percent of patients with a conversion diagnosis had "coexisting organic disease." Lewis and Berman (11) found that, in 30 percent of cases, diseases "of the variety conventionally diagnosed as organic" were diagnosed. Ziegler and Paul (12) reported that of sixty-six women hospitalized with a diagnosis of psychoneurotic hysteria twenty to twenty-five years prior to the study, twenty-two (33 percent) were later diagnosed as having a psychiatric disorder. Watson and Buranen (13), in whose study 25 percent of conversion disorder patients had systemic illness or coarse brain disease, wrote "the results appear to confirm the hypothesis that conversion reaction diagnoses often represent misdiagnosed physical disease." To summarize the above studies, there is an extremely high frequency of concurrent systemic illness, coarse brain disease, and psychiatric disorder in patients with conversion disorder diagnoses.

The following is an illustrative case of a patient who could readily have been thought to have a conversion disorder had the psychiatrist been less cautious in his diagnosis:

A fifty-three-year-old woman was admitted to a medical service because of a history of transient blindness and transient paralysis of the right lower extremity. By the time of her admission the vision and motor strength had returned to normal. The remainder of a thorough history, physical, and laboratory evaluation was unremarkable except for the observation that she readily became tearful when she discussed her symptoms. A psychiatric consultation was requested because of the tearfulness and because of the mysterious nature of her symptoms. The psychiatrist's history and mental status examination revealed only the tearfulness noted above, and his diagnosis was "history of transient blindness and hemiparalysis of unknown etiology; no psychiatric disorder."

Six weeks later the patient was readmitted for right hemiparesis associated with hyperreflexia, clonus, and a Babinski sign on the right. She showed emotional lability and severe motor perseveration. Lumbar puncture and evoked potentials supported a diagnosis of multiple sclerosis.

Regarding the systemic disorders found in patients labeled as having conversion disorder, Watson and Buranen (13) wrote, "The conditions most often mislabeled as hysteria appear to those involving degenerative conditions affecting skeletal, muscular and connective tissues, the spinal cord and peripheral nerves." Included among these are multiple sclerosis, dystonia musculorum deformans, transverse myelopathy, and thoracic outlet syndrome.

In one series Raskin et al. (14) found that the diagnoses made on patients for whom conversion reaction was considered in the differential diagnosis included "cerebrovascular accident, brain tumor, dystonia musculorum deformans, multiple sclerosis, phenothiazine reaction and transverse myelopathy." Epilepsy, particularly of the psychomotor type, should be included in the differential diagnosis (9, 15, 16). In reviews of neurological disorders mistaken for conversion disorders, multiple sclerosis is the diagnosis most prominently mentioned (11, 14, 17). Regarding psychiatric diagnosis found concurrently with conversion disorder, Guze et al. (18) wrote, "No psychiatric diagnosis was entirely free of patients with a history of conversion symptoms." They also reported that somatization disorder and antisocial personality disorder were found significantly more often among patients with conversion symptoms than among those without such a history.

In addition to the high prevalence of concurrent illness in conversion disorder, patients raising doubts about the validity of the conversion disorder diagnosis, a related question remains unanswered: What do the "pseudoneurologic" or other conversion symptoms represent?

Since the signs of conversion disorder are usually, if not always, identical with those seen in malingerers, one possibility is that the patient is malingering. Although any patient (particularly a sociopath) labeled as having a conversion disorder could be a malingerer, to this data there is no systematic research evidence that malingering routinely explains conversion disorders. The high prevalence of diagnosable medical illness in conversion disorder patients supports the conclusion that large numbers of conversion disorders are not malingered.

Another hypothesis is that the conversion reaction results from a conflict between an unconscious wish (e.g. to strike somebody) and an unconscious counterwish (e.g. that it is wrong to strike somebody), resolved by a process of "somatization," with the sign or symptom (e.g. paralysis of the "striking" extremity) "symbolizing" the wish and the counterwish (19). DSM-III explicitly accepts this notion. Its criteria for conversion disorder require that there be an antecedent event that evokes this unconscious conflict and that the patient obtains "secondary gain" (see page 422). There are significant problems with this hypothesis: (1) Unconscious conflicts are inaccessible to observation. (2) Medical illnesses are often preceded by stressful events (20), and stressful events do not distinguish conversion disorders from initially undiagnosed medical disorders (13, 14). (3) Regardless of the type of illness, the sick role (21) is associated with avoidance of activities that might exacerbate the illness.

Another hypothesis (22) is that the conversion disorder is a type of anosognosia, whereby the patient is unaware that part of his body is functioning normally. A hemiparalyzed patient might try to walk because he does not know he is paralyzed (Babinski's agnosia). Conceivably a patient might fail to attempt to move his left upper and lower extremities because he is unaware that they function normally. Thus what appears to be a motor dysfunction could be a gnostic dysfunction. This is consistent with the physical findings in patients with conversion disorder.

Unfortunately, the evidence for this hypothesis thus far has been modest. Several studies (22–24) have shown that a significant majority of conversion signs occur on the left side of the body, which is consistent with the association of anosognosia with right hemisphere dysfunction (22). A hypothesis that the left side of the body is more often affected because it is more "convenient" for the patient has been refuted, because the left side of the body is also more frequently affected in lefthanders (22). Although it has been shown that indifference to the affected part of the body ("la belle indifference") is not nearly as common in conversion disorders as was previously believed (11, 14), it occurs and is consistent with the phenomenon of anosognosia.

Finally, Flor–Henry (25) found a significantly increased frequency of EEG abnormalities in patients with somatization disorder, a condition with increased risk of conversion disorder. These EEG abnormalities were more likely to be located in the left side of the brain.

Given the uncertain validity of the conversion disorder diagnosis and the high frequency of concurrent systemic or psychiatric illness, the patient with symptoms and signs of conversion disorder should be treated as follows: As is the case for the diagnosis and management of any other psychiatric or medical disorder, the patient should receive a thorough history and physical examination, routine laboratory testing, and specialized testing of the system or anatomic region affected. There should be a vigorous search for a coexistent medical or psychiatric illness, which if present will determine the prognosis (4). Electroencephalography and CT or NMR scanning of brain or spinal cord, lumbar puncture, electromyography, and auditory, visual and somatosensory evoked potentials (26, 27) will often be valuable. Evoked potentials are the best means of diagnosing multiple sclerosis and reveal abnormalities in the majority of cases of multiple sclerosis (26).

It follows that the treatment of patients labeled with conversion disorder should be that of the concurrent medical or psychiatric illnesses, if one can be identified. If one cannot be found, the patient should be told that the cause of his problem cannot be determined, and he should be seen for follow-up examinations regardless of whether the signs and symptoms have spontaneously disappeared.

Psychogenic Pain Disorder

The *DSM-III* criteria for psychogenic pain disorder (see Addendum 1 below) are very similar to those of conversion disorder, and problems with the validity of the former are very similar to those of the latter. One recent study (28) demonstrated that 98 percent of chronic pain patients have a *DSM-III* axis I psychiatric diagnosis, and 37 percent had an axis II disorder.

Hendler *et al.* (29) employed thermography in 224 consecutive patients with no radiologic, neurologic, orthopedic, or laboratory abnormalities, who were diagnosed as having psychogenic pain, and found that for 19 percent the diagnosis was reflex sympathetic dystrophy, nerve root irritation, or thoracic outlet syndrome. Sympathetic nervous system dysfunction can easily be misdiagnosed as psychogenic pain unless thermography is employed. As is the case with conversion disorder, management includes a vigorous search for a "coexisting" psychiatric or systemic disorder, which itself determines the treatment and the prognosis. For intractable chronic pain for which no concurrent psychiatric or systemic illness, including depression, can be identified, a variety of therapeutic endeavors may be tried (see Chapter 10).

Hypochondriasis

DSM-III defines hypochondriasis as "an unrealistic interpretation of physical signs or sensations as abnormal, leading to preoccupation with the fear or belief of having a serious disease." *DSM-III* criteria for hypochondriasis are listed in Addendum 2 below. As is the case for conversion disorder and psychogenic pain disorder, the validity of the diagnosis as a discrete entity remains to be established. Kenyon (5, 30), in a literature review and a controlled study of 512 psychiatric patients with hypochondriasis, found that hypochondriasis was always secondary to another syndrome, usually depression.

An unexplained fact is that "Generally speaking, hypochondriacal symptoms as part of another syndrome seem to make the prognosis worse, as for example in depression" (5). The treatment of hypochondriacal symptoms is that of the underlying illness.

ADDENDUM 1   Diagnostic Criteria for Psychogenic Pain Disorder*

A. Severe and prolonged pain is the predominant disturbance.
B. The pain presented as a symptom is inconsistent with the anatomic distribution of the nervous system; after extensive evaluation, no organic pathology or pathophysiological mechanism can be found to account for the pain; or, when there is some related organic pathology, the complaint of pain is grossly in excess of what would be expected from the physical findings.
C. Psychological factors are judged to be etiologically involved in the pain, as evidenced by at least one of the following:
1. A temporal relationship between an environmental stimulus that is apparently related to a psychological conflict or need and the initiation or exacerbation of the pain
2. The pain's enabling the individual to avoid some activity that is noxious to him or her
3. The pain's enabling the individual to get support from the environment that otherwise might not be forthcoming
D. The pain is not due to another mental disorder.

*Source: J. B. W. Williams (Ed.), *Diagnostic and Statistical Manual of Mental Disorders*, Third Edition (*DSM-III*), p. 249. Washington, D.C.: American Psychiatric Association, 1980. Used by permission.

ADDENDUM 2   Diagnostic Criteria for Hypochondriasis*

A. The predominant disturbance is an unrealistic interpretation of physical signs or sensations as abnormal, leading to preoccupation with the fear or belief of having a serious disease.
B. Thorough physical evaluation does not support the diagnosis of any physical disorder that can account for the physical signs or sensations or for the individual's unrealistic interpretation of them.
C. The unrealistic fear or belief of having a disease persists despite medical reassurance and causes impairment in social or occupational functioning.
D. Not due to any other mental disorder such as schizophrenia, affective disorder, or somatization disorder.

---

*Source: J. B. W. Williams (Ed.), *Diagnostic and Statistical Manual of Mental Disorders*, Third Edition (*DSM-III*), p. 251. Washington, D.C.: American Psychiatric Association, 1980. Used by permission.

References

1. American Psychiatric Association Task Force on Nomenclature and Statistics. *Diagnostic and Statistical Manual of Mental Disorders*. 3d ed. (*DSM-III*). Washington, D.C.: American Psychiatric Association, 1980.

2. Cloninger, C. R. Diagnosis of somatoform disorders: A critique of DSM-III. In *Proceedings of Conference on Revising DSM-III*. Washington, D.C.: American Psychiatric Association, in press.

3. Slater, E. T. O. The diagnosis of "hysteria." *Br. Med. J. 1:* 1395–99, 1965.

4. Slater, E. T. O.; Glithero, E. A follow-up of patients diagnosed as suffering from "hysteria." *J. Psychosom. Res. 9:* 9–13, 1965.

5. Kenyon, F. E. Hypochondriacal states. *Br. J. Psychiat. 129:* 1–14, 1976.

6. Gatfield, P. D.; Guze, S. B. Prognosis and differential diagnosis of conversion reactions (a follow-up study). *Dis. Nerv. Sys. 23:* 1–8, 1962.

7. Molitch, M. E.; Reichlin, S. The amenorrhea, galactorrhea and hyperprolactinemia syndromes. *Adv. Int. Med. 26:* 37–65, 1980.

8. Whitlock, F. A. The etiology of hysteria. *Acta Psychiat. Scand. 43:* 144–62, 1967.

9. Stefansson, J. G.; Messina, J. A.; Meyerowitz, S. Hysterical neurosis, conversion type. Clinical and epidemiologic considerations. *Acta Psychiat. Scand. 53:* 119–38, 1976.

10. McKegney, F. P. The incidence and characteristics of patients with conversion reactions: 1. A general hospital consultation service sample. *Am. J. Psychiat. 124:* 542–45, 1967.

11. Lewis, W. D.; Berman, M. Studies of conversion hysteria: 1. Operational study of diagnosis. *Arch. Gen. Psychiat. 13:* 275–82, 1965.

12. Ziegler, G. K.; Paul, N. On the natural history of hysteria in women (a follow-up study 20 years after hospitalization). *Dis. Nerv. Sys. 15:* 301–6, 1954.

13. Watson, C. G.; Buranen, C. The frequency and identification of false positive conversion reactions. *J. Nerv. Ment. Dis. 167:* 243–47, 1979.

14. Raskin, M.; Talbott, J. A.; Meyerson, A. T. Diagnosis of conversion reactions: Predictive value of psychiatric criteria. *JAMA 197:* 102–50, 530–34, 1966.

15. Liske, E.; Forster, F. M. Pseudoseizures: A problem in the diagnosis and management of epileptic patients. *Neurology 14:* 41–49, 1964.

16. Niedermeyer, E.; Blumer, D.; Holsher, E.; *et al.* Classical hysterical seizures facilitated by anticonvulsant toxicity. *Psychiat. Clin. 3:* 71–84, 1970.

17. Aring, C. D. Observations on multiple sclerosis and conversion hysteria. *Brain 88:* 663–74, 1965.

18. Guze, S. B.; Woodruff, R. A.; Clayton, P. J. A study of conversion symptoms in psychiatric outpatients. *Am. J. Psychiat. 128:* 643–46, 1971.

19. Alexander, F. *Psychosomatic Medicine.* New York: Norton, 1950.

20. Holmes, T. Life situations, emotions and disease. *Psychom. 19:* 747–54, 1978.

21. Parsons, T. Definitions of Health and Illness in the Light of American Values and Social Structure. In Jaco, E. (ed.), *Patients, Physicians and Illness.* New York: Free Press, 1972.

22. Stern, D. B. Handedness and the lateral distribution of conversion reactions. *J. Nerv. Ment. Dis. 164:* 122–28, 1978.

23. Merskey, H.; Spear, F. G. *Pain: Psychological and Psychiatric Aspects.* London: Balliere, Tindall & Cassell, 1967.

24. Agnew, D. C.; Merskey, H. Words of chronic pain. *Pain 2:* 73–81, 1976.

25. Flor-Henry, P.; Fromm-Auch, D.; Tapper, M.; *et al.* A neuropsychological study of the stable syndrome of hysteria. *Biol. Psychiat. 16:* 601–26, 1980.

26. Green, J. B.; Walcoff, M. R. Evoked potentials in multiple sclerosis. *Arch. Neurol. 39:* 696–98, 1982.

27. Haldeman, S.; Glick, M.; Bhatia, N. N.; *et al.* Colonometry, cystometry and evoked potentials in multiple sclerosis. *Arch. Neurol. 39:* 698–701, 1982.

28. Reich, J.; Tupin, J. P.; Abramowicz, S. I. Psychiatric diagnosis of chronic pain patients. *Am. J. Psychiat. 140:* 1495–98, 1983.

29. Hendler, N.; Uematesu, S.; Long, D. Thermographic validation of physical complaints in psychogenic pain patients. *Psychosom. 23:* 283–87, 1982.

30. Kenyon, F. E. Hypochondriasis: A clinical study. *Br. J. Psychiat. 110:* 478–88, 1964.

CHAPTER 25

Sociopathy

Individuals with sociopathy (antisocial personality disorder, psychopathy) should not be admitted to psychiatric inpatient units unless they are suffering from an additional disorder such as mania, major depression, drug-induced psychosis, or alcoholic hallucinosis. Nevertheless, they frequently come to the attention of psychiatrists in emergency and consultation services and occasionally are inappropriately admitted to psychiatric services because of suicide or homicide threats or malingered illnesses. Problems presented by sociopaths are also discussed in Chapters 9, 13, and 19.

We employ the criteria for sociopathy of Feighner *et al.* (1), which are also descriptive of behaviors typical of people with the disorder:[*]

> A chronic or recurrent disorder with the appearance of at least one of the following manifestations before age fifteen. A minimum of five manifestations are required for a "definite" diagnosis, and four are required for a "probable" diagnosis.
>
> A. School problems as manifested by any of the following: truancy (positive if more than once per year except for the last year in school), suspension, expulsion, or fighting that leads to trouble with teachers or principals.
>
> B. Running away from home overnight while living in parental home.

[*] J. Feighner *et al.*, "Diagnostic Criteria for Use in Psychiatric Research," in *Archives of General Psychiatry* 26: 56–63, 1972. Copyright © 1972 by American Medical Association. Used by permission.

431

C. Troubles with the police as manifested by any of the following: two or more arrests for non-traffic offenses, four or more arrests (including tickets only) for moving traffic offenses, or at least one felony conviction.

D. Poor work history as manifested by being fired, quitting without another job to go to, or frequent job changes not accounted for by normal seasonal or economic fluctuations.

E. Marital difficulties manifested by any of the following: deserting family, two or more divorces, frequent separation due to marital discord, recurrent infidelity, recurrent physical attacks upon spouse, or being suspected of battering a child.

F. Repeated outbursts of rage or fighting not on the school premises: if prior to age 18 this must occur at least twice and lead to difficulty with adults; after age 18 this must occur at least twice, or if a weapon (e.g. club, knife, or gun) is used, only once is enough to score this category positive.

G. Sexual problems as manifested by any of the following: prostitution (includes both heterosexual and homosexual activity), pimping, more than one episode of venereal disease, or flagrant promiscuity.

H. Vagrancy or wanderlust, e.g. at least several months of wandering from place to place with no prearranged plans.

I. Persistent and repeated lying, or using an alias.

The *DSM-III* criteria for antisocial personality disorder incorporate many of the behaviors listed in the Feighner criteria and are probably just as useful in most cases. However, we hesitate to use *DSM-III* criteria in Veterans Administration or other compensation cases, because these criteria place too much emphasis on symptoms occurring prior to the age of fifteen, which are not likely to be reported by individuals claiming service-connected or accident-related psychiatric disability.

The overall prevalence of sociopathy is not known. Cloninger (2) estimates its population prevalence to be "no more than about 4%." It is known to occur in 2–3 percent of adoptees (3). In one outpatient series 15 percent of men and 3 percent of women had this disorder (4). It is more frequent among men than among women, in cities than in rural areas, and among people of low socioeconomic status (5). Its prevalence is greater for blacks (9 percent) than for whites (3 percent), but as Cloninger (2) writes, "The difference is not 'racial' in a genetic sense; when populations are matched for socioeconomic status, the racial difference disappears." The majority of sociopaths come from families in which parents were separated or divorced or in which one or both parents died when the patient was a child, deserted the family, or was alcoholic or criminal. Twin studies of criminals (the majority of whom are sociopaths) suggest indirectly that there is a genetic causal component to the disorder (6). Adoption studies of criminals also suggest a genetic causal component as well as nongenetic causes (3, 7). In families of sociopaths there is an increased frequency of sociopathy, Briquet's syndrome, alcoholism, and drug dependence (8, 9). Sociopaths tend to marry individuals with these latter four diagnoses (10).

Disorders that are more common among sociopaths than in the general population include alcoholism (11), drug dependence (2), drug abuse, conversion disorders (12), and venereal disease. The natural history of the disorder includes significant behavioral problems before age fifteen, including enuresis, fire-setting, cruelty to animals, running away from home, drug or alcohol abuse, truancy, fighting at school, suspension or expulsion from school, habitual lying, arrests, early age of sexual intercourse, promiscuity, prostitution, or minimal brain dysfunction/hyperactivity syndrome.

For some sociopaths there is a slight improvement in behavior in middle age (12). The life expectancy of sociopaths is diminished, with an associated increased frequency of deaths by homicide, accidents, or complications of drug or alcohol dependence (13, 14).

In the absence of superimposed illness the mental status examination is for the most part normal, but certain findings, predominantly in the areas of appearance and affectivity, are associated. These include a motorcycle gang style of dress, tattoos, needle tracks, and a swaggering gait. The patient is often glib and may convey a shallow warmth, but may also appear cold and callous (15). An initial compliance and superficial friendliness, if present, readily give way to irritability (15) when the patient's requests are not met, more so than for the average medical or psychiatric patient. Many sociopaths take the position that recent and past wrongs against them are a justification for their antisocial behaviors, and many convey a sense of entitlement (2). There is an increased frequency of nonspecific abnormalities on the electroencephalogram (16-18).

Sociopathy itself is not responsive to any treatment. Somatic treatments are of value only for the management of superimposed disorders. Lest an unrealistic expectation of therapeutic success be created, some patients will need to be told that they have a style of behavior (or a "personality disorder") that is not amenable to treatment; that they are responsible for their actions; and that as they get older they may develop more self-control and maturity. If the subject arises, they can be told that if they are contemplating having additional children, these children are at somewhat greater risk of developing a similar behavior pattern.

References

1. Feighner, J.; Robins, E.; Guze, S. B.; et al. Diagnostic criteria for use in psychiatric research. Arch. Gen. Psychiat. 26: 56-63, 1972.
2. Cloninger, C. R. The antisocial personality. Hosp. Pract. 13(8): 97-106, 1978.

3. Crowe, R. An adoptive study of antisocial personality. *Arch. Gen. Psychiat. 31:* 785–91, 1974.

4. Woodruff, R. A., Jr.; Guze, S. B.; Clayton, P. S. The medical and psychiatric implications of antisocial personality (sociopathy). *Dis. Nerv. Syst. 32:* 712–14, 1971.

5. Lunden, W. A. *Statistics on Delinquents and Delinquency.* Springfield, Ill.: C. C. Thomas, 1964.

6. Christiansen, K. O. A Review of Studies of Criminality Among Twins. In Christiansen, K. O.; Mednick, S. (eds.), *Biosocial Bases of Criminal Behavior.* New York: Gardner, 1977.

7. Hutchings, B.; Mednick, S. Criminality in Adoptees and Their Adoptive and Biological Parents: A Pilot Study. In Mednick, S.; Christiansen, K. O. (eds.), *Biosocial Bases of Criminal Behavior.* New York: Gardner, 1977.

8. Cloninger, C. R.; Guze, S. B. Psychiatric illness in the families of female criminals: A study of 288 first degree relatives. *Br. J. Psychiat. 122:* 697–703, 1973.

9. Guze, S. B.; Wolfgram, E. D.; McKinney, J. K.; *et al.* Psychiatric illness in the families of convicted criminals: A study of 519 first degree relatives. *Dis. Nerv. Syst. 28:* 651–59, 1967.

10. Guze, S. B. *Criminality and Psychiatric Disorders.* New York: Oxford University Press, 1976.

11. Robins, L. N. *Deviant Children Grown Up: A Sociological and Psychiatric Study of Sociopathic Personality.* Baltimore: Williams & Wilkins, 1966.

12. Goodwin, D. W.; Guze, S. B. *Psychiatric Diagnosis.* 2d ed. New York: Oxford University Press, 1979.

13. Robins, L.; O'Neal, P. Mortality, mobility and crime: Problem children thirty years later. *Am. Social Rev. 23:* 162–71, 1958.

14. Herjanic, M.; Meyer, D. A. Psychiatric illness in homicide victims. *Am. J. Psychiat. 133:* 691–93, 1976.

15. Tyrer, P.; Alexander, J. Classification of personality disorders. *Br. J. Psychiat. 135:* 163–67, 1979.

16. Arthurs, R.; Cahoon, E. A clinical and electroencephalopathic survey of psychopathic personality. *Am. J. Psychiat. 120:* 875–77, 1964.

17. Gottlieb, J. S.; Ashby, M. C.; Knott, J. R. Primary behavior disorders and psychopathic personality. *Arch. Neurol. Psychiat. 56:* 381–400, 1946.

18. Hill, D.; Watterson, D. Electroencephalographic studies of psychopathic personalities. *J. Neurol. Psychiat. 5:* 47, 1942.

CHAPTER 26

Malingering

Malingering is the simulation or fraudulent exaggeration of symptoms, or the deliberate production (e.g. heating a thermometer to produce "fever") of physical signs with fraud in mind. Factitious illness is the deliberate production of physical signs regardless of whether fraud is involved. Most factitious illnesses are malingered, but some are not; for example, some melancholics excoriate their skin when they are agitated.

Malingering is not rare. Among patients with certain diagnoses (e.g. sociopathy), the majority have malingered (1). An estimated 5 percent of World War II inductees malingered (2). Despite statements (2–4) that malingering is a sign of psychiatric illness requiring thoughtful, sensitive treatment, for the most part malingering wastes time and money (e.g. unnecessary hospitalization for malingered depression) and leads to unnecessary and often dangerous (e.g. diagnostic x-ray for feigned low back pain) medical interventions.

Manifestations

Some psychiatric symptoms, such as suicidal thoughts, depressive thought *content*, and hallucinations, are readily and frequently malingered. In Ganser syndrome (5, 6), an uncommon syndrome thought to be malingered

435

in some cases, a patient with no receptive aphasia or formal thinking disorder manifests "pseudostupidity" or "pseudodementia" by giving grossly incorrect answers (e.g. 2 + 2 = 5) to most or all questions posed to him. As new psychiatric syndromes (particularly those for which the criteria emphasize symptoms over signs) are identified, additional opportunities for malingering are created (7).

Malingering is not confined to psychiatry. There are case reports of malingered asthma (8); tuberculosis caused by intravenous injection of tubercle bacilli (9, 10); arthritis due to intra-articular injections (4); fever of unknown origin from heating a thermometer or drinking hot liquid before the temperature is taken, (11–13); thyrotoxicosis caused by ingesting thyroid hormone (14, 15); hematochezia (blood in the stools) from lacerations of the anus or rectum, or simulated by the patient using a syringe to draw blood from (phlebotomizing) an antecubital vein, and then squirting this blood into the toilet or stool sample container (16, 17); vaginal bleeding also caused by laceration or phlebotomy (18–20); hematuria or hematemesis simulated by phlebotomy (18); dermatitis caused by excoriation (21–23); cancer feigned by claiming a prior diagnosis of cancer (24); pheochromocytoma caused by injection of epinephrine (25); porphyria induced by ingesting antipyrine, an antipyretic agent with a high incidence of toxicity, which causes the urine to turn the color of cherry wine (26, 27); blindness (28); deafness (29); kidney stones (30); simulation of symptoms or production of factitious signs by a parent in a child (a form of child abuse) (31, 32); and anisocoria produced by unilateral application of mydriatic agents. In Munchausen's syndrome (33, 34) the patient repeatedly develops factitious illnesses, is hospitalized numerous times (sometimes hundreds), and willingly undergoes extensive diagnostic or therapeutic procedures.

Diagnoses Associated with Malingering

In the absence of extraordinary circumstances (e.g. feigned hallucinations by the "pseudopatients" in Rosenhan's social psychology experiment [35], feigned death in the presence of an enemy on the battlefield) malingering occurs primarily among persons with psychopathology, most commonly sociopathy. In one series of patients thought to be malingerers (2), 90 percent could be given one or more psychiatric diagnoses. The diagnoses most closely associated with malingering are sociopathy, drug dependence, and alcoholism (1–3, 36–40). Employing anonymous questionnaires, one of us (1) surveyed 322 patients and medical students on a medical center campus and found that self-reported malingering was significantly more common among the above-mentioned three diagnostic groups than among medical patients, surgical patients, medical students, and psychiatric patients with other syndromes (including Briquet's syndrome). Despite the temptation to think of it as such, there is no evidence as yet that Briquet's syndrome is a malingered illness (1).

Circumstances of Malingering

Malingering is more frequent when people are in extremely unpleasant circumstances such as prison or combat, are homeless, or have an opportunity (such as an accident) to claim compensation. Among people with factitious illnesses, there is a disproportionately large number of medical and paramedical personnel (11, 13, 18). Finally, people who have been identified as malingerers in the past are more apt to malinger again (8). Occasionally a hospital will post a notice on staff bulletin boards about a habitual malingerer. In all of the above-mentioned situations, the physician's index of suspicion should be higher, particularly if the patient is a sociopath or is drug dependent or an alcoholic.

Evaluation

Obtaining history from other sources may reveal falsifications. In some cases of malingered posttraumatic stress disorder, military records may reveal that the patient was never in combat or a prison camp (5). In two cases of "cancer pathomimicry" (24) the medical records at the hospitals where the diagnosis of cancer was supposedly made revealed no such diagnosis.

Other behaviors are consistent with a conclusion of malingering: (1) a patient recommending a particular treatment, typically a narcotic or anticholinergic or anxiolytic drug, early in an interview (e.g. "The only drug that works for my pain is Talwin."); (2) a patient refusing routine procedures, including the history itself (e.g. "Why do I have to go through all of this shit just to get some Valiums?").

Additional behaviors associated with malingering fall under the heading of "bad acting" or "lack of sincerity" (3). For example, an otherwise histrionic individual may describe a symptom in a blasé fashion, enticing the examiner to "discover" its importance. Or the patient may respond in an unnecessarily cautious fashion, as if he were being interrogated and not interviewed: "Yes, I guess I'd have to answer yes to that"; "Let me see. Yes. I'll give you a yes on that." Malingerers are less likely to express surprise or pleasure when the doctor anticipates some of his symptoms (e.g. "How could you have known I get pins and needles in my hands and feet when I get short of breath?"). Malingering should be considered in addition to Briquet's syndrome when there are no confirming physical or laboratory signs in the presence of extensive medical complaints.

Occasionally, when the patient is being observed by staff but thinks he is alone, he may stop his deception. For example, a patient with labored breathing due to factitious asthma may breathe comfortably when he thinks he is alone. In cases of factitious illness, staff may find paraphernalia (such as syringes or thermometers) used to induce the physical signs.

In other branches of medicine certain physical findings, diagnostic maneuvers, or laboratory tests may help. In auscultation of the respiratory tree in factitious asthma, wheezing is usually loudest over the larynx (8). Also, the inhalation of methacholine does not reduce forced expiratory volume. In factitious dermatitis, the lesions are typically on accessible skin surfaces, such as the left forearm in a righthander (41). In factitious "fever of unknown origin" the pulse rate may be much lower than expected from the temperature reading, and the fever pattern may not show typical diurnal variation (38). Strategies for diagnosing factitious fever include taking simultaneous oral and rectal temperatures, checking thermometer serial numbers, and taking the temperature of fresh urine specimens (42–44). The evaluation of fever of unknown origin should also include a thorough inspection of the skin for needle puncture wounds.

Excluding epileptics who also fake seizures, the EEGs of people feigning epilepsy show no spiking or other paroxysmal features, and prolactin levels do not rise. A more effective tool (if available) is continuous EEG telemetry with simultaneous videotaping of the patient's activities. For other types of malingered neurologic abnormalities in unsophisticated patients, findings may include hemianesthesia to the midline, stocking or glove anesthesia, and absence of pathologic reflexes, atrophy, or clonus. One maneuver in hemiparalysis is for the examiner to place one hand beneath the heel of the paralyzed foot with the patient lying in the supine position, and the other hand above the ankle of the functioning foot. He then asks the patient to elevate the "good leg" against the resistance of the examiner's hand atop the ankle. As the patient attempts this, if the "bad" extremity is not paralyzed, pressure will automatically be exerted against the examiner's hand beneath the heel of the "bad" foot.

Ophthalmologists have many tests for malingered blindness, most involving the patient's unwittingly having to see with his "blind" eye to produce a response that could only have occurred if the patient could see with that eye (28). For example, a tongue depressor is placed vertically in the midline 6 to 7 inches in front of a patient, who is instructed to read, with both eyes open, printed material placed 10 to 14 inches in front of him. A person with good vision in one eye and blindness in the other must move his head to read the printed material. A malingerer may not appreciate this and continue to read without head movement (28). Another strategy is to ask the patient to touch the tips of his index fingers together. A bilaterally or unilaterally blind person with normal position sense, spatial orientation, cerebellar functioning, and interhemispheric connection does this with ease; a malingerer with these functions intact may hesitate (28). In the evaluation of deafness, the use of auditory evoked potentials or pure tone delayed auditory feedback (29) may be very helpful.

In factitious thyrotoxicosis induced by ingestion of thyroid hormone, serum thyroglobulin levels are low or absent, I^{131} uptake suppressed, TSH levels decreased, and no ectopic thyroid tissue found on I^{131} body scan (14, 15).

Management and Disposition

Although malingering is socially unacceptable behavior, the malingerer still expects the physician to provide ethical care. And despite the fact that some malingerers refuse a complete examination, other malingerers angrily criticize the physician for perfunctory examinations. Thus, even when the physician suspects malingering from the outset, it is advisable to perform a conscientious evaluation.

Following the evaluation of the malingerer the examiner should tactfully summarize his objective findings and proposed treatments (e.g. "From my examination of your back, I don't find a fracture or muscle spasm or tumor, but if you're willing, I'd like to send you for an x-ray of your back to be sure. Of course too much x-radiation to your body can be dangerous, but I'm sure you want me to be as thorough as possible.")

Unless the malingered act is observed (e.g. the patient is seen to be heating a thermometer) or there is strong circumstantial evidence (e.g. secreted syringes or medications in the patient's clothes cabinet), usually the patient should not be told outright that he is faking, since he will try to save face. If he believes he is being wronged, he may retaliate by complaining, suing, or otherwise expressing his anger. One malingerer murdered several orthopedic surgeons who claimed that he was feigning back pain in a compensation case (45).

If the patient is to be confronted with the fact of observed malingering or solid circumstantial evidence, it should be done in a tactful and respectful manner that permits the patient to save face to a sufficient extent for him to comply with needed treatments of concurrent nonmalingered problems, to comply with recommendations for alternative methods of dealing with the circumstances that led to the malingering, or to accept the doctor's recommendation for discharge.

The physician's unwillingness to comply with unreasonable patient requests should be conveyed nonjudgmentally. For example, in response to an alcoholic, sociopathic patient's demand for alprazolam for the irritability and anxiety he feels when his needs are not being met, he might be told, "I can't prescribe alprazolam for you. It won't cure anything except alcohol withdrawal, and it's addicting. For you, it would be like prescribing an alcohol tablet, and in all good conscience I can't do that."

The physician should recommend all treatments that are appropriate, such as the referral of an alcoholic to Alcoholics Anonymous. If no treatments are appropriate, social interventions may help. For example, a homeless patient can be helped to find lodging, even if the lodging is a local mission, or a soldier with sociopathy could be granted his wish to be discharged from service in the form of an administrative discharge.

Where malingering is but one of several diagnostic possibilities following a complete evaluation, the physician should treat the patient as if he had a syndrome that does respond to treatment. For example, a clerk with a previously good employment history at a medical insurance company complained of hearing clear voices inside her head for several weeks, adding that this rendered her unable to work and that she was considering retirement "on disability." A thorough examination and extensive laboratory testing revealed no abnormalities. Possible diagnoses included phonemic paraphrenia and malingering, but the possibility of malingering was not mentioned to her. She refused electroconvulsive therapy as an empirical treatment for the hallucinations. She agreed to take haloperidol but discontinued several weeks later because of side effects and no therapeutic benefit. She then requested hospital discharge, remained on leave from work, and applied for a pension. While this was an example of a therapeutic failure, it was a reasonable approach for this patient.

In certain circumstances a malingering patient can be hospitalized for behavior modification. For example, a patient with malingered blindness can be hospitalized on an ophthalmology ward for "retinal rest." The patient is told his vision is likely to improve if his eyes are put totally at rest. He is then placed on bed rest in a room with no television, radio, or roommates, and his eyes are patched with patches that cannot be removed. No visitors are allowed, and staff visits are kept to a minimum. Kramer *et al.* (28) report that within several days this sensory deprivation is aversive enough to "restore" the patient's vision.

For factitious diseases that are not malingered, treatment must address both the underlying nonfactitious disorder and the secondary factitious illness. For example, for skin excoriations resulting from agitation in a melancholic patient, the patient should receive a course of ECT. But until the ECT has begun to take effect in reducing the patient's agitation, he should receive amobarbital sedation, his wounds should be dressed, and secondary infections should be treated. Some factitious disorders that are malingered will themselves be of sufficient severity to require treatment. For example, miliary tuberculosis produced by intravenous injection of tubercle bacilli will require vigorous antituberculous therapy.

References

1. Sierles, F. S. Correlates of malingering. *Behav. Sci. and the Law.* 2(1): 113–18, 1984.
2. Flicker, D. J. Malingering: A symptom. *J. Nerv. Ment. Dis.* 123(1): 23–31, 1956.
3. Garner, H. H. Malingering. *Ill. Med. J.* 128: 318–19, 1965.
4. Shurley, J. Factitious diseases. *Ann. Int. Med.* 90(2): 1328–41, 1958.
5. Ganser, S. J. M. On a peculiar type of twilight state. *Arch. Psychiat. Nervenkr.* 30: 633, 1898.
6. Goldin, S.; MacDonald, J. E. The Ganser state. *J. Ment. Sci.* 101: 267, 1955.
7. Sparr, L.; Pankratz, L. D. Factitious post-traumatic stress disorder. *Am. J. Psychiat.* 140(8): 1016–19, 1983.
8. Downing, E. T.; Braman, S. S.; Fox, M. J.; *et al.* Factitious asthma: Physiological approach to diagnosis. *JAMA* 248(21), 2878–80, 1982.
9. Jones, O. R.; Platt, W. D.; Amill, L. A. Miliary tuberculosis caused by intravenous self-injection of tubercle bacilli, treated successfully with streptomycin therapy. *Ann. Rev. Tuberc.* 60: 514–19, 1949.
10. Lemierre, A.; Amenill, P. Miliary tuberculosis following injection of tubercle bacilli intravenously in a human subject. *Bull. Num. Soc. Hosp. Paris*, February 1938.
11. Aduan, R. P.; Fauce, A. S.; Dole, D. G.; *et al.* Factitious fever and self-induced infection. *Ann. Int. Med.* 90: 230–42, 1979.
12. Hale, V.; Evseichick, O. Fraudulent fever. *Am. J. Nurs.* 43: 992–94, 1943.
13. Petersdorf, R. G.; Bennett, I. L. Factitious fever. *Ann. Int. Med.* 46: 1039–62, 1957.
14. Rose, E.; Sanders, T.; Webb, J. L.; *et al.* Occult factitial thyrotoxicosis. *Ann. Int. Med.* 71: 309–15, 1969.
15. Mariotti, S.; Martino, E.; Cupini, C.; *et al.* Low serum thyroglobulin as a clue to the diagnosis of thyrotoxicosis factitia. *New Eng. J. Med.* 307(7): 410–12, 1982.
16. Seijffers, M. J.; Welner, A. Massive rectal bleeding in a malingering patient. *Dis. Col. Rect.* 12(5): 347–51, 1969.
17. Daily, W. J. R.; Coles, J. M.; Creger, W. P. Factitious anemia. *Ann. Int. Med.* 58: 533, 1963.
18. Hustead, R. M.; Lee, R. A.; Maruta, T. Factitious illness in gynecology. *Ob. Gyn.* 5(2): 214–19, 1982.
19. Midgely, R. L. A case of menorrhagia. *Br. Med. J.* 1: 275, 1976.
20. Steinbeck, A. W. Hemorrhagia histrionica: The bleeding Munchausen syndrome. *Med. J. Aust.* 1: 451, 1961.

21. Herzberg, J. H. Self excoriation by young women. *Am. J. Psychiat. 134:* 320–21, 1977.

22. Hollander, M. H.; Abram, H. S. Dermatitis factitia. *S. Med. J. 6:* 1279–85, 1979.

23. Fisher, B. K.; and Pearce, K. I. Neurotic excoriations: A personality evaluation. *Cutis. 14:* 251–54, 1974.

24. D'Andrea, V. J. Cancer pathomimicry: A report of three cases. *J. Clin. Psychiat. 39*(3): 233–40, 1978.

25. Brandenburg, R. O.; Gutnik, L. M.; Nelson, R. G.; *et al.* Factitial epinephrine-only secreting pheochromocytoma. *Ann. Int. Med. 90:* 795–96, 1979.

26. Bunim, J. J.; Federmann, D. D.; Black, R. L.; *et al.* Factitious diseases: Clinical staff conference at the National Institutes of Health. *National Institutes of Health Clinic Staff Conference 48*(6): 1329–41, 1958.

27. Woodbury, D. M.; Fingle, E. Analgesic–Antipyretics, Anti-inflammatory Agents, and Drugs Employed in the Therapy of Gout. In Goodman, L. S.; Gilman, A. (eds.), *The Pharmacologic Basis of Therapeutics.* 5th Ed. New York: Macmillan, 1975.

28. Kramer, K. K.; LaPiana, F. G.; Appleton, B. Ocular malingering and hysteria: Diagnosis and management. *Surv. Ophth. 24:* 89–96, 1979.

29. Robinson, M.; Kasden, S. D. Clinical application of pure tone delayed auditory feedback in pseudohypococusis. *E.E.N.T. Monthly 52:* 31–33, 1973.

30. Sneed, R. C.; Bell, R. F. The dauphin of Munchausen: Factitious passage of renal stones in a child. *Pediatrics 58:* 127–30, 1976.

31. Rogers, D.; Tripp, J.; Bentovim, A.; *et al.* Nonaccidental poisoning: An extended syndrome of child abuse. *Br. Med. J. 1:* 793–96, 1976.

32. Meadows, R. Munchausen syndrome by proxy: The hinterland of child abuse. *Lancet 2:* 343–45, 1977.

33. Asher, R. Munchausen's syndrome. *Lancet 1:* 339–41, 1951.

34. Justus, P. G.; Kreutziger, S. S.; Kitchens, C. S. Probing the dynamics of Munchausen's syndrome: Detailed analysis of a case. *Ann. Intern. Med. 93:* 120–27, 1980.

35. Rosenhan, D. H. On being sane in insane places. *Science 179:* 250–58, 1973.

36. Phillips, M. R.; Ward, N. G.; Ries, R. K. Factitious mourning: Painless parenthood. *Am. J. Psychiat. 140*(4): 420–25, 1983.

37. Pope, H. G.; Jonas, J. M.; Jones, B. Factitious psychoses: Phenomenology, family history and long-term outcome of nine patients. *Am. J. Psychiat. 139*(11): 1480–83, 1982.

38. Naish, J. M. Problems of deception in medical practice. *Lancet 1:* 139–42, 1979.

39. Reis, R. K.; Bokan, J. A.; Katon, W. J.; *et al.* The medical care abuser: Differential diagnosis and management. *J. Fam. Pract. 132*(2): 257–65, 1981.

40. American Psychiatric Association Task Force on Nomenclature and Statistics. *Diagnostic and Statistical Manual of Mental Disorders.* 3d ed. (DSM-III). Washington, D.C.: American Psychiatric Association, 1980.

41. Ford, C. V. *The Somatizing Disorders: Illness as a Way of Life.* New York: Elsevier, 1983, p. 139.

42. Murray, H. W. Factitious fever updated: An editorial. *Arch. Int. Med. 139:* 739–40, 1979.

43. Ellenbogen, C.; Nord, B. M. Freshly voided urine temperature: A test for factitial fever. *JAMA 219*(7): 912, 1972.

44. Murray, H. W.; Tuazon, C. U.; Guerrero, I. C.; *et al.* Urinary temperature: A clue to early diagnosis of factitious fever. *New Eng. J. Med. 296*(1): 23–24, 1977.

45. Parker, N. Malingering: A dangerous diagnosis. *Med. J. Aust. 1:* 568–69, 1979.

INDEX